Public Health in Action:
Practicing in the Real World

Jan K. Carney, MD, MPH
Associate Dean for Public Health
University of Vermont College of Medicine
Burlington, Vermont

JONES AND BARTLETT PUBLISHERS
Sudbury, Massachusetts
BOSTON   TORONTO   LONDON   SINGAPORE

World Headquarters
Jones and Bartlett Publishers
40 Tall Pine Drive
Sudbury, MA 01776
978-443-5000
info@jbpub.com
www.jbpub.com

Jones and Bartlett Publishers
Canada
6339 Ormindale Way
Mississauga, Ontario
L5V 1J2
CANADA

Jones and Bartlett Publishers
International
Barb House, Barb Mews
London W6 7PA
UK

Jones and Bartlett's books and products are available through most bookstores and online booksellers. To contact Jones and Bartlett Publishers directly, call 800-832-0034, fax 978-443-8000, or visit our website at www.jbpub.com.

Substantial discounts on bulk quantities of Jones and Bartlett's publications are available to corporations, professional organizations, and other qualified organizations. For details and specific discount information, contact the special sales department at Jones and Bartlett via the above contact information or send an email to specialsales@jbpub.com.

Library of Congress Cataloging-in-Publication Data
Carney, Jan K.
    Public health in action : practicing in the real world / by Jan K. Carney.
        p. ; cm.
    Includes bibliographical references and index.
    ISBN-13: 978-0-7637-3447-3
    ISBN-10: 0-7637-3447-0
  1. Public health. 2. Medical policy.
    [DNLM: 1. Public Health–United States. 2. Public Health Administration–United States. WA 540 AA1 C283p 2006] I. Title.
    RA427.C37 2006
    362.1–dc22
                                                                                2006000373

6048

Production Credits
Publisher: Michael Brown
Associate Editor: Kylah Goodfellow McNeill
Production Director: Amy Rose
Associate Production Editor: Daniel Stone
Associate Marketing Manager: Marissa Hederson
Manufacturing Buyer: Therese Connell
Composition: Graphic World, Inc.
Cover Design: Anne Spencer
Printing and Binding: Malloy, Inc.
Cover Printing: Malloy, Inc.

**WA
540
AA1
C2p
2006**

Printed in the United States of America
10 09 08 07 06   10 9 8 7 6 5 4 3 2 1

To My Family

Table of Contents

Contributors

Peter D. Galbraith, DMD, MPH, started the Vermont Dental Care Program, operating mobile dental clinics, which serve children throughout Vermont. Later, as Chief of the Bureau of Health Promotion for the State of Connecticut Health Department, he worked to develop environmental risk assessment programs in Connecticut and other states, and served as an advisor to the U.S. Environmental Protection Agency and other federal agencies. In Connecticut, he also worked with others to create the HIV/AIDS Program, and later held the position of State Epidemiologist in the Vermont Department of Health.

Margaret A. Moran, MEd, is Director of Planning and Development, Community Health Centers of King County, Washington. She has held positions as County Health Administrator in Benton County in Corvallis, Oregon, and Deputy Commissioner of Health at the Vermont Department of Health, in Burlington, Vermont.

Patricia A. Nolan, MD, MPH, is Clinical Associate Professor at Brown Medical School, Department of Community Health. She served as Director of Health for Rhode Island from 1995–2005.

Preface

As a teacher of public health, I am always looking for new and better ways to teach public health and reach my students. A physician in Vermont once told me that he had learned about the field from watching "public health in action", and this notion became the idea behind this book. In health fields, case-examples are often used to illustrate the application of scientific knowledge to real life, and some of the best teachers tell stories, use real-life examples, and are able to capture lessons in a way that illustrates what they are trying to teach. In public health, we are faced with many challenges and the urgent need to best teach health professionals, students, and individuals in public health practice. Some of our greatest current and future challenges—preparedness for bioterrorism, pandemic influenza and emerging infectious diseases, stopping the obesity epidemic, furthering progress against smoking, alcohol abuse and drugs, preventing chronic conditions in an aging population, eliminating health disparities, and many others, will only be addressed through public health efforts that are comprehensive, sustained, and effective.

Although I have been teaching for many years, I have spent much of my career in public health practice, and served as Vermont's health commissioner for more than a decade. There, I learned that in order to succeed, science has to be put into practice; partnerships are essential to solve public health problems, and the ability to communicate clearly is essential. I observed and participated in many public health issues, from policy to practice, and in Vermont, one case of an illness, or one concerned citizen, was just as important as an epidemic or large public hearing. The aspects of public health that were most challenging were also tremendously rewarding, and I continue to be grateful for having the opportunity to work with many dedicated colleagues in public health, from all backgrounds and disciplines.

This book is organized into four parts: Part One, Fundamentals, includes basic concepts for public health practice. Part Two, Issues, includes examples of public health issues, how they were addressed, and the tensions at play. Part Three, Strategies, discusses approaches that have contributed to successful efforts in areas of public health. Part Four, Challenges, looks at continuing and future challenges, and further emphasizes key approaches in public health. Most of the stories are from Vermont, but also included are contributions from public health in Oregon, Rhode Island, and Connecticut, from the perspective of different issues and types of public health practice. Most chapters begin with a story, experience, or example followed by a brief summary of the teaching perspective for public health practice.

Public Health in Action: Practicing in the Real World is intended to provide stories, examples, and experiences of how issues and challenges in public health are faced in the real world. In public health, we struggle in our day-to-day work to continue to answer the question of how we know if our efforts have succeeded and the public is healthier. We are challenged to balance short-term crises with progress on longer-term issues, to find new and better ways of solving problems, and to communicate more clearly and effectively. But at the heart of public health, we are all teachers, whether through formal lectures or courses, conducting and explaining research, talking to community groups, to the media, or most importantly, through our actions to improve the health of the public.

PART I

Fundamentals

CHAPTER 1

How Do You Know
If You Have Succeeded?

I stood at the podium and looked out over the audience. I could see more than 150 people, many from healthcare, education, public health, and the legislature, joined for our conference in the well of the House. The décor was always impressive: Freedom and Unity–our state's motto behind me, red carpet, wooden desks in concentric semicircles, white pillars supporting a large balcony. Large windows were framed by heavy draperies. The podium was elevated, where the House Speaker usually stood when the legislature was in session. They weren't in session yet, as it was December and they didn't reconvene until January and we were, for the first time, having a conference in the Statehouse. My team worked hard to get to this point. We had developed measurable goals and objectives based on those for our nation; it was our blueprint for public health–*Healthy Vermonters 2000*.[1]

A year earlier, I had approached a broad-based advisory group for Vermont that drew its membership from state government, the Vermont legislature, and academia. I asked this group to choose public health priority areas and individual objectives for Vermont, based on the health promotion and disease prevention objectives for our nation–*Healthy People 2000*.[2] I asked the group to consider the "size and severity" of our public health problems, "costs," and the "potential for prevention."[1] Eleven priority areas were chosen, and working groups from both the public and private sectors selected several objectives within each priority area from the 15 to 20 listed in *Healthy People 2000*. Although all the national objectives were important, the ones chosen for Vermont reflected the most pressing needs. Priorities involved changing the behavior of individuals, changing the environment, and delivering clinical preventive services in a variety of health care settings.[1]

Now, as I stood at the podium in the House, I talked about our collective goal to improve the health of our citizens by the year 2000 and beyond.[3] I spoke about our process–it was the first time that the state health department had reached outside its walls to help set public health goals for the state. I told the audience that the document was initiated by the Vermont Department of Health, but it was the work of many organizations. I told them that to succeed in addressing these public health problems, it would take more than the government. Many public health problems are "societal problems," and their solutions require support from "broad sectors of our society."[1] My words, in many instances were the introduction to *Healthy Vermonters 2000*, setting the stage for public–private partnerships. The collaborative efforts of many groups and organizations were needed to address such large and challenging public health issues as smoking, cancer, heart disease, and children's health. All required an intense focus, widespread support, and a multidisciplinary public health approach to achieve their improvement. For these issues, there was simply no magic bullet, no simple intervention, no quick cure. It would take the most current science and our best collective and sustained efforts to bring about the more difficult changes in habits and behavior that were related to so many chronic conditions.

I used the analogy that few of us would dare to drive in a city where we have never been before without a map. First of all, we would probably get lost. And even if we knew where we wanted to end up, we would really have no idea of how close we were to getting there. Measurable goals and objectives, relying on data, would help us focus and chart our course. This conference was the launching point for *Healthy Vermonters 2000*. The audience was engaged, and more importantly, it stepped forward to join us in our work of public health.

A few years earlier, when I became responsible for all the public health activities and programs in Vermont, I wondered how we would know if we succeeded in promoting public health, if the health department's work was successful, and if I was successful. A trusted senior manager who had much experience in public health told me that when running large organizations some people picked one or two things to focus on, as it was not possible to change or understand all the details—it was the steering the ship to a slightly modified course theory of managing. For me, this didn't seem to be enough. I thought about all the issues—access to health care, infant mortality, smoking, infectious diseases, environmental health—how would we know if we were doing better? How could I explain, to my own staff, to legislative committees, to the general public, how we knew if the health department was doing its job? Was public health getting better or worse? How did we know? Our mission statement was great for creating organizational unity, but it was too broad—we protected and improved public health—to serve as a measuring stick. I didn't want to have to speak about actions and programs and process; I really wanted to know if what we were doing, how we spent our time and resources, and what I did was making a difference.

The answer, I decided, could be found in results, outcomes, and real information about which public health issues were priorities. How did we compare to national figures? How we were doing over time? Was our health getting better or worse? There was a model at the national level—*Healthy People 2000*[2] that provided benchmarks and targets for the year 2000, and later for 2010. Large consensus groups had looked at broad areas of health, such as heart disease, access to health care, cancer, environmental health, diabetes, and many others, and set measurable goals and objective—targets for the next 10 years. The 10-year goals were a balance between what was ideal and what was feasible, and the broad range of areas gave states the ability to pick and choose priorities that were most pressing in their state. The idea was appealing to me, as it applied epidemiology—the language of public health—in a practical way to help focus resources and prioritize our efforts.

The challenges, however, in shifting towards this type of focus were not minor; programs and work done by health departments had constituencies—

advocacy groups that worked to see that the programs were still present and well funded. If you asked staff why certain programs were done, you might get answers such as "We've always done that," "The federal government gives us money to do that," "An advocacy group lobbied to have it put in our budget," or less commonly, "It is part of our core responsibilities." At that point, programs, work, budget numbers, and priorities were not linked to measurable goals or areas. And there was the even more difficult challenge of making a 10-year goal and work plan feasible in a 2-year election cycle. It would be more expedient to create short-term changes in such an environment. But that would not have addressed my original question of how we knew whether we were making a difference in improving the health of the citizens of our state.

In addition, if we were to use results as a means of measuring our success in dealing with such health issues as access to care, diabetes, cancer, smoking, that meant we had to monitor progress in issues and efforts well beyond the traditional responsibilities and jurisdiction of the health department. We had to work with private-sector entities, nonprofit organizations, other government entities (often very challenging), hospitals, doctors, nurses, schools, law enforcement, advocacy groups, and the public. Our success with public health issues would be defined not only by how we did our job, but also by how well we worked with other groups, organizations, and individuals in focusing on public health priorities.

I had been on the job about a year when I decided we wanted results—provable results. We wouldn't always have data for everything, but we had more information already than nearly any department in the government, and if we were able to organize it, it would help us see where we needed to focus our efforts, resources, and collaborative strategies to improve health. We would also have to go outside the health department, although constrained by limited resources, to form partnerships in many areas to focus our collective resources on public health issues.

I enlisted the help of a capable manager, who was knowledgeable and respected in his field. I gave this person the task of overseeing the process of looking at the national goals and objectives for public health, *Healthy People 2000*, looking at all the data we had—from birth and death certificates to ongoing surveys about risk behaviors—and picking out the most pressing areas and measurable goals and objectives for Vermont. An advisory committee was formed, including health department staff from different programs and outside experts from academics, nonprofit organizations, and other groups. Part of the strategy in bringing in outside people and organizations was to begin to develop and institutionalize the relationships that were needed to take on big, important, but complicated, public health issues.

The advisory group had to consider the size and seriousness of the problem, costs, and the potential for prevention.[1] Finally, I gave my staff a limit as to how many areas and goals and objectives they could choose. It would be too easy to pick a long list that encompassed all, and my fear was that such a document would just end up on the shelf, similar to plans I had seen from other places. The debates needed to occur, and priorities needed to be set. Based on expertise from inside and outside the health department, the national priorities, and Vermont data, we were going to set Vermont priorities, and come up with an ambitious, but achievable list of priorities, with goals and measurable objectives. We used *Healthy People 2000* to create our first *Healthy Vermonters 2000,* with a Vernon dairy farmer, standing with an axe next to his woodpile of split wood, pictured on the cover. It was the beginning of our work to know whether or not we would succeed in making progress in many areas of public health.

I liked the image of a roadmap. This was the beginning of a new journey, and using our map, we now knew where we were and where we needed to go if we wanted to improve the public's health.

REFERENCES

1. Vermont Department of Health. *Healthy Vermonters 2000.* Burlington, VT: Vermont Department of Health; 1992.
2. U.S. Department of Health and Human Services. *Healthy People 2000.* Available at http://www.cdc.gov/nchs/about/otheract/hp2000/hp2000. htm. Accessed on September 30, 2005.
3. Pfeiffer B. Project lists ways to improve the health of Vermonters. *Rutland Daily Herald.* December 4, 1992; 11.

CHAPTER 2

Act Swiftly to Protect the Public's Health

We had experience with meningococcal disease over the years, and the events were often sudden and caused public alarm. One weekend I was at home, and I received a call from a state legislator. A child had been diagnosed with meningococcal disease and the community was terrified. She asked if someone from the health department would come and talk to the people there. Later, I discussed the situation with our epidemiologist on call. A nurse epidemiologist was slated to attend a meeting with concerned parents at the school. Meanwhile, other epidemiologists had been doing their job. After receiving notification of the disease and confirming the diagnosis, epidemiologists in the Burlington main office worked with local physicians and nurses. They investigated the situation, spoke with physicians caring for the child, and made sure that all close contacts were identified and received preventive antibiotics.

In a different year, in another part of the state, a newspaper reported that a high school student had died from meningococcal meningitis,[1] triggering an investigation by the Vermont Department of Health and calls to the health department offices local to the incident. Antibiotics were given to very close contacts of the student, and an informational letter was distributed. But waves of questions and concerns from parents about how the disease spreads continued and remained an issue in the local paper. A health department epidemiologist explained to the reporter how the infection is spread and how contagious it is.[1,2]

After another isolated report, at yet another different time, I was at my desk, when the phone rang and it was the governor on the line asking me whether or not we should put out a press release to the entire state regarding the meningitis issue. A child had been diagnosed with meningitis, and appropriate steps had been taken including antibiotics given to close contacts. I explained to the governor how the disease was spread, and said that a statewide press release was not needed. The local community had already been informed, this was most likely a solitary event, and we did not want to cause a statewide panic. The governor understood and agreed.

In Vermont, there is a list of diseases required to be reported to the state health department by law, and about five confirmed cases of meningococcal disease are seen each year.[3] From 1997 through September 2002, there were 29 cases of confirmed *Neisseria meningitidis* infection in Vermont, a rate of 0.8 per 100,000 population, compared to the United States rate of 0.8–1.3 per 100,000. Most counties of the state were impacted, and there were no outbreaks. Nearly half of all cases occurred in December through February. Patients had meningitis, bacteria found in the blood, pneumonia, or a combination. About 8% died.[3]

Meningococcal disease is a bacterial disease cased by the bacterium *Neisseria meningitidis*. Meningococcemia is a serious blood infection cased by the bacteria, and meningitis, an inflammation of the membrane that covers the brain and spinal cord, can also be caused by this bacterium. It is known that some individuals "carry" the bacteria in the back of their throat and do not become ill, and the infection is most contagious in those with close household contact or direct contact with oral secretions.[4,5] Rapid diagnosis and treatment with antibiotics are important, and generally cases reported to the health department were single instances, rather than an outbreak of several cases. It was unusual for more than a single case to occur in a community.[4]

According to the CDC, each year 1400 to 2800 people in this country get meningococcal disease, 10–14% die (about 300 people), and as many as nearly 20% of survivors have permanent disabling conditions.[5]

In 1998, a cluster of meningococcal disease cases that occurred in Rhode Island prompted an investigation of meningococcal disease in New England.[6] Although the situation described in Rhode Island did not meet the exact criteria for an outbreak of this disease[7] but involved nine cases, a statewide vaccination program for people aged 2 to 22 years old was carried out. The CDC reported that from 1993–1998 less than 1% of meningococcal disease cases were outbreak associated, and most were sporadic.[6]

Fortunately, there has been progress in the vaccine approved in January 2005 and recommended by the CDC. Called meningococcal conjugate vaccine (MCV-4), the vaccine protects against groups A, C, Y, W-135, but not serogroup B, and is recommended now for routine vaccination of young adolescents.[5,8] Although there are concerns about supplies of the vaccine, as it is newly approved, the CDC has a goal within three years of making this routine beginning at age 11. College freshmen living in dormitories are at higher risk for the disease than young adults of the same age. Although all children are not yet vaccinated for this, and vaccine development has continued, it doesn't protect against type B, which accounts for about a third of the cases, and more than half in young infants.[5] Recommendations for college students have been published previously by the CDC.[9]

Although uncommon, meningococcal disease is serious, because it begins with common symptoms, but can progress rapidly and kill within hours.[5] It is this severity and rapidity of meningococcal disease that causes such intense public concern. Some of the most difficult tasks that face epidemiologists and public health nurses responding to the report of a sick child or young adult diagnosed with meningococcal disease is to promptly investigate, identify close contacts, ensure those needing precautionary antibiotics get them, and then explain how the disease does and does not spread. The notion that an infection that can progress so rapidly and sometimes causes death is not as contagious, according to the CDC, as the common cold or flu[10] simply defies logic, particularly when a young adult has died. It is difficult, if not impossible, to understand, and even more difficult to communicate at a time when a child who was previously healthy is now in the hospital and very ill.

Some of the most important work done in these situations, after the immediate tasks are completed, has been the willingness of an epidemiologist or public health nurse to go to the area of the state where a child has been ill and talk to parents in a group in a school or in a community setting. Concern by community members, parents, and school officials is understandable, and such public health efforts can greatly help preventing community chaos and unnecessary widespread antibiotic prescribing or vaccine administration.

It is essential to act swiftly to protect the public's health. Whether a disease outbreak, environmental threat, or public health hazard, one of the key measures of success in public health is how swiftly and effectively the public is protected. Preventing and controlling infectious diseases is a cornerstone of public health practice. A health department cannot be credible without being able to perform this core activity of investigating and preventing epidemics and the spread of disease in an efficient and effective manner, consistently, every time there is a need. You cannot sit and count cases; you must act, and in this situation, at the first indication that disease is present. Picture a healthy child or young adult with a cold, then a rapid illness requiring hospitalization, all within hours. When a child or young adult has meningococcal meningitis, it is a terrifying moment for a family and the surrounding community.

So what can you do in public health? How can you be prepared to act swiftly in situations that are not common, but when they occur are emergent and potentially devastating? Ensure your disease surveillance system works, both the formal and informal means of communications. States have laws requiring the reporting of infectious diseases, but often, there are little or no funds available to evaluate how effective the reporting systems are (except in retrospect, after an outbreak). You need to have a system in place that you can depend on so you can act quickly at any time, day or night, evening or weekend. A call from a doctor or nurse before the laboratory test results are even in that meningococcal disease is being considered can give you a little time to prepare fully to respond in a rapid way.

The way that you as a public health official communicate when there is *not* a crisis, and your ongoing relationships with laboratories, hospitals, doctors, nurses, and within your own department will determine how well and quickly you can respond when a crisis *does* occur. Move fast. Confirm the diagnosis, find the contacts, and recommend the proper preventive medication to those who need it and not to those who don't. Explain the disease and how it is spread to the family and the community. Be available, and have someone capable go to the community where the child lives. Sometimes an entire school will need attention. Follow the situation closely. Keep the phone lines open. Don't be afraid to seek consultation from experts in infectious diseases or from the CDC, if you need it. If your work is swift and competent, you will do your job to protect the public.

REFERENCES

1. Montany G. Meningitis was cause of death. *Caledonia Record.* April 17, 1995.
2. Montany G. Risk of meningitis is small. *Caledonia Record.* April 20, 1995;4B.
3. Vermont Department of Health. *Meningococcal Disease in Vermont: 1997–September 2002.* Burlington, VT: Vermont Department of Health. November 2002 Disease Control Bulletin. Available at http://www.healthyvermonters.info. Accessed April 11, 2005.

4. Vermont Department of Health. *Meningococcal Disease Fact Sheet.* Burlington, VT: Vermont Department of Health; September 1999. Available at http://www.healthyvermonters.info. Accessed April 11, 2005.

5. CDC. National Immunization Program. Meningococcal conjugate vaccine. ACIP Recommends meningococcal vaccine for adolescents and college freshmen. Available at http://www.cdc.gov/nip/vaccine/meningitis/mcv4/ mcv4_acip.htm. Accessed on April 11, 2005.

6. CDC. Meningococcal disease. New England 1993–1998. *MMWR* 48:629–633.

7. CDC. Control and prevention of meningococcal disease and control and prevention of serogroup C meningococcal disease: evaluation and management of suspected outbreaks. *MMWR.* 1997:46(no-RR-5).

8. Center for Biologics Evaluation and Research. Product approval information. Meningococcal polysaccharide (serogroups A, C, Y, and W-135) diphtheria toxoid conjugate vaccine. Washington, DC: U.S. Food and Drug Admini-stration; January 14, 2005. Available at http://www.fda.gov/cber/approvltr/mpdtave011405L. htm. Accessed April 11, 2005.

9. CDC. Prevention and control of meningococcal disease and meningococcal disease and college students: recommendation of the advisory committee on immunization practices (ACIP). *MMWR.* 2000:49(No. RR-7).

10. CDC. Meningococcal disease: general information. Available at http:// www.cdc.gov/ncidode/dbmd/diseaseinfo/meningococcal_g.htm Accessed on April 11, 2005.

Know How Your House Is Built

During my scheduled budget testimony to the Senate appropriations committee, there was an ongoing discussion about the high number of inmates in Vermont prisons, the growing problems of alcohol and drug use, and the health and social problems common with young adults. One senator asked me if there should be a Department of Addiction. Another on the committee asked if there should be a Department of Prevention. Another asked about a Department of Juvenile Justice. I did my best to answer the health-related parts of their questions, but it occurred to me that in this forum, a structural solution was felt to be a logical fix to the health and social issues we were facing. Solutions that would rearrange government programs were a feasible work product in this environment, as the pace of the decision making and legislative process sometimes had the potential to lend itself to the immediate crisis, and ways to fix it. But the problems that provoked the questions were much deeper, with both health and social roots, and the answers were indeed to try and prevent addiction and crime in young adults; it was just that creating a new department was unlikely to be the ultimate remedy. The committee was trying to find a solution, to improve what was a complex and difficult problem.

There have been other examples of this in the legislative process. A Health Care Authority was created in Vermont to address access to health care; this was during the time of intense public debate (both nationally and in Vermont) about access to health care. The Health Care Authority later became part of the Banking and Insurance Department. Was this a mistake? Not necessarily. It was a response to a cry for better health care for our citizens. During the same time period, national health reform did not pass Congress, but extensive debate occurred in Vermont. Access to health care was greatly expanded, particularly for children, but not necessarily because of any structural changes in our government.

What is behind this architectural approach to solving problems? In a legislative environment, it represents one approach to take action on an issue, and such an approach may sometimes be indicated. Alternatively, responses could include better communication between government agencies, more focus on the outcomes or results, rather than the process, and better understanding of the root causes of the issues we face in public health. Such issues, such as alcohol and drug abuse, have multiple determinants and deep roots, requiring cultural change, and longer-term multidisciplinary solutions. Also, solutions to such problems may involve more than one government department, and they often require much more than just the government for a solution. It is hard to imagine that a Department of Childhood Obesity could really prevent children from being overweight, without a much more comprehensive response not limited to the public sector.

The nation's health departments—state, county, and local—represent quite a mix of structures and responsibilities not to mention their relationships to not only the CDC but also other federal departments. Does this matter? Does it matter what form public health takes in a given state? Does it matter whether you call the department "Health" or "Public Health" or a human service agency? In contrast to the earlier work by the Institute of Medicine that focused on the role and responsibilities of the governmental public health agency in public health,[1] more recent work has shifted to examining the responsibilities of academia, health care, business, the media, and communities in public health, in addition to the work of governmental agencies.[2] Public health looks, works, and acts differently in different places, encompassing different issues, in departments and programs with different names. More importantly however, progress in areas of health also vary, some experts contending that such variations represent "public health opportunities in waiting."[3]

What matters for those in practice is to understand what the biggest public health issues are, now and in the future, and how you are positioned to affect them. When we're at home, unless we've designed and built our house, we rarely think about how the support walls, foundation, or overhead lighting were put into place. In public health, we need to understand our structure and roles and responsibilities, not in and of themselves, but to address our most pressing problems in the best way possible. There is no perfect structure, and it is not likely that one uniform structure or creating new structures every time the issues change will necessarily result in solving the problems.

In Vermont, there are no autonomous county or local health departments. This allows easier coordination of efforts around the state through 12 local, but state run, public health offices. It is an efficient model where connections between centralized and decentralized programs can use limited resources in the most effective way. Public health nurses are the backbone of the statewide system and often function in a way where they act as generalists, able to shift focus to be able to better address public health issues as they change, over time, from day to day, week to week, and year to year. These public health nurses help in emergencies—floods, ice storms, and natural disasters. They serve as environmental designees, working with town officials and community members to find solutions to environmental problems and questions. In Vermont, there are also volunteer town health officers who are appointed and who have public health authority to deal with public health hazards and risks, but who also have other occupations outside this role. Public health nurses work with these volunteer officers with such things as cases of rabies, failed septic systems in mobile homes, rental housing, mercury spills, and when dealing with other agencies, such as the state environmental department. Public health nurses function in a similar capacity to help prevent infectious disease outbreaks. Called "epi designees," these nurses receive training from health department epidemiologists to be able to provide the local arm of disease investigations. They help with West Nile virus surveillance, work with health providers to make sure children receive up-to-date preventive care, and distribute potassium iodide to residents near the nuclear power plant. These nurses are part of the statewide team of law enforcement, emergency medical services, health care, and public health that prepare the state against bioterrorism. They interview the public in their own communities, when necessary, to gather information about a specific issue, such as smoking, or to help develop a health plan for the state.

Such a public health system, depending on the broad skills and flexibility of local public health staff, particularly public health nurses, has served effectively in Vermont, being able to be local but statewide at the same time—connected, but responsive to local community needs. Such a flexible system can facilitate effective and efficient responses to new and changing public health issues with training and ongoing communication. The downside, if there is one, is that these individual districts of the state can't advocate for more funding for an issue in their area outside of the state health department budget process—they can't fly solo in the budget process.

Where is Medicaid or mental health located in the state hierarchy of public health? What about long-term care? In Vermont, Medicaid is separate from the Department of Health, but using a collaborative process, the health department had a critical role in defining preventive services for children. The department that housed the Medicaid program was a critical partner in efforts to provide prenatal care and health insurance to children.

In different states, public health may have autonomous county and local health departments, be a cabinet department, be part of a super agency of human services, be called a "bureau" or a "department" or an "agency," and include or not include programs that are important to public health such as mental health, health care services, environmental or occupational health, long-term care, or Medicaid. Is one structure ideal? Is it necessary to have all these items under the purview of public health in order to improve public health?

There are many different forms and structures of public health and many ways to improve health outcomes. There are trade-offs, advantages, and disadvantages to each. Large service programs may, as demands increase, siphon away critical funds for core activities and essential public health services needed to address future issues, such as promoting healthy behaviors, monitoring health status or the population, preventing epidemics, or providing sound public health policy and planning. In contrast, a department with no direct service constituency and resultant advocacy groups may be at a disadvantage in the legislative process and competition for funds. The size of the department may make managers less nimble and able to respond quickly to new problems, necessary to gain and maintain public credibility. Separate local and county health departments have different ways to advocate for funding, to set priorities, and to communicate. And government alone, without partnerships with business, academia, health care, health organizations, communities, and the media, will have a tough time being able to deal with complex health issues, such as emerging infectious diseases, aging of the population and chronic conditions, obesity, and uninsured populations, without understanding who to work with to improve health conditions in communities.

It is essential to know how your public health house is built. Do you have a strong legal foundation, walls with sufficient data, a roof with adequate staff to keep it from leaking? Who are your neighbors, and how well have you gotten to know them? Whether your responsibility is at the program, state, county, or local level, what are the strengths and weaknesses of your community partners, and how well have you identified and prioritized health issues and outcomes? If you know how your house is built and where its strengths and weaknesses are, it will help you as you work to get your job done and get results in public health.

REFERENCES

1. Institute of Medicine. *The Future of Public Health*. Washington, DC: The National Academies Press; 1988.
2. Institute of Medicine. *Committee on Assuring the Health of the Public in the 21st Century. The Future of the Public's Health in the 21st Century*. Washington, D.C.: The National Academies Press; 2003.
3. McGinnis JM. Health in America—the sum of its parts. *JAMA*. 2002;287:2711–2712.

CHAPTER 4

You Must Earn Credibility

In my early years as health commissioner, one of the largest hospitals in the state claimed that it had a bed shortage; there were too many urgent patients and not enough beds. The issue had become a public one with news coverage. It was also a sensitive issue because of the need to accommodate capacity for health care, without a surplus of hospital beds, and the attendant cost of maintaining and staffing them. I was in the statehouse, and entered the governor's ceremonial office, the office sometimes used by the governor during the legislative session. Seated at the large oblong table at the far end of the room were some of the governor's staff and advisors. The governor told me that she needed to know whether the hospital had enough beds or needed more. Such decisions were under scrutiny both from an annual budget perspective, called the Hospital Data Council, and through the Certificate of Need process, a lengthy process that reviewed new health care services or additions to existing ones, to try and promote an efficient health care system and stem the rate of rise of health care costs.

I said that I would review our department's information and provide some further guidance. The governor then asked how long it would take. Not really knowing all that it would entail and having a strong sense of urgency for the results, I replied about a week. I couldn't help but notice the facial expressions of those around the table, and wondered what they were thinking. At least from their expressions, and the fact that I was relatively new, they seemed skeptical that I could answer the question in that amount of time.

On the drive back to the office, I thought about what my next steps would be. As soon as I got back to the department, I spoke to the individual in charge of health planning and relayed to him the question at hand. He said he would get me the information as quickly as possible. What came back was an encyclopedic and nearly unintelligible mass of health planning bureaucratic information—many seemingly convoluted assumptions and jargon, all in a lengthy report. When I complained that it needed to be more clear and simpler, my health planner told me that this was how the governor would have to understand it, because it was complicated. After carefully reviewing all the materials, it appeared that the hospital had a "blip" in the number of admissions; this was not a reason to permanently increase their bed capacity in an emergency fashion.

I spent part of the next couple of days summarizing the situation as best I could in plain language, and delivered the report to the governor's office. It provided more information in a timely manner, and I was subsequently asked about many other health issues.

A number of years later, the education commissioner, a brilliant individual who had a vision for a new system to assess student performance in our public school system, was working diligently to educate the legislature on his vision and its importance for Vermont students. Somewhere during the legislative session, it was noted that in the education department's budget a substantial error had been made in their budget numbers.[1] This became the subject of legislative discussion, and it also became public. Think about it, a math error from the state department responsible for ensuring the education of our students in math (and many other disciplines). Although the education department continued to make strides and finally implemented its vision, it experienced a rocky time that session and its credibility suffered.

You must earn credibility. You need to deliver information in a timely fashion, in a way that the person asking for it will be able to use it, and you must communicate it clearly. In the case of the questions about hospital beds, the response from my health department staff gave me a major clue as to what I needed to do to enhance the credibility of the department's work and make public health issues more important to the administration, the legislature, and the public. Although there may be some risk, it is sometimes necessary to "stretch" your abilities and those of your department if there is an opportunity for public health. The governor's response told me that I was right on the mark, able to respond in a time frame needed. This opened the door for more assignments and more opportunities to bring public health issues to the forefront.

In the case of the education department, there was a moment of damage to its credibility; though not lasting, it made progress toward their goals difficult in the short term. Many people trained or working in public health think that knowing your field is essential. It is, but it isn't enough. If you are responsible for running a state, county, or local department or program, or just about anything else related to health, it really doesn't matter how medically smart or knowledgeable you are if you can't manage your program or agency. If you can't keep a budget or manage the smallest details, why can you be trusted to manage the bigger issues? It doesn't matter how smart you are if you can't keep your own house in order.

How do you know if you have gained credibility? Often, it means being asked to do more work. Proving that you are capable with a timely response, an effective program, and especially by improving health outcomes may mean that you are asked to be involved in larger and more complex issues. It may mean that the legislature asks you to fix something that they are struggling with. It may mean that you have opportunities to work in a way to influence policy on a public health issue. But it is not easy to get there, and it takes ongoing attention to detail. Ideas are not enough; actions and results speak volumes. You must also earn credibility with your own staff and your colleagues in public health, whether they work in your own department or in another health-related organization, profession, or schools. And of course, you must have credibility with the public if you hope to make inroads in the largest and most complex areas of public health.

Sometimes, it is a crisis, real or perceived, that triggers a public health question, and it is far too easy to place energy and efforts on urgent problems at the risk of never dealing with the important and complex issues that affect the health of the public.[2] The major work that needs to be done in public health is as much about long-term and nonemergent issues as it is about immediate needs. The challenges of changing behaviors to reduce smoking, improve nutrition and physical activity, and reduce alcohol abuse are critical leverage points to improve public health, yet require long-term, comprehensive, and sustained efforts. If you haven't gained credibility on the urgent issues, you may never get to the larger and more complex ones that require broader societal involvement and multidisciplinary strategies, such as efforts to prevent obesity and related conditions. The response of the health department to immediate questions and issues, whether a health planning question, a press call, taking care of an individual citizen's concern, or a response to a disease outbreak, if done in a timely manner and in a form that can help the person asking the question, provides an opportunity to enhance credibility, and future opportunities to improve public health.

REFERENCES

1. Zentz A. Accounting problem discovered in January. *The Burlington Free Press,* April 3, 1992;4B.
2. McGinnis JM, Foege WH. The immediate vs. the important. *JAMA.* 2004; 291:1263–1264.

CHAPTER 5

Fighting HIV and AIDS—Finding Community Leaders in Public Health

Dr. Peter Galbraith

"Syringe exchange programs (SEPs) can help prevent blood-borne pathogen transmission by increasing access to sterile syringes among IDUs and enabling safe disposal of used syringes. Often, programs also provide other public health services, such as HIV testing, risk-reduction education, and referrals for substance-abuse treatment."[1] Although this makes a great deal of sense in 2005 when this article was published in the CDC's *Morbidity and Mortality Weekly Report* (MMWR), there was no such consensus in the mid-1980s when the New Haven, Connecticut, Mayor's Task Force on AIDS began a community-organizing venture to create a needle exchange program, addressing the connection between HIV transmission and injection drug use (IDU) that was not so obvious to those addressing these epidemics.[2]

Advocates from the New Haven, Connecticut, Mayor's Task Force, who were early pioneers in the United States for needle exchange programs (NEP) were told:

- Drug addiction is a criminal problem, not a health issue.
- Drug addiction is morally reprehensible.
- Sharing of needles is an accepted ritual in the drug community.
- A state-approved NEP will send a mixed message and deter addicts from entering treatment.
- A NEP will reduce funding for drug treatment.
- Addicts can not and will not change their behavior.
- You distribute bleach for cleaning needles, you don't need needle exchange.
- The local police will stand in the way of success.
- I can't support this legislation without appearing to be "soft on drugs."
- The governor is clearly against it.
- We will create a mecca for drug users in a city already overwhelmed with injection drug use.
- It simply makes the drug problem worse.[2]

As the HIV/AIDS epidemic emerged in the United States, one of the earliest patterns of cases was in New York City and neighboring counties including

New Haven. The epidemic was described as moving up a corridor formed by Interstate HighwaysI-95 and 91.[3]

AIDS was made a reporting requirement to the Connecticut Health Department in 1983 at a time when the cause of the disease was unknown. Nevertheless, early information suggested that it was blood borne and sexually transmitted. Cases were seen among injection drug users, sexual partners, and those receiving blood transfusions.

It became clear early in the epidemic that AIDS transmission through the sharing of infected needles was a significant source of new infections. As the New Haven AIDS initiative began to distribute bleach for cleaning shared needles, it was obvious that more aggressive action was required to slow the progress of the epidemic.

Connecticut, as in 10 other states where substance abuse was a major issue, required prescriptions for the purchase of clean needles in a pharmacy. Repealing the law and passing legislation that would permit the distribution of clean needles were bold tactics that had not yet been successfully implemented in the United States.

In 1987 New Haven AIDS cases were having a disproportionate impact in the African-American and Hispanic communities. Thirty-five percent of the AIDS cases in Connecticut through 1987 were African-American, and 16% were Hispanic. African-Americans constituted 12% of the state population at that time and Hispanics 4%. At the time, IDUs represented 26% of the AIDS cases.[3] By 1990 the percentage of AIDS cases that were IDU had increased significantly as had the percentage of cases that were African-American and Hispanic.

Implementation of a needle exchange program required extensive planning and consultation with community members, including support and resources for local leaders and organizations; Connecticut's first educational and services organization, the AIDS Project New Haven; and subsequently the Mayor's Task Force on AIDS. The task force was created by local community leaders and was a source for innovative ideas, such as reaching out to injection drug users starting with the distribution of bleach and progressing to clean needles in 1987. This was at a time when the president of the United States still had not acknowledged publicly that there was an AIDS epidemic.

Local leaders began to discuss the possibility of creating a needle exchange program despite the recent failure of a similar effort in New York City. It was clear that the role of the African-American churches was critical to exploring and potentially implementing these prevention measures. In early discussions with some African-American church leaders and other leaders in that community, it became clear that giving out free clean needles was not going to be easily accepted. The struggle to prevent substance abuse and to treat those that were addicted was enormous, and the thought of facilitating easier access to needles was a concept that created understandable resistance. Even if enabling legislation was passed, implementation and success were dependent on community support.

During this period the state experienced an example of what can happen when you act without community support. A new health commissioner, an African-American and former dean of the University of Connecticut School of Allied health decided that the health department staff did not have adequate representation from minority groups. The commissioner, in a process with no request for proposals or bidding, selected a minority firm from Maryland and awarded them half of a recently appropriated state fund of $2.5 million to develop a prevention initiative directed at minority communities.[3]

After a year of nonperformance and substantial community unhappiness as well as an exposé in the major Connecticut newspaper, the *Hartford Courant,* department minority staff took over and implemented a successful prevention initiative using local contractors and advocates who knew their community.

Factors that made for success in gaining legislative and community support included the leadership of a local respected expert, Dr. Ed Kaplan, a professor, Sher Horosko, and Elaine O'Keefe whose community organizing skills were a significant asset in reaching out to local African-American churches and many others. Local leaders successfully used many of the principles of community organizing. They had to reach a wide spectrum of the community including IDUs, leaders in the criminal justice system, the drug treatment sector, local police, and others. The community needed to be convinced that a needle exchange program would not only reduce HIV infection but the use of drugs as well.[2]

Another factor that facilitated community acceptance was a decision to not force the issue. There had to be community acceptance and respect for a full range of views. There had to be a shared vision with a candid and clear presentation of the science as it was understood at the time combined with extensive attention and resources applied to building relationships in the community.

Developing a shared vision[4] for the implementation of a needle exchange program in Connecticut had to have the support of a wide array of community members, not just people willing to go along. A sense of commonality in the community of advocates and government officials needed to be created. One person's vision of a prevention initiative can be imposed, as with the contract described above; however, a shared vision is a vision that many are committed to because it fits with their personal vision. A shared vision takes time to develop and to emerge.[4]

The spirit of connection that is critical to developing a shared vision, such as a commitment to implement a needle exchange program, is fragile and requires nurturing. Identifying potential advocates and leaders, developing relationships, and extensive consultation were required and essential. Ultimately, what gained support from community leaders were the relationships and shared vision as well as a commitment to use the distribution of clean needles as a mechanism to reach out to IDUs not only to prevent the spread of HIV by use of contaminated needles, but to bring at-risk people into the system and ultimately into substance abuse treatment when and if they were ready. Knowing the science or the applicable public health intervention is less than half of the challenge. Building relationships, one at a time, brings success.

REFERENCES

1. CDC. Update: Syringe Exchange Programs–United States 2002. *MMWR.* 2005;54:673–676.
2. O'Keefe E. Altering public policy on needle exchange: the Connecticut experience. *AIDS & Public Policy Journal.* 1991;6:159–164.
3. Melchreit RL. *Connecticut History.* 1997–1999;38(1):44–55.
4. Senge P. *The Fifth Discipline.* p205–230.

CHAPTER 6

How Do You Know If a Population Is Healthy?

If you go to your doctor for a checkup, or for an illness, he or she may ask you some questions, ask more details in certain areas, and perform a physical examination, usually starting from head to toe, and focusing on areas where you have problems. If you have pain in your stomach, there will be more questions about your eating and bowel habits and a more thorough physical examination of your abdomen. There may be blood or X-ray tests, depending on how serious your complaint is and what the doctor finds after questioning and examining you. Depending on your age and sex, there are recommendations for immunizations, regular checkups, blood pressure checks, mammograms, colon cancer screening, or other health screening tools to make sure you are healthy. For doctors, we know or have a systematic way to tell whether or not an individual is healthy. But how do we measure the health of a population? How do we know if a population is healthy, or unhealthy, or if their health is getting better or worse? What measures and tests do we choose? How can we compare them? What do we do with the results?

There are published articles, particularly from the Centers for Disease Control and Prevention (CDC), about defining health status.[1] However, the difficulty is that we are usually measuring disease, not health.[2] Measures of death, because they are so universally available, are commonly used. Measuring morbidity, such as hospital discharge rates for diseases or conditions, disease rates of infectious or communicable diseases, or the number of screenings performed for breast, colorectal, or cervical cancer may be helpful in your profile. Rates of immunizations for children and adults, as well as surveys of percentages of the population that smoke, wear safety belts, use too much alcohol, or exercise may be included.

There are many measures that are commonly used and plenty of room for flexibility to fit the profile to the population or location in which you are interested. Rates of health services, particularly preventive care, are often used as a proxy for rates of illness. Although we do track measles, we track childhood immunization rates as a proxy for many other infectious diseases, because of their high rate of success in preventing them.

When you define the health of a community, it is important to read what has been published, what others have said and done, but before you look at your first death rate, it is important to think about how you might use the information you are collecting. If you want to look at the health of an entire state and compare it to other states, you may limit yourself to measures easily and readily comparable to ones already gathered in other states. If you want to look within your state, you may want to look at measures comparable between counties or towns. You need to decide what to compare to and what geographic boundaries to use. You need to decide what type of comparisons to report—by age groups, by sex, by trends over time—and the descriptive epidemiology using person, time, and place.

How do you want to compare the information? If you compare health status indicators to a statewide average, you may get a different picture than if you compare to the national *Healthy People 2010* goal, or in Vermont, the *Healthy Vermonters 2010* goal.[3]

In Vermont, public attention was called to diabetes by showing that nearly all Vermont county death rates from diabetes were statistically significantly greater than the *Healthy Vermonters 2000* goal, though when comparing them to the state average, they weren't all that different. Similarly, when looking at adult smoking rates, they were very similar all over the state, but all were much greater than the 2010 goal, making something that was the same everywhere in Vermont a top priority for action.

What measures you choose and consistently report will determine the focus of your subsequent public health efforts. Rates of food and waterborne illness varied by county, and by highlighting this we focused attention on these conditions. If your purpose is to focus on public health and prevention, define the health of your population in those measures that must be impacted to improve health. Death rates from common illnesses that represent leading causes of death, such as heart disease, cancer, stroke, lung disease, diabetes, suicide, and that have a preventable component should be included. A focus on tobacco, diet, and exercise will help prevent many chronic conditions[4,5,6] in the future. Likewise, if one of your goals is to prevent unnecessary hospitalizations from these conditions and help advocate for higher quality health care, hospitalization or hospital discharge rates should be used, and for such diseases as diabetes or asthma, these may be an important measures. Habits and behaviors related to smoking, alcohol use, physical activity, seat belt use, obesity, and hand washing, might be measured, in men and women, for different ages. Measuring access to health care, particularly preventive health care, will focus attention on prevention. Such data can also act as a proxy for future illness immunization rates for young children and older adults; adequate prenatal care, clinical breast exams and mammograms, and access to primary care all give clinical links to public health measures. When the CDC published national death rates for breast cancer, we saw that Vermont had one of the highest death rates; this was the first step in our efforts to improve access to screening and reduce breast cancer deaths. Despite the fact that at that time we couldn't tell whether the deaths were due to Vermont having more breast cancer than other states or due to inadequate access to health care, the data helped focus attention on the issue and helped define the problem and its potential remedies.

When it is important to focus on a specific population, such as women, men, adolescents, children, refugees, or other populations or age groups, reporting this specific data will help define priorities as well as focus on the unique health issues of a specific population. How you define the population geographically is also important. Measuring health at the state level or national level can be too distant. It is far too easy to believe that such health issues are not happening close to home. Local problems, when described with only statewide or national data, may seem too distant, too remote, and seem like someone else's problem. National comparisons are broad, state comparisons a little smaller, and the clear definition and presentation of community health status is a powerful tool to focus attention, and, if presented clearly and thoughtfully, it can propel community action towards health. By letting the data speak for itself, problems of drug addiction or lead poisoning can be identified without laying blame. Sometimes when you see the health profile (and it really can paint a picture of the health of your community), you just can't ignore it; more likely, you are motivated to be part of the solution. Seeing the health of the community in the form of local health statistics brings the issues closer to home and closer to action.

Reporting and mapping rates of diseases, habits, or preventive services by hospital service areas (or health care areas if primary care services are attached to hospital catchments areas), relates these measures, and their improvement, at least in part, to the health care system. Reporting health status measures along government agency boundaries or by local health or human service districts may give the false impression that improving the measures is the sole responsibility of government programs. Reporting by town or county boundaries, often following both geographic and political lines, may be more neutral and allow easier conversations with local legislators who are important to work with at the local level as well as at the state level in developing health policy.

Define health status using standard measures, as well as incorporating unusual measures that may be needed in specific regions. For example, certain infectious diseases were found in some Vermont counties more than others, and using such measures helped focus community attention on preventing these diseases. Tuberculosis was not as common in Vermont as in other states, but pertussis was a growing concern, as was chlamydia.[7] Although a low-prevalence state, and before reporting HIV became a requirement, a map that showed reported cases of AIDS in every Vermont county was important in dispelling the myth that AIDS was a problem only in urban areas.[7]

How do you know if a population is healthy? You measure it, looking at both those universal and unusual indicators that can tell you where you are and where you should be going. Such health status indicators, or health outcomes, can tell you whether you've got a clean bill of health or if you and your community are in need of some regular public health attention.

REFERENCES

1. CDC. *Consensus Set of Health Status Indicators for the General Assessment of Community Health Status—United States. MMWR.* 1991;40:449–451.
2. Turnock BJ. Public Health: What It Is and How It Works. 2nd ed. Gaithersburg, MD: Aspen Publishers, Inc; 2001:43, 331.
3. Vermont Department of Health. *Healthy Vermonters 2010.* Burlington, VT: Vermont Department of Health; 2000.
4. McGinnis JM, Foege, WH. Actual causes of death in the United States. *JAMA.* 1993;279:2207–2212.
5. Mokdad AH, Marks JS, Stroup DF, Gerberding JL. Actual causes of death in the United States, 2000. *JAMA.* 2004;291:1238–1245.
6. Mokdad AH. Letter: Correction: Actual Causes of Death in the United States, 2000. *JAMA.* 2005;293:293–294.
7. Vermont Department of Health. *The Health Status of Vermonters 1988–1993.* Burlington, VT: Vermont Department of Health; 1995; pp. 22–23.

7

Be a Guest in Their Home

Beginning every January, the legislature worked Tuesday through Friday all the way to May, occasionally June. It was not uncommon, particularly when important bills were discussed by multiple committees over many weeks, for me to be urgently requested to appear before a committee looking at the details of a controversial bill or one that had substantial opposition. During one winter, I was sitting at my desk when I got a call asking if I could be at the appropriations committee meeting in an hour. "Come right down," I was told. "The bill is being held hostage." The Comprehensive Clean Indoor Air bill, the law that would prohibit smoking in the common areas of public places, was stuck in the appropriations committee.

The health department and other coalition members were on alert to potential mischief once the bill's opponents sent the bill to the appropriations committee. It had passed out of the health and welfare committee after much support and testimony from advocates, from the Vermont Coalition for Clean Indoor Air, and from our department, including myself. This law, if passed would be one of the most comprehensive in the nation at that time; it was critical to our efforts to reduce exposure to environmental tobacco smoke and to change the culture around smoking, a major part of our strategy to reduce smoking in Vermont. Opposition efforts to kill or derail the bill included trying to slow it down, getting it sent to other committees so that it would stall, time running out, or it being seen as costing too much. In this case, the appropriations committee had questions about costs of enforcing and implementing the bill. There was no time to do anything but pick up my papers, get in the car, and drive to Montpelier, not quite an hour away. During the drive, I tried to mentally review the key points of why the bill was important, what difficult questions I would be asked, and how I might answer them. Despite the fact that I did this, and did my best to be prepared, I never could predict everything they might ask, and I had to have background knowledge of health details always in my head. I had to be able to think on my feet, or in this case, while I was sitting in the hot seat, the chair where testimony was given. The chair of the committee looked directly across the table at me and began his questions.

This was the appropriations committee, and the topic was budget impact. Some of the bill's advocates in the building heard what was happening and had come to observe. I always started out by giving a very brief statement, my health rationale for the bill. This served to put into context the questions asked, keep the focus on health, and ensure a strong health statement in the event that print or television reporters were present. Then, I tried my best to answer the committee's questions. I could not always tell if I was successful right away. Sometimes the committee voted out the bill while I was there. Often, they put it on hold for more testimony or to be voted on another day. In this case, after testimony and advocacy from me and others, the bill did move out of the committee and made it to the floor of the House for debate. The law later successfully passed. It was a critical juncture in our efforts to reduce smoking in Vermont.

In stark contrast to my previous work in health care settings, where the daily shift routine of a hospital followed a time-pressured regimen, the clock of the legislative process had its own keeper. I watched as others became frustrated as their committee testimony was interrupted by a ringing bell that signaled committee members going to the floor of the House to debate and vote on the budget bill. Hearings were scheduled and rescheduled. The time posted on the door of the committee room was sometimes accurate, and often an estimate, depending on what issue was pressing. There was always conversation going on in the hallway that was as important, if not more important, than the formal conversations in the committee room.

From the moment you entered the statehouse, you saw the marble floors, the ornate staircase, and the impressive House and Senate chambers, you realized that you were somewhere important, somewhere that felt as if much history had passed long before you were there and was still being made, sometimes quietly, sometimes with great noise and argument, and at a pace and with a system all its own.

Citizen legislators, some new, some that had represented their communities for years or decades, carried out their work in committees, hallways, the cafeteria, and after hours, in hearings and small meetings, in impassioned defense or opposition to a bill—a bill that would start or add to a foundation of the framework for how we lived in our state. In our citizen legislature, it is not uncommon to be in a committee room with a nurse, a farmer, a self-employed business owner, an attorney, a teacher, and a community member. There are 30 senators and 150 representatives total, and committees are small and meeting rooms even smaller.

I was a guest in their home. My first impression never changed. I quickly learned to bring work to do. I learned where the phones, computers, and fax machines were. I learned who had the most recent drafts of bills. And I learned that if you were serious about getting a bill through, you had better be prepared to know your stuff, be ready to spend time at the statehouse, and be willing to talk with people when they had time, whether in their committee, at lunch, at a hearing or after hours. I had to drive from Burlington to Montpelier several days each week during the legislative session. Testimony for the budget was scheduled in advance, and committees had a format that they expected every department in the executive branch to follow. Other testimony was sometimes scheduled ahead, and committee chairs, usually of the health committees, would sometimes let you know what bills they were working on as priorities, when they would probably get to them, and when they wanted you or a member of your department to provide testimony. When there was time to prepare, it was helpful to make sure we knew the background of each legislator on the committee, their education and occupation, their experience, and what part of the state they were from. Our local health offices could provide us with information about current health issues or concerns in their areas, to help anticipate questions from the committee members.

Sometimes, however, the pace was more chaotic, with testimony scheduled the day before, or even the same day, and testimony before several committees during the same day. There was no changing this, and every invitation to speak on an issue was an opportunity to speak about public health. During the fall, administrative agencies and departments were asked for priorities—bills that were needed, policy initiatives, legislative language that needed changing—for consideration as part of the governor's legislative agenda. I learned to keep these requests simple and to include priorities only. If you had 10 bills that you needed, you had better consider which few were most important, because the work required to successfully pass a bill was extensive, the process complex, and your time was spent not only advocating for bills that you felt were important, but responding with testimony to virtually every bill that had the word "health" in it. There were not enough hours to do all this.

Interest and commitment to health was high. For example, after the CDC redefined lead poisoning and published a policy statement making this a national public health priority, helping to pen new bills was part of our prevention effort during several legislative sessions. These bills became part of the governor's priorities, which helped us gather support for their passage. We found sponsors for these priorities, legislators from the House or Senate who would introduce the bill and support efforts to have it be discussed. If possible, it was best to find multiple sponsors, from both political parties, and if the bill had sponsors from the health and welfare committee, it increased the likelihood of it being taken up. Many groups and individuals were doing the same thing, and the total number of bills introduced was very large, but the number taken up for discussion much smaller, and the number passed a very small proportion. It was critical to try and get a needed bill on the calendar for discussion in the committee. In the health and welfare committees, index cards held the bill number and title. They were tacked up on the wall in columns that identified whether they were introduced and sent to this committee, under discussion, or passed out of the committee after testimony, discussion, and a vote.

Lobbyists were always present in the statehouse, formally testifying, monitoring bills of interest, or talking to key legislators about issues they were advocating, such as health care, the environment, or other issues. It was important for myself and my staff to be available, when not in the statehouse, and to provide information in an accurate and consistent way to whoever asked. Although working for an administration of a governor of one party, it was expected that we provided information to whoever called. It happened on more than one occasion that I received calls requesting information from two legislators from different parties arguing on two different sides of the same bill. It was our job to provide the information, in an objective way, to both, as quickly as possible.

In the cafeteria, a legislator with a pile of French fries on his plate, looked up at me standing behind him, next in line, and told me that he didn't eat these very often. I agreed that was a good thing. The role of public health spanned beyond the health and welfare committees. Although much time was spent in health committees, it was also spent in other committees, because of the nature of public health issues. We spoke to agricultural committees on rabies prevention; appropriations committees about proposed budgets; education committees about the health of our youngest citizens, the school health curricula, and the quality of indoor air in schools. I spent time in the Senate finance committee, when called to testify about a bill that would allow wine tasting in convenience stores, and spoke about its potential negative impact on health. I visited the Senate and House judiciary committees to help determine the disciplinary standard for physicians as the legislature changed responsibility for regulation of medical practice. I sat in the well of the House for debates on important health issues, sometimes simply to provide moral support to a representative who was anticipating opposition of a health-related bill. Over time, my staff and I were almost everywhere, seeing the inside of many different committee rooms, as the health issues changed, and their roots and solutions spanned many disciplines.

Watching and participating in the legislative process gave an incredible view of the way that laws are made in Vermont. The process was often unpredictable. In the areas of public health where laws were needed, I did my best, as did others in the department, to work with many other groups and organizations and to be available to the legislators by phone or be present at their committee meeting, whether scheduled in advance or in an hour. I spent as much time watching and listening as I did talking. I got to know many different legislators, with many different political views. I spent time in many committees and talked about health in hallways, balconies, bathrooms, and the cafeteria. I learned that just because someone has opposed all your efforts in one area, such as tobacco, didn't mean they would not support other areas such as professional regulation, immunizations, or making tattoos safer.

In the 2005 Vermont legislative session, 728 bills were introduced, 42 became laws, and the length of the session was 84 days, as compared to 65 in 1995. There were nearly two registered lobbyists for every lawmaker.[1] But each time the process was unique. I gave testimony and helped many bills in different areas of health get passed: large bills and small bills, bills that expanded access to health care, bills that better protected confidentiality of health information, strengthened the regulation of medical practice, and improved the quality of indoor air in schools. We helped pass bills that linked health and housing policy in an effort to prevent children from being poisoned by lead. We helped pass bills to prevent children from becoming smokers and to change the culture around tobacco use. I testified against bills that could adversely impact health, directly or through unintended consequences, and provided information related to the scope of practice of health care providers.

When I sat in the balcony with other administration officials during the governor's annual State of the State Address, I watched previous governors march in, officials sworn in, and heard speeches that were sometimes broad and far reaching and sometimes much more pragmatic. At these times, as when I sat in the back of the House of Representatives during important debates on health issues, I sometimes felt like I was seeing what would later be called "history." I felt the same way as I watched the governor sign important health bills, ones that would be seen years later as building a foundation to reduce smoking in children, preventing contagious diseases, improving our ability to fight cancer, or expanding access to health care. Such work was a part of my job, and it provided an important view of how our government worked. I was fortunate to be a guest in their home.

REFERENCES

1. Remsen N, Staff. It's over, but not really. *The Burlington Free Press.* June 5, 2005;1A.

CHAPTER 8

How Do You Keep the Balls in the Air?

My first office was a shoebox-shaped, off-white aged space with a couple of windows in a building long outgrown by the burgeoning programs and responsibilities of public health. After years of planning, one winter the entire health department, except for the lab and the morgue, moved into a new office space in the downtown area. The scheduled move coincided with a measles outbreak, and some of us spent much of the time in our new office space sitting on a newly carpeted floor with no furniture, just a phone and a fax machine, doing our job. My office in the new building had window space spanning the upper half of two walls on the third floor of the building. The top of cathedrals, office buildings, and parking garages could be seen, and there was a view of Lake Champlain and the Adirondack mountains in the distance.

After a couple of weeks, looking out the window as I spoke on the phone and after seeing a plane fly across the distant sky, I began to mentally categorize my busy days as "air traffic controller" days. From the moment you entered in the office, phones rang, people entered and exited, papers flew, and discussions and decisions were measured in seconds and minutes, not hours or days. There was a possible outbreak. An environmental investigation was beginning, and public health nurses were helping coordinate at the local level. A citizen wrote with a health question. There was a legislator on extension 80 calling to complain about something the environmental health staff did. Phone calls were taken standing up, as people came in an out of the office, papers swooped away, papers dropped in front, and of course, the press was always calling. One week, I had three television interviews during the workweek on three different issues. I thought this seemed busy until the October after September 11, 2001, when anthrax scares took hours out of each day.

Most of us have seen a juggler, keeping three, four, five or more balls, pins, or plates moving in the air and never hitting the ground. When you are at your desk reading a letter from a worried citizen and the phone rings with a senator wondering why your inspectors made them throw out all the meat at their booth at the county fair in his county, and your epidemiology field officer comes in to tell you about a possible outbreak, and then there is a question about mercury in fish, and . . . the press calls about who knows what, and then it's already afternoon, and . . . How do you keep all the balls in the air? How do you deal with the immediate threats, prioritize the issues, and make time to think about next week, next month, and the next decade? How do you survive the day, the year? More importantly, how do you make sure you stay focused on priorities for health?

If there were a simple, quick, uncomplicated answer, then health officials wouldn't be changing every few years. The reality is, it is tough, and you have to work to focus on balancing short-term and long-term goals, the moment's crisis, the day's issue, the week's work, and the plan for the decade. So how do you start? You have to be conscious of the fact that if you live only in the short term, you may never take on the most important, complicated, long-term issues for the public's health. And if you focus only on strategic long-term planning, your department, program, and likely you, will be obsolete.

You must figure out how to do both. Public health is a dynamic and ever-changing field, with a mix of short-term and long-term thinking required. Some days are busier than others, those are the days you feel like an air-traffic controller. For the day-to-day crises, it is essential to learn how to prioritize. Things that make people sick, today and next week, take precedent over the senator's call (though you will still need to place the call as soon as possible). Talk to your epidemiologist and find out why she thinks this is an outbreak, due to what, and what steps you must take in the next minutes and hours. The fish question is next, and involves balancing a message to the public that may cause them to limit consumption of certain fish due to concerns about mercury but won't cause them to stop eating fish altogether.

Next, call in your field food inspector (sanitarian), and ask him what happened at the fair. He explains that the meat at the fair booth had been sitting out all day in the hot sun, unrefrigerated, and he made the booth owner throw out the entire batch, and even after he explained why, because people would get sick, the vendor was still mad and called his senator. Thank him for doing his job, and calmly call the senator, and explain to him about the risk of food-borne illness after the meat has been in the warm temperature for too long, and tell him how you will provide education to the fair officials and send an inspector down the morning the fair starts next year, so this won't happen again, and the vendors will know more about food safety. Find out the reporter's deadline and what she was asking about, and then take a breath before the phone rings again, or another staffer comes to see you. A regular meeting to focus on developing a new chronic disease program begins when you are interrupted by a phone call. The rest of the day is similar.

How do you prepare and be comfortable about all this? You must know your field. You must know what you know, and more importantly, what you don't, but where you can find it–fast. You must develop and have complete confidence to make prompt, correct decisions that will protect the public. You must also know your staff, what your staff knows, what they don't know, and when to call a colleague, when to call CDC, or when to call your mother. (I often asked my mother what she and her friends were reading and where they were getting information about health. I would then read the same things, so I would know more about issues that were of interest to the public).

But you also have to make time for long-term thinking as well. When driving the hour-long distance to the state capital, during the busiest time of year when the legislature was in session, I would think about the longer term during these quiet car rides. It was during such a moment that I decided we needed to focus on outcomes, develop a way to measure our progress and the health of the public, and put in place long-term priorities. I decided that to take on the toughest, most complex public health issues would take an effort bigger than a single person, department, organization, or group. It would take all of them, and much public focus.

My long-term thinking quickly evolved into *Healthy Vermonters 2000*[1] and later into *Healthy Vermonters 2010*,[2] a set of priority areas, measurable goals and objectives, and outcomes in key priority areas of health. While other places and organizations may have different issues, the idea of prioritizing efforts though measurable goals was the best way I knew to impact public health in a positive way, to not only deal with the short-term issues, but get beyond them. Such a framework, whether you call it a plan, a blueprint, or a roadmap, gives you a context for your efforts.

In addition, on an annual basis, I wrote down what was accomplished during the previous year, and what were the goals, objectives, and issues that I wanted to address in the next one. Sometimes it included a recap of the legislative session—did we get all the bills passed that we needed? Were they strong enough? Did we get blindsided by any issues? How were we doing at our long-term priorities, the complicated ones: access to health care, smoking, cancer? What data did we have this year and what were the trends over time? Any new issues on the horizon that aren't already on the list?

I always kept our list of Healthy Vermonters priority areas, our 10-year plan, in my head as I read the paper, drove back and forth to the legislature, and experienced a chaotic workday, looking for opportunities to move one of our priorities to the top of the list, but more importantly, staying conscious of the long term while we dealt with the short term, and keeping a focus on the big picture, even during a day's crisis.

It was important to be flexible, nimble, and able to pivot, as immediate crises happened, sometimes, with dramatic shifts in new public health issues, such as West Nile virus and other emerging infectious diseases. But it was also necessary to keep focused on longer-term progress on chronic illness, habits and behaviors, and other public health needs that don't gain the immediate attention that outbreaks of diseases or vaccine shortages do, but that are critical when you look at the changing demographics of our population and longer-term goals. The challenges and approaches to changing habits and behaviors, to prevent obesity, smoking, and alcohol and drug use all involve comprehensive and multidisciplinary approaches that must be sustained.

So how do you keep the airplanes from colliding? How do you keep the balls in the air? I learned a variety of ways to not only survive the day, but to get done what needed to be done. We all had to know our field and have strategies to keep learning. Learning to make decisions promptly when necessary and sleeping on those that you could (and knowing how to sort out the difference) was a part of it. Bringing staff into your decision making creates a culture of problem solving. I always made health decisions first, and then figured out how to get them done.

It was also important to learn to be comfortable with ambiguity. There was never enough time for another study and more data. You had to decide, based on what information you had at the moment, especially in urgent situations or public health emergencies. But despite the fact that time may be lacking and data even more so, data was essential to public health efforts, and it was important to be thinking about what kind of data would actually provide useful information, this data giving us hints about what directions to take and when to take them.

If public health were simple, we would all be healthy. But the most important thing is not shy to away from taking on a health issue because it is big and complicated, like preventing smoking or childhood obesity, when your days may be spent dealing with short-term crises. Most of the leading causes of death are, in reality, habits and behaviors that will require long-term public health prevention strategies.[3,4,5,6] You need to develop an approach that will fit side by side with your short-term demands to give you a starting point to focus on longer-term issues, to begin to make progress. And while you are busy thinking about all this, you have to remember to answer that letter from the worried citizen.

REFERENCES

1. Vermont Department of Health. *Healthy Vermonters 2000*. Burlington, VT: Vermont Department of Health; 1992.
2. Vermont Department of Health. *Healthy Vermonters 2010*. Burlington, VT: Vermont Department of Health; 2000.
3. McGinnis, JM, Foege WH. The immediate vs. the important. *JAMA*. 2004;291:1263–1264.
4. McGinnis JM, Foege WH. Actual causes of death in the United States. *JAMA*. 1993;270:2207–2212.
5. Mokhad AH, Marks JS, Stroup DF, Gerberding JL. Actual causes of death in the United States, 2000. *JAMA*. 2004;291:1238–1245.
6. Mokdad AH. Letter: Corrections: Actual causes of death in the United States, 2000. *JAMA*. 2005;293–294.

CHAPTER 9

Strike While the Iron Is Hot

In the period from 1990 to 2001, 44 cases of measles had been confirmed in Vermont. From 1994 to 2001, there were 10 cases confirmed, 60% occurring in individuals exposed outside of the United States.[1] In 1993, there were 28 cases of measles confirmed, most in children who had gotten only a single dose of the Measles, Mumps, and Rubella (MMR) vaccine.[1] Second doses of MMR have since become the standard practice because of the vaccine's efficacy of only 95% and the fact that measles is so contagious.[2] Much effort was spent, with epidemiologists, public health nurses, and many others holding second-dose clinics in doctor's offices, schools, and other locations. An immense response and a great deal of activity was required to prevent uncommon but serious complications. Publicity was high and offered opportunities for parents to check their children's immunization status.[3]

During February 1993, a resident student at the University of Vermont was confirmed with measles. The news report added to the growing number of cases reported in Vermont's largest county.[4] The university worked with the health department and began second-dose measles vaccine clinics for students, staff, and faculty who were not immune. In February, nearly 2250 people received vaccination against measles. A second clinic was scheduled and expected that 1000 more students, faculty, and staff might need the MMR vaccine.[5]

The Centers for Disease Control and Prevention (CDC) had noted that in 1993 there had been a 99% decrease in reported measles cases for the first half of the year, as compared to 1990. The measles in 1993 mostly involved school-aged children who had one dose of MMR vaccine, as compared to the situation observed from 1989 to 1991 in which many cases involved younger children and unvaccinated children in urban areas.[2] Vaccine coverage likely increased in response to the outbreaks, and the CDC reported higher levels of vaccination in 1991 (83%) than in 1985 (61%) for 2-year old children. In addition, the CDC noted that risks for both school-aged and college-aged entering students could be reduced through offering and enforcing vaccination with second-dose MMR vaccine in both these age groups.[2] In addition to the availability and recommendation for vaccines, requirements for vaccinations prior to school entry have contributed to the decrease of disease. The current concern was because measles was so contagious and because of potential complications that were more common in children under 5 years and adults over 20 years of age. About 6% to 20% of individuals with measles experienced a complication such as an ear infection, diarrhea, or pneumonia, and more rarely, encephalitis or death.[6]

During this time, we reviewed our immunization laws and regulations and discovered that our authority did not extend past high school.[7] Vermont law said that a record or certificate of immunization issued by a license physician or health clinic is needed for school enrollment as a student in a Vermont school. The health department usually consults with the state education department to establish which immunizations are required and what should be given at which age. This allows the requirements to be updated as new vaccines are shown to be effective. In Vermont, the decision to require certain vaccines was often made when such vaccines were available and able to be distributed through the immunization program. The most important part of the law, though, was in the section that allowed for school exclusion of a person (not exempt from the requirement) who does not comply. This provision, after appropriate notice, provided the ability for school boards to exclude individuals in the event of contagious diseases. The practical problem was that the current immunization requirements and exclusion provision only applied to public, private, or parochial kindergarten, elementary, or secondary school.[7]

In a college or university, where large numbers of students lived in dormitories and attended classes together, there was no provision to exclude them from school or to require appropriate immunizations for contagious diseases. No matter what was required for children, there was no way to attach it to college aged students under our current law. Why was this a problem? Students in Vermont colleges and universities might come from many different states and locations around the country, and as long as measles was a problem in or outside the United States, as it had been in the recent past, it could be a potential problem that quickly became a much larger problem if groups of students who needed to receive a second dose of vaccine to be protected were not covered.

Given what had just happened at the university, we knew we had to act fast. With the advice of our legal counsel and legislators, a bill was introduced during the first week of March to the health and welfare committee in the House. It was a "committee bill," meaning that the entire committee had sponsored it. It amended the part of the immunization law that defined schools to include postsecondary schools and include the same language in the school exclusion section. There was brief testimony given: information about immunizations, measles, and why the gap in the law needed to be mended. Legislators were well aware of the measles that had been seen in Vermont this year, and the publicity and public health response for both young, school-aged children, and university students was widely noticed. The law that passed had gone through the House and Senate and been approved by a conference committee, in the third week of April, record time for complete passage of a bill.[8] The only controversy came about when questions were asked about including colleges that did not have resident students and the timing of the implementation. These were handled with further discussions to make sure that concerns were addressed. Fortunately measles activity slowed in Vermont as it did in the rest of the country, and the changes in the immunization law helped us in our efforts to be best prepared for the future.

It is never a simple task to get a law passed in public health, even one that is simple, focused, and urgent. Health issues are often complex, and anticipating them sometimes goes against human nature—if it is not a crisis or emergency, the immediate relevance may not be clear and compelling enough to put it ahead of all the other priorities in all different areas of the government. Prevention efforts designed to anticipate problems before they happened or a situation before it worsened, were difficult and required much proactive, clear, and thoughtful education. However, an emergency, serious outbreak, or other near crisis—especially if it was well publicized—had everyone's attention and made it much easier to update laws or fill gaps.

Sometimes, you must be ready to move when the opportunity arises. In this case, children with measles in Vermont and a case at the university made us discover a serious gap in both our public health immunization law and our ability to prevent and control such situations in the future. Despite the fact the session was already well underway, we moved quickly, with the administration's blessing and legislatures' strong support, and shepherded a simple, but much needed bill[8] through the legislature in a short period of time to better protect public health in the future.

REFERENCES

1. Vermont Department of Health. *Measles.* Burlington, VT: Vermont Department of Health; January 2001. Disease Control Bulletin. Vol. 3, Issue 1. Available at http://www.healthyvermonters.info/dcb/012001.shtml. Accessed March 17, 2005.
2. CDC. *Measles, United States, First 26 weeks, 1993. MMWR.* 1993;42: 813–816.
3. Ring W. Vermont measles outbreak is most severe in nation. *The Burlington Free Press.* February 20, 1993;1A.
4. Geggis A. UVM to get shots: 12th measles case confirmed in county. *The Burlington Free Press.* February 13, 1993;1B.
5. University of Vermont. Measles clinic enters second week, now at UVM student health center. Burlington, VT: University of Vermont; February 22, 1993. News release. Available at http://universitycommunications.uvm/ newsarchives/ h.%20spring-summer%201993. Accessed March 29, 2005.
6. CDC. *National Immunization Program. Measles—What you need to know and frequently asked questions about measles.* Available at http://www.cdc.gov/ nip/ diseases/measles/vac-chart.htm; www.cdc.gov/nip/diseases/measles/ faqs.htm. Accessed June 20, 2005.
7. Vermont Statutes, Title 18 Chapter 21 Communicable Diseases, Subchapter 4. Sections 1120 Definitions, 1121, Immunizations required prior to attending school, 1123, Immunization rules and regulations, 1126, Noncompliance.
8. Acts of the Vermont Legislature 1993-1994. Act No. 75. An Act Relating to Immunizations in Post-secondary Schools. Available at http://www.leg.state.vt.us. Accessed March 17, 2005.

CHAPTER **10**

Respect the Unwritten Rules

During a particularly tough budget year, one of the members on the House appropriations committee questioned me about my health department budget, asking, "But, Commissioner, what about trees?" I respectfully told the committee that I could not speak for trees but that I could only speak for health. What the legislator meant when he asked that question was this: considering the responsibility the committee had to look at the budgets for all the state departments, and that the state budget could not fund all budget requests, if my budget *was* funded, how would the legislature handle the shortfall that would probably occur elsewhere? Such were the challenges and responsibilities of the appropriations committees. Our challenge was getting a budget through that could protect and improve the public health.

Every year, usually in February, we were scheduled to appear before the House appropriations committee to defend our budget. The legislature began in January, received the governor's budget address in mid-January, then took up what was called the "budget adjustment," any unforeseen budget needs for the current fiscal year. Usually, I was not at these hearings, as our budget rarely exceeded what we were allowed, or appropriated, for the year. Usually, the types of things that would cause budget pressure were unexpected increases in caseloads, more people needing assistance in human service programs, or sometimes, in our case, more people in need of treatment services for alcohol and drug addiction, a problem that had grown in recent years. Departments or agencies that had programs that provided assistance to people, food supplements, health care, health insurance, child care, or similar programs had a greater likelihood of having an unforeseen budget need. Having too many unexpected needs made people wonder (both the people that you worked for and also the legislature) if you knew how to do your job. Were you estimating what you would need over the next 12 months or not being precise enough? Sometimes adjustments were unavoidable, caused by a sudden change in needs for certain populations, an especially tough winter, a sluggish economy, or increased demand for specialized services such as drug treatment.

The budget process that preceded the legislative session was often intense and competitive. In our case, the health department was part of a "super agency," the Agency of Human Services, rather than a cabinet department reporting directly to the governor. That meant that first there was a haggling process within the agency, and then another round with the governor's office, called the "fifth floor," because it occupied the fifth floor of an office building in Montpelier, just a short walk from the statehouse.

The budget process started with the baseline of the past year's budget and went up or down from there. Depending on the economic forecasts, how the state's revenues were coming in, and other factors, the budget "exercise" might start with level funding, a 2% increase, a 5% decrease, or so on. It was a challenge to manage this within the department in a way that was realistic without unnecessarily alarming staff about being able to do their jobs, or wonder if they would still have one. It was difficult explaining to staff when we had to do a large decrease exercise, that it would likely not happen, but that we still had to do it. My view was that we needed to understand our priorities all year long, not just at the time of the budget process, which usually started in late summer or early fall and culminated with the governor's budget being finished just before December holidays.

In regular meetings with senior managers, called division directors, which happened every few weeks, I tried to understand on an ongoing basis what their needs and priorities were. We worked hard to successfully apply for and receive federal grants in our priority areas, as state funds were always limited. Our focus on outcomes and measurable goals and objectives to improve public health, called *Healthy Vermonters 2010,* was designed to help us be as efficient as possible, by creating partnerships to improve health outcomes, as well as focus our priorities for grant applications. Although the budget process was usually the same time each year, predictable in its process and format, sometimes a decision would be made, revenues would be off track, or something else outside our purview would become a priority, and we would have to have a budget exercise submitted within one to three days, with a sizable reduction. If there were a crisis in Medicaid, not under the direct control of the health department, there could be budget repercussions in our department, because we were part of the same agency. Likewise, even though not a direct reduction, a reduction in another department that we worked with, such as game wardens for rabies, or the state police on bioterrorism preparedness, could result in an impact on public health. In such severe situations, there was not enough time to have more than a cursory management meeting, or talk to directors by phone, so it was essential for me and my budget staff to understand priorities across the departments and programs on an ongoing basis, to help us make the best decisions possible, with the least negative impact on public health.

There were different budget strategies used by different state department commissioners. Some utilized the "Washington monument" strategy–putting sacred programs that had a political constituency or provided services to people, at the top of the list, with the theory that no agency secretary or governor's office staff in his or her right mind would reduce funding for these things, and your program would be spared. Unfortunately, those higher up sometimes called the bluff, and the commissioner was left with a hole gutted somewhere else in his department, from a decision made by someone else, or the monument ended up on the governor's recommended budget reduction to the legislature and the commissioner or department head was left to face the appropriations committee and explain why this decision was being made. I preferred, no matter how draconian the budget exercise, to think in terms that if it really were to happen, how we would deal with it in a way that had the least negative impact on the public's health, both in the short term and the long term. This was another reason why it was so important to have measurable outcomes, to help define priorities, and to apply for grants.

The one time I did propose putting a Washington monument on the chopping block, when the state had the longest, deepest recession it had in a long, long, time, it was because it needed to be there. The program involved a chest clinic for granite workers that had been in the health department for many years. Although important, there were other ways to carry out these activities in a traditional health care setting, and cutting this program would allow us to continue to protect and improve the health of our citizens who most needed our help.

But the budget process is never easy, and many times we were prepared to put a few of our 12 district offices on the list to be cut. These offices were the focal point for local public health in Vermont, but the budget forecast was grim, and there was no place left to cut. We were down to the core programs that protected public health and improved health for the future. Vermont's public health system depended on the 12 district offices around the state, as there were no autonomous county or local health departments. Not only were the public health nurses in the districts our eyes and ears for community health, they were able to extend our resources, not only by having a generalist function, but also by preventing disease outbreaks from getting worse by serving as "epidemiology designees," by helping to investigate environmental contaminants as "environmental designees," and by helping prevent pregnant women from smoking, through various prenatal programs. A reduction in this part of our workforce represented a worst-case scenario for public health, and through many years of budget preparation, though they may have been on the list for the exercise, they were never the target of massive cuts.

We always had to make clear in writing the impact of any reductions whether for a "hurry up and cut" type of budget exercise or the usual one. It was important to be as precise as possible, and define in clear terms, what a reduction would do. Those departments that provided health care to citizens, such as in the area of mental health, could cite reductions in patient visits for children and adults. In public health, in the areas of our core responsibilities, such as monitoring the health of the population, we had to be more cautious. If we put a statistician on the chopping block, he or she would be cut, as the competition between long-term investments in understanding health, as important as we felt it was, could not compete with short-term direct clinical services. So if something was important to our core mission and focus, for both the short term and long term, we didn't put it on the list.

We rolled up our sleeves, and made our best case for the budget to the agency, trying our best to show why it was important to public health. Sometimes the agency was sympathetic, but other times, the pressures of providing services in tough economic times was so tough that it was a victory to get even a small increase in the budget, sometimes to get even a level-funded budget.

When the haggling at the agency and the fifth floor was over, the governor's budget was put to bed before the New Year, and the governor's budget address was delivered in January. The legislature may have similar or different priorities, depending on the composition and year, but by and large, the governor's budget was the biggest predictor of the state budget. There were changes here and there, sometimes frank disagreements over funding and policy, but these made up a relatively small proportion of the overall state budget. The best chance of adequate funding was to be an effective as possible in the "inside" budget process, the one that occurred before the governor's budget was finished and delivered to the legislature for their work.

We could expect to go for about a 2-hour session in the House appropriations committee in February, and after the entire House passed the budget with its changes and sent it over to the Senate, we could expect to spend about the same amount of time in the Senate appropriations committee in March. Although the House and Senate made some changes, the vast majority of the budget that ended up for the year came from the governor's original budget. This was not to minimize the impact of either the House or Senate, but budgets from last year were the starting point for the current year's discussion and debate, and the governor's budget carried incredible weight in the process.

The process was similar each year, and each year there were new challenges. The unwritten rule was that you haggled during the time your budget was prepared—making your best case for maintaining, adding, reducing, or adjusting your current budget based on your best predictions about what health issues would change in the coming year. Then, once your budget was set and became the governor's budget, it became your job, as a part of the administration, to defend it. After that, you had to learn to live within your means and not be a regular participant in the budget adjustment process asking for additional funds.

Sometimes, this was really tough. Advocacy groups sat in the committee rooms, listened to your testimony, and had an opportunity to testify before the same committee and tell them when your budget as presented just wasn't enough: there would be more needs for people living with HIV and AIDS, additional respite services needed for parents of children with special health care needs, or more money to fight smoking. It is natural to want all the funding available, but part of my job was to set priorities and manage all of public health, which was always a difficult and challenging balancing act. This risk of putting too much into immediate public health services was that you might not be anticipating longer-term and emerging health issues. Committee members would ask you if you couldn't just use a little more in these areas, and despite the temptation to use the wink and the nod, because the tape was always running, you had to follow the unwritten rules. Besides, a budget representative from both the agency and the fifth floor were always sitting in the committee room listening to your testimony as well.

How can you do your job if you can't advocate for health in this public setting? You can, and you must, but you need to play by the rules. Part of the challenge of running a public health agency was the responsibility to deal with all the issues, balance short-term crises and long-term needs, continue to provide immediate help as well as think about the future, and all in a world with limited resources. Credibility with those you work for was an essential quality that helped when it was time to haggle every year. Relationships with advocates had to be ongoing and efforts cooperative. One of the agency secretaries that I worked for always said that advocates served as the conscience of government and of the budget process.

A health official also has a responsibility to advocate for public health. In a similar way, a skilled public health official learns to advocate on a regular basis through the issues that are made public, educating the public around key issues and priorities, and efforts to educate the people he or she works for on a regular basis, through memos and meetings, as well as ongoing relationships with legislators. One of the governors I worked for once told us in an extended cabinet meeting to educate the public, and the legislature would come around. Tough to do, but he was right.

I wasn't always happy during the budget process; it was tough, not always rational, and required quick thinking. But I did learn to respect the rules, and I learned to always haggle. There were always tensions at every step of the way, because of the intense competition for limited resources. During a severe recession, we saw improvement in some health outcomes, despite the fact that there were fewer state funds, because we sharpened our ability to apply for grants in priority areas. And because it was so tough for everyone, it also made groups inside and outside the government work together toward similar goals. However, that was not always the case. The prioritization of resources for programs and needs and the challenges of meetings the needs over time, setting priorities, balancing short-term and long-term needs, all while respecting the unwritten rules but still advocating at every opportunity, was one of the toughest challenges in public health.

11

Always Stay on the High Road

Tobacco was the leading preventable cause of disease and death in Vermont and the focus of much public health and legislative activity. The Master Settlement Agreement, negotiated by many attorneys general, brought never-seen-before funding to public health. However, where there is money, there may be controversy. In Vermont, a task force was established to make recommendations to the governor and legislature on the fate of the funds. One recommendation was to create an independent board to administer the funds, outside the department of health, outside of any current government agency. The rationale from some of the members of this group was that these funds would be better protected and independent from any adverse influences that might occur if located in an existing state department or agency.

Of course, we at the health department disagreed, arguing that the accountability for public health issues should be in the public health agency, who with meager funding, was leading the effort to reduce youth smoking, an effort already showing results. If smoking was not a public health issue, what was? A disagreement ensued. Unfortunately, any public disagreement also had the potential to hurt public health. If there was disagreement, why spend any money at all? Why should so much money really be spent on preventing kids from starting to smoke and helping adults to quit? A public disagreement had the potential to create a wedge, one large and wide enough to allow talented lobbyists to influence the outcome, or the disagreement could become a distraction that would take away an incredible opportunity to raise awareness and develop a way to reduce smoking for the longer term.

Our real worry was that a new independent agency would be slow, a potentially disastrous outcome when there were suddenly more funds than were ever seen before to fight a public health problem. The pressure to achieve results would be incredible. Tobacco prevention and cessation efforts would have to be credible and each year compete against such areas as housing, human service, health care, and environmental needs. Although there was academic representation on the task force, who emphasized that reducing smoking would take time and should be carefully evaluated, our point of view was that virtually no government program was carefully evaluated, and we would now be judged against a far different standard. Not that this careful approach was a bad thing, but it was simply not customary for the legislature to spend money on evaluation when there were people in need of mental health services, health care, heating assistance, and many other competing priorities. We had been successful in public health in presenting data and outcomes to legislative committees, so much so that within a few years, the committee members were coming to us asking for data; however, this was certainly not universal compared to the universe of state agencies and departments.

The simple fact was that the legislature met every year, was elected every two, and would expect with large investments to see large results, and fast.

Our other worry stemmed from what we knew, as advised by the Centers for Disease Control and Prevention, about how best to reduce smoking. A public health approach, using our best practices, relied on the many day-to-day relationships that existed to implement a consistent and focused, short- and long-term approach to improve a measurable outcome. In this case, our goal was to cut smoking in half by the year 2010, an ambitious but achievable goal. Our partners would include the usual doctors, nurses, hospitals, and the University of Vermont, but would also include insurance companies, to pay for smoking cessation; schools, to implement science-based curricula to prevent young people from starting to smoke; other state departments, such as the department of liquor control, to continue strong enforcement of Vermont's tough access laws; and many other groups and organizations, particularly nonprofit entities, parents, and the administration and legislature. We just couldn't see how a new independent board could quickly develop such partnerships and implement programs in a way that would meet the legislative and public expectations. We believed that we could do more to reduce smoking, and do it much faster.

The disagreement about the responsibility for the issue continued, and it was clear that we were the minority view. Although we made the points, in public meetings, in interviews or when asked by the media, that funds should not be spent on a new bureaucracy, we worked hard to frame this disagreement to creating more public attention on our leading health issue–tobacco. In interviews we emphasized that all of us agreed that a top public health priority was that smoking needed to be reduced. All of us agreed that our programs should be developed and evaluated based on the most current science-based approach. Really, the only areas of disagreement were the need to create a new independent board, and the total amount of funds required to reach the goal of cutting smoking in half by the year 2010.

At the statehouse ceremony where the final task force report was released, with task force members and children in attendance, I was still a minority voice on this issue. After the presentation and summary of the report and recommendations, media questions came to many of us, many directed at me, attempting to create controversy. I worked hard to sidestep the differences, and highlight the importance of reducing smoking and our commitment to deal with what I called "public enemy number one." Although it was obvious that the disagreement would spill over into the legislative session, where such decisions would be made, the current opportunity was to continue to get the message out about the importance of smoking as a public health issue, to position our group to success in a competitive environment.

This was the high road, as ultimately it wasn't about the form of a new bureaucracy or not, it was about reducing smoking: making sure children never started to smoke, and that all adults who smoked had the benefit of the most current means to try and stop. It was about health, public health, and it was, at the time, the most tremendous opportunity to solidify, in a comprehensive and sustained manner, our efforts to impact the public's health by reducing smoking. The controversy, about this aspect of the use of funds went on too long, and it was frustrating for myself and public health staff who had worked so hard with such meager funds to get results. But the controversy, in this case, was also an opportunity, as long as we stayed on the high road, to protect the funds from competition from other sources not related to public health, which was something happening in other states. Ultimately, public health funds came to the Department of Health with an evaluation and review board created (with critical and independent functions), and smoking has continued its decline in young people in Vermont. And perhaps the most important and compelling reason for keeping to the high road was that the public debate, framed around the issues, increased the public's education and support for reducing smoking.

Always stay on the high road. That's the side of the issue that includes no complaining, finger-pointing, whining, excuses, or saying something bad or insulting or demeaning about someone or their work. The high road is sometimes like a path in the forest that is hard to find and follow, and some days if you find it, you may not see anyone around for miles. But as difficult as it is, it is important to find it and stay there. When someone says something negative about you, your work, or your department to your face, in a public meeting, or to the press, respond with a positive comment. Find the path back to the issue at hand. Our debate was really, after all, about reducing smoking. Talk about the issue and why it is important and why you are trying so hard to improve it—talk about public health. Stay on the high road. You'll never regret it.

CHAPTER 12

Have a Code of Ethics

In recent years, attention has been focused on disclosure of financial interests by authors of articles in peer-reviewed journals. The same is true for presentations to national professional meetings. Recent controversy surrounded the question of what constitutes "conflict of interest" and what role it plays in the recruitment and retention of scientists at the National Institutes of Health, and more importantly, how such policies impact the credibility and reputation of the world's leading biomedical research institution.[1] The development and implementation of such rules struggle to balance cooperative work needed between scientists and industry against the real or perceived conflicts that can occur when the relationship involves substantial financial arrangements. In public health, groups such as the American Public Health Association have published a code of ethics for public health with written principles about the ethical practice of public health and its rationale.[2]

For public health workers in a government environment, there often exists general personnel policies and procedures, as was true in the state of Vermont.[3] Such guidance was used for all employees of the state; those termed "classified" as well as those "exempt," "appointed," or "temporary" were expected to abide by required employee conduct. Such guidance prohibits employees from accepting compensation from people other than their employer for work related to their job. In addition, employees were prohibited from any activity that would be determined by the department head to be in conflict with their job responsibilities or with the responsibilities of the department or agency where they work. Vermont's policy also notes that the "appearance" of improper activity or conduct may be a conflict of interest and instructs employees to find out about whether any activities could create potential conflicts before doing them.

As commissioner of health, every two years following my appointment or reappointment, I had to sign a State of Vermont Code of Ethics Acknowledgement, stating that I had read the Executive Code of Ethics[4] and agreed to adhere to it. The Executive Code of Ethics, promulgated by the governor as an executive order for gubernatorial appointees, an order not requiring legislative approval, was important to the operation of our state government. This Executive Code of Ethics defined conflict of interest, payments, gifts, and favors, what was included and excluded, and contained written ethical guidelines that were designed to "instill public trust and confidence,"[4] and included a detailed code of conduct.

Why are considerations of conflicts, both real and perceived, so important? In the government, such codes of ethics and conduct were designed to ensure that public officials were making decisions in a way that was fair and impartial based on the issue at hand and not influenced or to appear to be influenced by factors that were unrelated and that might possibly result in personal gain. Taken as a whole, with the many department and agency heads that made up our state government, it was necessary for the public to have confidence in the people that were making important decisions that impacted the lives of the people in our state and that there were expectations of integrity, impartiality, and fairness—a tone set from the top.

Conflicts of interest and real or perceived improprieties all create a distraction to the ongoing effective work of a department or agency and have the potential to create irreparable damage that impacts credibility and the ability to carry out the department's mission for a long time.

One of the first of a handful of written policies that I implemented in the Department of Health was a code of ethics. It was short and simple and included a reference to the more general conduct required of all state employees. Although no breaches had occurred that damaged the reputation or credibility of the department, I felt that it was important to send out an expectation that such conduct, especially conduct or activities that could create the appearance of conflict, must be prevented. I wanted the issue to be at a conscious level for all health department staff.

An obvious example in public health of a conflict of interest would be an asbestos regulatory worker or a restaurant inspector moonlighting as a consultant for an environmental remediation company or as a food-service consultant. Or if the individual responsible for investigating hospital licensing complaints was also being paid by the hospital to provide worker training to its employees, the impartiality of the decisions made would be undermined and leave any public confidence in the resulting work in doubt. These types of hypothetical situations would not likely be a problem, because they are so blatant; rather, it is the gray situations that are the most problematic. For example, imagine a public health nurse working part-time at a community health agency (even though her usual job has nothing to do with the health agency's work). This could inadvertently appear as if the nurse is influencing referrals to the agency. An *appearance* of conflict exists because of the dual employment. Such appearances can be potentially as damaging, if not more damaging to the credibility of the department and its work, because such appearances and suspicions can be insidious, and not always immediately obvious. And once the conflict or the apparent conflict is noticed, it is too late to fix, and the ensuing questions about organizational credibility are often damaging and tough to repair.

If you think about how difficult it is to lead health efforts in a community, to gain resources within the tough environment of the administration and in the legislative process, to withstand controversy in remedying a public health issue, then you realize every ounce of credibility is needed in individuals and in entire organizations. Conflicts of interests and potential conflicts must be brought to consciousness, identified early, and prevented. For this illness, there is no cure, and we asked managers to submit requests for outside employment and explain why conflicts were or were not present. Often this prompted discussion, sometimes rejection of these requests, sometimes firm boundaries, but the goal was to identify these situations early and prevent problems later on. Fortunately, we never had the hypothetical asbestos worker, restaurant inspector, hospital licensing staff, or public health nurse be a part of a situation that created any real or perceived conflict.

In addition to code of ethics for appointees, employees, and organizations, there is another level of ethics as well. At a career day forum at the school of public health that I attended, I participated in a panel designed to inspire current students about their future careers in public health. All of the panel members talked about the challenges of their respective jobs. One of the areas that I mentioned was the importance of a department code of ethics. One of the other panel participants spoke more personally and directly–about when you go to work, that people buy your services–but not you–and made the distinction to the audience. Simply stated, a code of personal ethics is the place where your allegiance is. A code of personal ethics wasn't necessarily something written down; sometimes it is just a consciousness about where your loyalty is, what the boundaries are, and what lines you will never cross.

What does this mean in public health? I interpreted his advice as stating "Be conscious of always making health decisions first." When we are in school, in public health, medicine, or other careers, our interests and goals may be simple. But sometimes it gets more complicated in the real world, especially when making unpopular decisions, that need to be made to protect health. Health decisions may have consequences, even if made in the most practical way, and there may be tensions between health, economics, and industries. Decisions that protect health may have costs, or are sometimes simply unpopular. Fish advisories protect public health by limiting consumption of fish and thus the intake of mercury in children and pregnant women, but such limits may not be popular with the fishing industry. Following a 1996 outbreak of E. coli 0157:H7 associated with apple juice,[5,6] the Food and Drug Administration's regulations to increase the safety of fruit and vegetable juices and the requirements for warning labels on all untreated juices were not especially popular here, but the regulations were followed and implemented to protect the health of children. Some decisions are difficult and have to be made and carried out in the real world, but they are necessary for health. In public health our service is to the public. I always felt fortunate to have worked with individuals whom I respected because of their integrity, love of Vermont, and interest in improving health.

In public health, in a department whose mission it is to protect and improve the public's health, it is always essential to focus first on what is the health issue, what is the best course of action to protect the public health, and how to best accomplish it in the real world. I always tried to consider every problem, every issue, and every challenge in this light, and I always felt that it was my job to define the health risk or problem and the potential options to improve the situation and protect health, and then figure out how to get it done, in the context of real-world challenges. Making sure that rat carcinogens in stinky tubing didn't end up in maple syrup in a state where the maple industry is a cornerstone of the culture took some fast thinking, swift actions, great science, and hard work to make sure there was no risk to the public (there wasn't).

The concept of a code of ethics is an important one. It gives you, in an ongoing way, your frame of reference and makes sure you and your organization are not slowly moved downstream by a new current, blown in the breeze, caught up in the heat of the moment, the noise of the crowd, or otherwise distracted from your primary allegiance to public health. At every level, being conscious of your responsibilities and obligations and making sure you have a code of ethics for your organization will enhance your credibility and help you to be more effective in your job.

REFERENCES

1. Steinbrook R. Standard of ethics at the National Institutes of Health. *N Engl J Med.* 2005;352:1290–1291.
2. American Public Health Association. *Public Health Code of Ethics. Principles of the Ethical Practice of Public Health.* Available at http://www.apha.org/ codeofethics/ ethics.htm. Accessed May 4, 2005.
3. Vermont Department of Personnel. *State of Vermont Personnel Policies and Procedures. Employee Conduct.* Montpelier, Vermont Department of Personnel; December 15, 1996. Number 5.6. Available at http://www.vermontpersonnel.org/employee/ policy.php?id=pm56.htm. Accessed Novemeber 22, 2005.
4. State of Vermont. Executive Code of Ethics, Executive Order No. 8-91. Montpelier, VT: 1991.
5. U.S. Department of Health and Human Services. FDA proposes new rules to increase safety of fruit and vegetable juices. *HHS News.* Washington, DC: U.S. Department of Health and Human Services; April 21, 1998. P-98.
6. U.S. Department of Health and Human Services. Warning labels required on all untreated juices. *HHS News.* Washington, DC: U.S. Department of Health and Human Services; September 8, 1998. P98-25.

CHAPTER 13

You Must Be Ready for Anything

In public health, one of our core duties is to respond to disasters. What distinguishes a public health emergency from a disaster is a matter of degree and judgment. Natural disasters, earthquakes, floods, and other weather-related events are often unpredictable or, if predictable, occur with great intensity and little warning. One March, during an early spring thaw, in less than a few hours much of Montpelier, Vermont's downtown, our capital city and home of our statehouse, was covered with flood water from an ice jam. The flood destroyed businesses but fortunately resulted in no loss of life.[1] Before 7 A.M., a large ice jam on the Winooski River broke loose and dammed the river. Within moments the river banks had overflowed and water backed up into the streets. Basements and cars were flooded. The first warnings rang out, and evacuations of residents and workers began. The governor declared a state of emergency within an hour and the National Guard was called to assist fire, police, and emergency workers. Electricity was shut off, and an estimated 200 downtown buildings were flooded.[1]

Public health workers were involved in the response as part of the state emergency management effort, which was part of the department of public safety, the government department overseeing the state police and emergency response. Health department involvement included emergency medical services, environmental health, and food and lodging (sanitarians) expertise. Eight thousand gallons of fuel oil leaked into the floodwaters, further contaminating streets, basements, and everything else covered by the floodwaters.[2] After the immediate emergency efforts, questions arose about cleanup, safety of water and food, and restoring flooded areas. Food that came into contact with floodwater had to be discarded, along with food stored in containers with screw caps and flip tops, and canned foods had to be carefully disinfected.[3] For individuals, restaurants, food banks, and many others this was a tremendously difficult time, and the effects were seen for long afterward. Although not the primary response agency, public health had a role to ensure that clear information was provided regarding food and water safety, with the prevention of food and waterborne illness a primary goal. We also had to assure that adequate sanitation precautions were taken. The flood occurred rapidly, caused extensive damage and loss of property to the historic downtown, and required both an immediate and sustained response.[2]

In January 1998, an ice storm blanketed Northern New England and parts of Canada with several inches of ice. Maine, Vermont, New Hampshire, parts of New York state, and Canada were impacted. Thousands were without power and more than 3 million Canadians were without electricity for days after the storm.[4] Five hundred members of the National Guard were summoned to help 20,000 residents in Chittenden County, Vermont's most populous county.[4] Schools, businesses, and government offices were closed for several days, and many people were "iced in" their homes, without power. Six Vermont counties were declared federal disaster areas, and Burlington, Vermont's largest city lost nearly half of its trees.[5] The weather service felt that the geography of the region was responsible for the concentration of freezing rain: the Green Mountains trapped the cold air in Northwest Vermont and northern New York.[6] The intense rain over the several-day period created thick accumulations of ice, causing tree branches to bend down and break, snapping the already sagging power lines. In some cases, huge blue sparks from power lines were mistaken for lightening. Tree limbs fell; roads were closed due to debris and falling power lines. The airport was closed and lost power. A state of emergency was declared in Vermont and New York, and more than about 35,000 people had no electricity in the northwest counties of Vermont. Even some radio stations went off the air. Communications through Vermont Emergency Management was used, and the weather service reported that cell phone communication was not effective due to the large volume of calls. Utility companies looked for additional workers to help with the overwhelming demand.[6] More than 3 million people in the northern New England states and two Canadian provinces were without electricity. Alternative heating carried risks of fire and carbon monoxide poisoning.[6]

Although the weather service had some warning, in public health there really was no way to adequately prepare for the prolonged freezing rain and layers of ice that caused power outages and treacherous roads. The potential health dangers of power outages had been publicized: food in an unopened refrigerator would stay cool for about four hours, and refrigerated food should be discarded after being at room temperature for two hours or more,[3] but such precautions had to be continually repeated to the public to prevent food-borne illness.

Many of us were stuck at home, iced in, with no way to access the health department, located in the city of Burlington. Employees living close by could walk there, but I was stuck in my house, on a hill, looking down a driveway obscured by frozen tree branches from trees that lined the driveway. Even if the branches were clear, the steep ice-covered driveway and long rural road were impassable. Phone and electricity were still working, and I directed staff to make a phone and communications tree with critical employees. Health protection was the name of the health department division that handled much of the responsibility for these situations, but responsibilities included staff in other divisions as well: communications and public affairs, public health nurses and staff in the district offices throughout the state, epidemiologists and food safety experts, and emergency medical services staff.

This makeshift effort continued until power was restored, trees cleared, and roads made passable. Emergency management, federal agencies, law enforcement, and emergency workers did their best to communicate and quickly restore essential services and provide public information regarding instructions and possible dangers during the storm. As power was gradually restored, people slowly recovered their routines, though the damage to trees, homes, and power lines continued for a long time. I turned on the TV to see the news, still iced in at my home and saw a person from a local grocery store being interviewed and the store selling foods, likely spoiled from the power outage and lack of generator power. We contacted available health department sanitarians, who visited the stores to assure all spoiled food was discarded, not sold, to make sure the public would not become ill from the exodus out of their homes, when conditions improved slightly, to buy perishable food supplies.

As one of its core duties, public health has to assist in the response to disaster. In writing about the public health risks of disaster, the Institute of Medicine highlights the importance of interdisciplinary preparedness, communicating to the public, and paying particular attention to vulnerable populations, such as children or the elderly.[7] Although infrequent, the response to each disaster must be rapid, and our attitude must be that we can be ready for anything. Each situation is different, and the response required may be immediate with emergency workers, or during the time of cleanup and recovery, or both. In floods and ice storms, there needs to be careful attention to potential public health hazards from loss of power and use of alternate sources as fires and woodstoves for heat. In addition, preventing illness from contaminated drinking water and food, both through public education and vigorously ensuring that grocery stores, businesses, and others providing food to individuals are consistently following public health guidelines. The response required by the ice storm was a new situation; usual communication strategies could not be used because the office was not accessible. The creativity and dedication of staff to figure out ways to perform required duties prompted a follow-up effort to make sure such adaptive responses and contingencies were understood and communicated throughout the department. This type of thinking, based on the rapid response of health department staff, as well as their flexibility and creativity, was helpful later when response plans for potential bioterrorism attacks were developed, and again in the aftermath of September 11, 2001, during a time of uncertainty and white powder scares.

Such severe floods were fortunately uncommon, and such an ice storm might not be seen again for a long time, but the lessons from the responses were important: be ready to protect the public from the next disaster, whenever it came, whatever it comprised, in the future.

REFERENCES

1. City of Montpelier, Vermont: The Flood of 1992, Chronology. From Ice and Water: the Flood of 1992, Ice and Water Committee. Available at: http://www.montpelier-vt.org/flood/1992/chronology.htm. Accessed March 3, 2005.
2. City of Montpelier. *Montpelier Flood Hazard Mitigation Plan: 1998.* Montpelier, VT: Montpelier Department of Planning and Development; 1998: 40. Available at http://www.montpelier-vt.org/flood/FloodPlan1998.pdf. Accessed March 3, 2005.
3. CDC. *Emergency Preparedness and Response, Food Safety.* Available at: http://www.bt.cdc.gov/disasters/floods/food.asp. Accessed March 3, 2005.

4. CNN Website. January 10, January 13, 1998. Available at: http://www. cnn.com. Accessed March 2, 2005.
5. Vermont Department of Forests, Parks and Recreation. *The Ice Storm in Vermont.* Available at: http://www.state.vt.us/anr/fpr/forestry/ice/icevt. htm. Accessed March 2, 2005.
6. National Weather Service. *The Ice Storm and Flood of January 1998, Service Assessment.* Bohemia, NY: U.S. Department of Commerce, National Oceanic and Atmospheric Administration, National Weather Service, Eastern Region; 1998.
7. Institute of Medicine. *Public Health Risks of Disasters.* Washington, DC: The National Academies Press; 2005:1–6.

Don't End Up in the Recycling Bin— Communicating Health Information

I watched during testimony in the House health and welfare committee at a critical juncture of testimony on a lead prevention and screening bill. I sat in one of the folding metal chairs along the wall of the committee room and listened as different people testified. There was tension between those promoting the mandating of lead screening by passing a law, and those supporting that programs be put in place, parents and health providers educated, and barriers removed to children getting tested, which was our position. We felt that just requiring something didn't necessarily make it happen, and it could even provide a false sense of security. Increasing lead screening was not going to happen without understanding how to get it done, and if you understood how to get it done, why tell people they have to do it? Just show them how, and make it easy for them. However, in some other states, there were laws passed that mandated children be screened for lead, and some of the testimony advocated this approach for Vermont. There was clearly a disagreement as to how to go about making sure all children in Vermont were best screened for lead poisoning, and this was an important part of the bill.

A national environmental group spokesperson was testifying to the committee by speaker phone from a remote location. This was not uncommon, when the committee had additional questions, and was reviewing key sections of a bill. At this point they literally rewrote language, or asked for suggested language; this was the final stage of crafting a bill, just prior to it being voted on, and usually out of the committee. It was also not uncommon for persistent lobbying to result in a section being brought up again for one final committee discussion.

Now, on the other end of the phone, the individual speaking, a strong advocate and expert in her field, was reiterating her strong advocacy for her position, referring to a voluminous document that sat in front of committee members. I sat in my metal folding chair and watched facial expressions and body language as the speaker went on and on, over the speakerphone. The committee thanked her for her testimony, the speaker phone cut off, and the committee discussion continued. I noticed movement at the far end of the table, near the committee chair's seat, and watched as one of the committee members at the end of the table, took the thick paper handout, and dropped it into a recycling bin near the table. The discussion continued for a short time, but ultimately, the speaker's recommendations were not followed.

What had happened that day stuck in my memory as I subsequently prepared testimony for various legislative committees. Even though the person testifying was credentialed and articulate, the large handout was discarded, literally ignored by the committee. It was too long, too verbose, too single-spaced, just too much to be absorbed in that form at a critical decision point. Even at the beginning of the discussion of a bill, a long, detailed report is probably not the form that will get attention or reviewed at a later date. Legislators are busy. They must read and prepare for votes on all kind of issues, rapidly scanning bills, introducing their own based on constituent needs, proposing amendments, and spending time understanding, addressing, and affecting health issues, both large and small, through their committee deliberations. They try their best to understand all dimensions of the issue at hand, and usually listen very carefully, and ask detailed follow-up questions. For example, sometimes the health and welfare committee wants an overview of a department's budget, even though they are not the money committee, to see if spending and priorities are consistent within a department budget. But in order to do this work, in a citizen legislature, with legislators from all types of backgrounds working from January through May each year, each committee member must be able to get information in a form he or she can use to make complex, rapid, and accurate decisions in what may later become the law.

Legislators may be administrators, nurses, doctors, lawyers, teachers, farmers, parents, business owners, employers, employees, or any one of many and varied backgrounds in education, experience, and work. In Vermont, House members sit on a single committee, and in the Senate, they sit on two. If they haven't understood the issue during the committee discussions and done their homework on a bill, when it is voted out of committee it will be debated on the floor of the House or Senate, and must withstand scrutiny from other representatives or senators. So, in order to impact the process, when a bill is taken up by a committee, it is absolutely essential for you to give legislators information in a form they can and will use. Simple is elegant. Shorter is better. A picture, graph, or visual is worth many pages of text. The data should speak for itself. And you should be able to present whatever issue you are discussing in a way that any citizen can understand. Clear information, presented in a form that is helpful to the committee, will not guarantee that your idea or position is supported, but may get you invited again to the table. And that is the beginning.

During this committee hearing and bill markup, I was delighted that the very intelligent, credentialed, knowledgeable, and energetic speaker on the other end of the speakerphone went on and on, accompanied by a tome, that was largely recycled, because no matter how many pages the speaker had typed and faxed, the proposed approach would not work in Vermont, and the committee understood that. She helped make our case with her presentation.

There were other examples of the need to successfully communicate in my day-to-day work. As a member of the administration, I was appointed by a secretary, with approval of the governor. One of the things I had to learn was how to get information up the ladder, fast. Phones were great in an emergency, but often, you got a staff person. We always, in addition to our agency secretary, our immediate boss, had a liaison in the governor's office, a key staff person who was another link to a department. What I asked and needed to understand, instead, was what form did the secretary and governor like for information. That way I could prepare for weeks, months, and years ahead, in how I was thinking, and how we needed to get new issues on the table, and also develop a relationship for those urgent, sometimes controversial issues, that created immediate tensions.

There was a document that went every week from secretaries to the governor called the governor's weekly report. It was a report that the governor read that summarized work of the administration departments and impending problems. It was for both good news and clouds on the horizon. I realized that it provided an opportunity over time, to provide health information. During my early years as health commissioner, I wrote several paragraphs about important health issues, smoking in women, breast cancer, and many other issues to provide background for something we might later want to propose. It required a discipline, in an environment that was usually way too busy for typing, but over time it paid off. One paragraph was perfect, two was okay, and with three you were bordering on hitting the recycling bin. I stopped writing long memos, complete with references. When I got pages of my weekly report submission back with handwritten notes in the margins of paragraphs, I realized that this was the form to use and I made sure to stick with it. We wrote a mix of good new and impending problems, and upcoming issues. Of course, for big issues, there were meetings, but between them, this was a consistent way to communicate with the busiest person in Vermont government.

The form of your information must fit the function it will serve, whether the information is for legislators, governors, senior administration officials, doctors and nurses, the press, parents, or the public. All are busy and if you want to have an impact and get your message across, you must not only know your material and understand the issue and how to approach it, but you must also be able to communicate in a way that can be easily understood and your information utilized. If you want to get your message across, you must avoid the recycling bin. That is the first step to getting your health issue on the table, up the ladder, or out of the legislative committee.

15

The Press Is Not Your
Enemy or Your Friend

Nationally, in the early 1990s, there was a renewed focus on preventing childhood lead poisoning, as the Centers for Disease Control and Prevention (CDC) had lowered the lead level that defined poisoning because of scientific evidence that showed potential adverse health effects at levels previously thought to be safe.[1] This statement from the CDC changed policy direction for lead, and it shifted the focus of public health efforts to prevention, including screening and public education. We were busy developing a public health approach that included working with doctors, nurses, parents, advocates, and others. We worked to set goals, raise awareness, focus public attention, collect data, apply for grants, work with the legislature to pass needed laws, and screen children in free clinics throughout the state. Reducing the percentage of Vermont children with elevated lead levels became a top priority.

The Vermont Department of Agriculture had decided to be very proactive and test some maple syrup for lead in the spring of 1994. Wisconsin had been the first state to do this and, in keeping with the national focus on reducing lead exposure in children from every source, took steps to ensure the quality of their products. In 1992, tests in Wisconsin syrup had found a sample with levels as high as 2500 parts per billion, and their state health agency subsequently advised against lead solder in any equipment used to make maple syrup.[2]

During the time when the agriculture department was conducting tests in Vermont a newspaper reporter filed a request for the testing results under the provisions of the Vermont Access to Public Records Act. Such records were found to be public records and later became material for a front-page newspaper article in the fall.[2]

Our relationship with the agriculture department was always an interesting one. In recent years, we had several issues in common, from rabies to food safety and other animal and human health concerns, which made a strong working relationship essential. Although quarterly meetings between departments staff helped identify and anticipate joint health and agriculture issues, sometimes there were still surprises. Lead tests from 34 of the estimated 2500 maple syrup sugar makers in Vermont found 5 with elevated lead levels, 1 with a level of 1923 parts per billion.[2] We talked with the agriculture department and quickly worked to interpret the impact of their testing on public health, and, given the importance of maple syrup in Vermont, we also prepared to respond to what would undoubtedly be a very public issue.

The October front-page article, with the top headline "Syrup Checks Find Lead" was lengthy and talked about the wide range of results, and that new lead tests were in progress. The agriculture commissioner told the reporter that the highest level was found in syrup from a homemade preheating apparatus that was constructed with lead solder, and the syrup produced contained lead at a level that translated to 29 micrograms of lead in each tablespoon, nearly five times the six microgram per day maximum recommended by the United States Department of Agriculture.[2] Sugar makers and representatives from their associations who were interviewed tried to put the issue in perspective and emphasized that warnings against using lead solder had been in place for several years and that most of the state's syrup was made by larger producers who had already modernized their equipment.[2]

There were no real standards or guidelines for lead in syrup, as there were in drinking water and blood tests for children. Our toxicologist and risk assessor calculated, using a model from the Environmental Protection Agency[3] and based on estimated syrup consumption on pancakes by children, what the health effects would be from consuming syrup with lead at different levels. The agriculture department had tested only a small number of producers and was conducting further tests. We had previously seen a severely lead poisoned child from drinking large amounts of apple cider produced in a maple syrup evaporator that contained lead solder,[4] but the cider was acidic, and the child had consumed large amounts over a long time. This issue was different, and although more extensive testing was needed, as well as health recommendations to reduce lead from all sources, we also needed to keep our focus on lead-based paint and screening children for lead poisoning.

The press got around to calling me the day before the lead in maple syrup article would run. I explained my concerns, why it was important to determine with additional tests how big a problem this really was, and about the calculations used by the health department to determine health impact. Then the reporter asked me if I was going to limit syrup consumption for me and my family. I told him that my family and I enjoyed maple syrup several times a week and would continue to do so, but I also made sure that my children were screened as we recommended. He got it. Later, the same day, another reporter called to ask about sources of lead and childhood lead poisoning, as there would be another article about lead poisoning in the same paper.

There was an opportunity to get the public health message out again. In Vermont, the presence of lead-based paint in our old and aging housing stock was the biggest concern and the focus of much of our public health approach. I reiterated our recommendations to have all young children screened to help prevent childhood lead poisoning. The reporter also interviewed a local pediatrician and parent, and using information from the CDC, wrote a detailed article giving information about sources of lead poisoning, health effects, the importance of screening and the public health recommendations in Vermont.[5] This article ran side by side with the article about lead in maple syrup, helping to put the syrup issue into perspective and providing another opportunity for public health education about lead poisoning.

Following this, the agriculture department conducted further testing and adopted (and later updated) an action level for lead in maple syrup.[6] They continue to work with the maple industry on this issue and with researchers at the University of Vermont.[7]

The press is not your enemy or your friend. To be successful in public health, you must develop a professional relationship with the press. They have a job to do, and you have a job to do, and where those roles intersect, the result can be very powerful for education about public health issues. You must have a proactive strategy for your agency, department, or public health organization. One of the most powerful tools in public health is public education—not shouting about every issue, or becoming embroiled in every momentarily popular health controversy, but making a conscious effort to educate professionals, communities, and the public about health. This is never easy, and sometimes you have to respond quickly when there are health questions or a crisis. But even during those moments when you have to act fast, there may be opportunities to talk about public health and reiterate your public health message. Some articles are controversial and some aggravating, and sometimes you just have to remember that people recycle their newspapers. But, despite these moments, as you formulate your responses to reporters the opportunities to provide important public health information should always be considered. We always tried to work with the press openly, honestly, and consistently, by returning calls and respecting deadlines, because every opportunity to talk with the press, even when the issue was controversial, was an opportunity to talk to the public about public health.

REFERENCES

1. CDC. *Preventing Lead Poisoning in Young Children: A statement by the Centers for Disease Control and Prevention.* Atlanta, GA. United States Department of Health and Human Services, 1991.
2. Howland J. Syrup checks find lead. *Burlington Free Press.* October 5, 1994; 1A.
3. U. S. Environmental Protection Agency (EPA). *Integrated Exposure Uptake Biokinetic (IEUBK) Model for Lead in Children.* Washington, DC: EPA; 1994. Available at: http://www.epa.gov/superfund/programs/lead/products.htm. Accessed November 11, 2005.
4. Carney JK, Garbarino KM. Childhood lead poisoning from apple cider. *Pediatrics.* 1997;100:1048–1049.
5. Blackburn M. Children most at risk from 'silent disaster.' *Burlington Free Press.* October 5, 1994; 6A.
6. Vermont Agency of Agriculture. *Food and Markets. Lead Testing Resources.* Available at: www.vermontagriculture.com/lead.htm. Accessed May 18, 2005.
7. Proctor Maple Research Center. *Research Highlights, 2005.* Burlington, VT: The University of Vermont; 2005. Accessed May 18, 2005.

CHAPTER 16

When You Think You Have Seen It All, Look Again

The Department of Labor and Industry, who administered the Vermont Occupational Safety and Health Administration Program (VOSHA), announced more than $750,000 in fines had been levied against a medical waste disposal facility in Vermont's largest county.[1] Occupational health inspectors from the department of health had been working for several months along with safety inspectors from the Department of Labor and Industry inspecting problems at the facility. There were 42 citations of violations,[2] most related to protection of workers from diseases such as hepatitis and HIV, called blood-borne pathogen standards. From the investigations, it was clear that workers had repeatedly come into contact with material from medical and animal waste that was potentially infectious. In addition, training and protective equipment was lacking.[1]

The publicity around this facility was intense and repeated. Our involvement was related to our role in Vermont's Occupational Health and Safety Program (VOSHA). Vermont was one of the states with a state program, and occupational health inspectors were located in the department of health, but the overall program responsibility was located in the Department of Labor and Industry. In this case, the inspection process was detailed and lengthy and the violations so horrendous that one newspaper article wrote that "state officials were told by one unidentified worker that a bin of used hypodermic needles broke over his head, an experience the worker compared to 'acupuncture'."[3] Because the violations had been so serious and because the VOSHA process could be lengthy, especially if the company appealed the findings, we also negotiated a type of voluntary enforcement agreement, called an Assurance of Discontinuance[4], that required the company to pay for medical exams for workers, because of their repeated contact with medical waste and possible exposure to infectious diseases. Although this type of agreement is filed with the court, it was not clear whether many employees would ultimately participate, but it was an additional action that we could take with our public health authority, while other enforcement actions were ongoing.

The company was not without previous controversy and problems. The facility had gotten permits and began to operate in 1991, despite protests from local citizens and environmental groups.[3] After much ongoing controversy around permits and operations of its incinerator, it installed an autoclave in the mid 1990s. The incinerator had the capacity to treat up to 36 tons of waste daily. It served both medical and veterinary facilities. One third of the waste was incinerated and two thirds was treated in a large autoclave.[5] In 1998, the Agency of Natural Resources, Vermont's environmental agency, had an agreement with the company for penalties related to air and water emissions from the plant that totaled $250,000, the largest single penalty for an environmental violations.[6] Heavy metals and dioxins had been found in the fluid from the waste after sterilization.[5] After the large occupational health and safety fines, the company changed management, but was ordered to close on an emergency basis because of ongoing pollution.[5] Within three days, the facility was open again, after the company challenged the enforcement order,[7] but agreed in February 1999 to relinquish its permits and close for good, after further violations of previous environmental enforcement agreements.[3,6]

Just when you think you've seen it all, look again. There was no way to describe the violations impacting the workers at the plant but horrendous, and it was clear we were all bothered by what we saw and what had happened. It finally took three separate state agencies, using their full authority over a prolonged time period to deal with the problems at the facility. Despite ongoing efforts to improve management, and the constructive nature of many of the enforcement agreements, there were continued problems, and the plant ultimately closed. Public health has a broad scope, one that may require protecting health of many different populations, including workers, and may require persistence and working with other agencies until the issue is resolved.

REFERENCES

1. Vermont Department of Labor and Industry. Safety medical systems fined $762,200. Montpelier, VT: Vermont Department of Labor and Industry; September 8, 1998. News Release. Available at: http://www.state.vt.us/labind/Press/smspress.htm. Accessed July 28, 2004.
2. U.S. Department of Labor, Occupational Safety and Health Administration. Inspection: 302365028, Safety Medical Systems, Inc. Available at: http://www.osha.gov. Accessed July 28, 2004.
3. Bazilchuk N. Incinerator to close for good. *Burlington Free Press.* February 6, 1999; 1A.
4. State of Vermont, Chittenden County, Chittenden Superior Court Docket No. 1150-98. Assurance of Discontinuance, Acceptance and Order, September 28, 1998.
5. Bazilchuk N. State shuts Colchester incinerator. *Burlington Free Press.* January 23, 1999; 1A.
6. State of Vermont, Agency of Natural Resources, Enforcement Division. *Recent enforcement actions. March 1–June 1, 1998; December 1, 1998–March 3, 1999. Available at: http://www.anr.state.vt.us. Accessed June 17, 2005.*
7. Bazilchuk N. Judge rules SMS may reopen. *Burlington Free Press.* January 26, 1999; 1B.

CHAPTER 17

If the Public Doesn't Understand It, It Won't Happen

One of the first public reports I reviewed was a report on testing for dioxins in Lake Champlain prepared by environmental health staff. I read it, and it was indeed very technical. The media had requested copies of the report, and I instructed the staff to write a brief one-page or less abstract summary to put on the cover page, something clear and easy to understand by individuals with no scientific or public health training. The newspaper reporter used what was in the summary for an article in the local paper. No factual errors, clear information, and no time spent trying to correct incorrect information that was our doing.

The visual image of taking any of our documents, publications, reports, educational materials and walking outside the front door of the health department, and handing it to the first person who walked by and having the person be able to read the information and understand it became the way I thought about our communication in public health. It was, of course, more complicated than that, depending on the issue and the group we were trying to reach, but the principle was the same. Our fish advisories for mercury in Vermont waters were as specific as possible and written in different languages. We put specific anti-smoking messages on radio stations that were popular with the group we were trying to reach. We prepared short documents and summaries for legislators about health issues and developed a similar approach when I was preparing my budget for the intense and competitive testimony during the legislative process.

Over time, as we developed short- and longer-term strategies to educate the public and policy makers about public health, we began to create documents using our data to show where we had been, where we were, and where we needed to go, along with the information about how we needed to get there. The first plan for cancer prevention and control was just 16 pages, and the size of a folded sheet of paper, but many of its ambitious goals were accomplished in just a few years. Our first cancer registry report was different from many other states, and took complex data and put it into context, explaining about the leading cancers and cancer killers, screening tests, risk factors, and more. We developed reports and short publications about health: the health of our communities, our health goals for the years 2000 and 2010, progress reports, reports of vital statistics, cancer reports, reports of women's health, men's health, tobacco, lead, mercury, immunizations, diabetes, and alcohol. Although the goal was to let the data speak for itself, charts with our health status in a specific area, such as adults who are physically active on most days of the week, showing where we were and what our goal was, would invariably prompt questions about what people could do, why was it important to their health, how were we doing compared to the nation, or New Hampshire. We anticipated these questions and tried to provide guidance, based on science, best practices, and common sense.

It was a way for us to put issues on the table, to promote and be involved in the discussion. A concise report and plan for diabetes framed the problem and our goals and objectives in areas of public awareness, access to services, patient self-care, clinical practice, professional education, and surveillance (as well as references) in about a dozen pages.[1] When people think of government reports, they may think of big, voluminous, black-and-white documents in small print or something not very readable (though we know that many of our national public health documents and reports are not like this at all), so we made our reports short, inexpensive, colorful, and clear. Our tobacco report "Vermont Best Practices to Cut Smoking in Half by the Year 2010"[2] helped us in the legislature, as well as educating the public at a time when there was debate as to the amount, need, and use for funds for tobacco prevention and control. (A copy of this report was requested by a woman, using a child's voice on the phone, who finally admitted to our public relations staff that she was calling on behalf of a tobacco company.)

There are also tremendous benefits of clear public health communication during urgent issues. At no time was this more challenging than during the white powder scares following September 11, 2001. As white powder was being found everywhere, along with real anthrax threats being seen in Washington and elsewhere, these situations were ones that created real worry and concerns from the public. White powder was discovered by citizens in a magazine in their mail, prompting a local law enforcement and health department response, and a white powder incident closed the Immigration and Naturalization Services building.[3] Papers carried headlines and articles of Vermont scares and national cases, and there were moments when it was difficult to focus on anything else.

When a baggage handler found a substantial amount of white powder on an airplane from Detroit that arrived in Burlington, Vermont, local and national attention became focused on our response. The largest newspaper in Vermont had a picture of the plane and an article about the cases in Washington all on the same page. During these white powder investigations, we learned an approach to communicating with the public that helped us with this as well as other issues. The ability of our national media to get the word out promptly and accurately when there is a major event is incredible; however, if there are inconsistent messages that are promoted nationally and internationally, not only does it cause confusion, but creates worry.

We began to get calls during Vermont's white powder scares and the national anthrax letters about areas discussed on the national press that were confusing, and we watched a report about testing for anthrax in the environment and on the use of nasal swabs for rapid diagnosis that were inaccurate. As the calls came in, we began to monitor national news stations in order to proactively put out statements to Vermont media about areas of confusion created by national news. We worked with infectious disease experts and our epidemiologists to advise physicians not to prescribe Cipro as a preventative antibiotic as a precaution and advised the public why it was not a good idea to take or ask for this or other antibiotics when not indicated. The specifics of laboratory testing, and how long it took for an accurate test to determine if a white powder was anthrax or not, were explained, as well as the use of nasal swabs for epidemiologic purposes. We did our best to address the issues that had become confused in the national press, not because of any intentional effort, but because of the many people trying to speak on the issues and the pace at which it was all happening.

During these days, particularly when white powder was found on the airplane, the phones rang constantly, with local and national inquiries, and it took immense amounts of time to keep up with the questions each day. We began issuing a statement on the Web site for any news and pointing callers to this. It was a consistent message, with the most current and accurate details, and often it was enough for reporters who just wanted an update, and saved much time. The articles that resulted, even though we still answered many calls and also did many interviews, were factual, accurate, and timely and contributed to our efforts to provide the best possible communication to the public.

The dual strategy of providing daily communication during these events, as well as utilizing Web technology to facilitate rapid response to inquiries and maximize the use of our small staff, helped us get our job done. It was so effective that we utilized this same approach for serious disease outbreaks, such as Legionnaire's disease and during our efforts to educate people about West Nile virus. Issues such as influenza and bioterrorism preparedness were also amenable to such an approach. One news article written during the anthrax scares talked about how most Vermonters remained calm despite these events.[4] That was our goal, and we did our best to accomplish it by providing regular communication and developing quicker and better methods to get the information out.[5]

Involving the public can also help you get your work done. Asking the public to report dead birds as part of surveillance efforts for West Nile virus, raising awareness about symptoms of pertussis (it was not uncommon to receive reports of whooping cough from patients themselves), or looking for blue-green algae, were some examples where public education efforts made it easier for the public to access information about public health and helped to address these problems.

Because most organizations have limited budgets for this work, it is important to integrate these principles into practice. Are you an effective teacher of public health, whether communicating to doctors, nurses, parents, the legislature, or the public? Can you translate the scientific basis of a complex issue and write it on an index card? Can you talk about the issues, and put them into the context of public health duties and responsibilities? Can information be understandable to the person you are trying to reach? Clear communication is also an opportunity to build credibility for public health. Over time, it can create more educated public and policy makers, and it enhanced our ability to have the best chance we could to do our job.

Health communication can help in many aspects of public health, especially disease prevention and health promotion at the individual and population level.[6] We know in public health practice, that health communication skills are critical to our success in improving health. Communication is a critical theme in every area of public health—whether giving health warnings to protect the public, explaining data and reports, answering questions raised by the interest of the public and media in many aspects of health, or implementing systematic health communication strategies to promote healthy behaviors. In many ways, public health practitioners must be skilled communicators—translating complex scientific facts and findings into language understandable by the public and specific audiences.

Everyday there are news reports of new scientific findings in science and medicine. On the one hand, the intense interest of the public and media in health is tremendous, and provides opportunities, often at just a moment's notice, to get an important health message out, or reinforce one you have been saying over and over. On the other hand, unlike years and decades ago, individual studies, sometimes conflicting, are presented way before they are folded into the scientific consensus' recommendations on an issue, and have the potential for confusion. A strong and consistent message can be a powerful one that repeated and heard over time, through many different venues, targeted to specific situations, and refined and focused, can shape and promote healthy behaviors. Changing misperceptions around smoking was a conscious and well-developed countermarketing effort, using tobacco settlement funds and professional experts to change the perceptions of smoking created by tobacco advertising. Many times, however, there is neither budget nor time to orchestrate concerted media campaigns, though when able, they served to buttress public health efforts in improving access to prenatal care, reducing youth smoking, and encouraging Vermont women to get mammograms.

Public health officials need to take time to develop strategies to incorporate the science and principles of health communication into every document and opportunity. The danger of not doing so is to risk mixed messages, having the media get it "wrong" because you didn't explain it "right," wasting time, and losing your hard-earned credibility in the process. Clear communication is essential to public health practice, but it can't be a program or isolated event—it must be a way of thinking. If the public can't understand it, chances are it won't happen—whether it is mothers asking about lead poisoning, questions about where to get a test for HIV, women calling to sign up for cancer screening, calls to a quit line to help stop smoking, or what to do with a dead bird. If the public can't understand you, you are missing an opportunity to improve public health.

REFERENCES

1. Vermont Department of Public Health Diabetes Control Plan. Burlington, VT: Vermont Department of Health, 1998. Available at http://www.healthyvermonters.info/hi/diabetes/pubs/diabctrl.shtml. Accessed November 11, 2005.
2. Vermont Department of Health. Vermont Best Practices to Cut Smoking Rates in Half by 2010. Burlington, VT: Vermont Department of Health; 2000.

3. Silverman A. Anthrax scare closes INS. Vermont incident among 8 reports. *Burlington Free Press.* October 14, 2001; 1A.

4. Remsen N. Vermonters respond to threat with a guarded calm. *Burlington Free Press.* October 19, 2001; 1A.

5. Carney JK, Howland J Jr, Erickson N. Bioterrorism: Public education using the internet. Abstract presented at the American Public Health Association 130th Annual Meeting, Philadelphia, PA, November 2002.

6. U. S. Department of Health and Human Services. *Healthy People 2010.* Chapter 11, Health Communication. Available at: http://www. healthypeople.gov/document/HTML/Volume1/11HealthCom.htm. Accessed February 23, 2004.

18

Listen to the Children

Vermont's Attorney General, along with the attorneys general from 47 other states, sued the tobacco industry and according to the November 1998 Master Settlement Agreement, Vermont was scheduled to receive nearly $30 million dollars each year for at least twenty-five years. The governor and legislature agreed on the creation of a Tobacco Control, Prevention and Cessation Task Force (called the Tobacco Task Force for short) that would develop a spending plan for Vermont. Task force members included State senators and representatives who had been active in tobacco advocacy and health, a public health advocate, experts in prevention and cessation research from the University of Vermont College of Medicine, the attorney general, the commissioner of education, a low-income advocate, and me. The task force met through the summer and fall, and a series of public forums were held around the state to gather public input about how the money should be spent. The idea was that the task force would have a plan for the legislature, such that there would be advance preparation and planning prior to the legislature convening in January, when budget discussions would commence. Strategically, it was to get ahead of the intense and sometimes tumultuous debates that occurred when additional funds were available. This settlement was not a usual occurrence and it was anticipated that there would be much advocacy for a variety of different uses for these funds.

The task force met over a dozen times and had an extensive and well-publicized effort to gather public input. Six forums were held around the state, and a youth forum was attended by over 200 students in grades 5 to 12. In addition, members of the task force received many letters that provided additional suggestions.[1] In the course of the public discussions, one group of young citizens captured my full attention, a class of students from a small elementary school in Randolph, Vermont. During the fall, coincident with the public forums and much media publicity about Vermont's use of the settlement fund, I received a packet of letters, handwritten by students in a sixth-grade class at the Randolph Village School, outlining their thoughts about what Vermont should do with the settlement money.

Some children who wrote had family members who smoked and were worried about their parents' health. One letter suggested that there should be anti-smoking commercials and that before they were developed, that we should talk to kids like them, because (diplomatically stated) the current ones were dull and didn't work as well as they could. Kids, the letter said, could help tell us what would get kids' attention.[1] Another idea was to show x-rays of smoker's lungs to every kid. A suggestion was made to increase the fines for stores that sold cigarettes illegally to children. One writer expressed hope for the future - that no kids would smoke.[1] Children were supportive of our efforts and from their suggestions, knew that smoking was bad for their health, and understood how important it was to keep kids from starting to smoke.

One child asked me to write back and said that we should save all the money until we had enough to buy the tobacco industry. He suggested turning the factories into something else so that there would be no more cigarettes and cigars. Then, he reasoned, people would have to quit smoking. [1]

In the midst of our efforts to allocate Vermont's share of the Master Settlement Agreement, we received much wise and original advice from children who would be impacted by the decisions that we made. I read the letters over twice and wrote a letter back to each child. Children touched upon many areas recommended by the CDC in the development of comprehensive tobacco control programs.[2] Many suggestions, such as better enforcing laws to prevent illegal sales, making sure help with quitting was a priority, and using focus groups of young people to help develop anti-smoking ads all became part of the way the program was ultimately designed and implemented. (Unfortunately, we were unable to buy the tobacco industry.)

Later, after the task force had concluded and final legislation passed, the newly-created 13-member Tobacco Evaluation and Review Board included 2 youth members, who would have a critical role in developing and implementing this program.[3] Although still sparse, articles from the scientific literature highlight efforts to evaluate the impact of youth empowerment in tobacco programs.[4-6]

At a time when we were trying to develop the best possible tobacco program, a teacher recognized an opportunity to add children's ideas to the discussion, and these honest and insightful suggestions stuck with me as we worked to reduce smoking. Nowhere is the thinking so honest and the perspective so clear as how children see the world, including public health. On this issue, smoking, what I called over and over again, our "top priority" or sometimes "public health enemy number one", a single classroom of children's voices helped shape our efforts. I was glad that they wrote.

REFERENCES

1. Blueprint for a Tobacco-Free Vermont: Final Report of the Tobacco Task Force. Montpelier, VT: Vermont Tobacco Task Force, 1999: 28, 33. Available at http://www.leg.state.vt.us/tobacco/finalreport.pdf. Accessed March 28, 2005.
2. Centers for Disease Control and Prevention. Best Practices for Comprehensive Tobacco Control Programs. Atlanta, GA: US Department of Health and Human Services; 1999.
3. Acts of the 1999-2000 Vermont Legislature. Act 152 (H842). An act making appropriations for the support of government. Available at www.leg.state.vt.us. Accessed March 28, 2005.
4. Holden DJ, Messeri P, Evans WD, Crankshaw E, Ben-Davies M. Conceptualizing you empowerment within tobacco control. *Health Educ Behav*. 2004: 31(5): 548-63

5. Ribisl KM, Steckler A, Linnan L, Patterson CC, Pevzner ED, Markatos E, Goldstein AO, McGloin T, Peterson AB; North Carolina Youth Empowerment Study. *Health Educ Behav.* 2004: 31(5): 597-614.
6. Dunn CL, Pirie PL. Empowering youth for tobacco control. *Am J Health Promot.* 2005: 20(1): 7-10.

PART II

Issues

CHAPTER 19

Anthrax and Airplanes

It was nearly midnight, and I had just drifted off to sleep when the phone rang. It was a health department manager, calling to tell me that there was a problem in a plane at the Burlington International Airport. This was October 2001, the same month when members of Congress received envelopes containing anthrax and many samples of white powder had come to the health department laboratory from a variety of places. It was a frightening time. The public and health department laboratories all across the country were flooded with white powder samples from all over. Without laboratory testing it was not possible to tell which were real, which powders were hoaxes, and which were just white powder.

A baggage handler had found a significant amount of white powder in the cargo hold while luggage was being removed from a jetliner arriving from Detroit. Airport security had called local police, the state hazardous materials team, and the health department. The FBI was also called. Passengers arriving had been taken to a seating area at one of the airport gates and an epidemiologist arrived to interview individuals and make sure all contact information was obtained. Health department staff provided advice regarding any need for decontamination and arranged for the department of health laboratory to receive samples for testing.[1,2]

The next morning the health department received many calls from concerned citizens. This was happening in the context of local and national white powder scares and finding real anthrax. A man in Florida had died with a diagnosis of inhalation anthrax.[3] CNN reported a fifth and then a sixth case of anthrax infection—a CBS News employee and a postal worker from New Jersey—both diagnosed with cutaneous anthrax,[4] more treatable and less lethal that the inhaled form. Reports of anthrax made national news when national news media and senators, including the senate majority leader, were targeted. Then anthrax was diagnosed in a postal workers.[5] Rewards were offered. The FBI investigated links between the New York and Washington, DC, form of anthrax,[6] as national public health officials issued warnings for physicians to be on alert for diseases caused by bioterrorism.[5]

In Vermont, about 20 samples of suspicious powders from around the state were being tested, and the number of scares and white powder incidents increased, causing a frenzy.[2] The state public health laboratory could perform a quick visual inspection of the powder under low magnification and look for spores. However, more reliable culture methods, though slower, were needed to determine the presence or absence of anthrax bacteria. The testing took 72 hours, and despite the growing concern of the public, there was no faster way to do it. I spent my time giving press interviews[2] and checking in with our lab and epidemiologists about the testing and whether or not individuals on the plane would be at risk.

One question we had was: could the powder find its way from the cargo hold to the cabin where passengers were seated? Was the ventilation of the cargo hold connected to the cabin? I listened to one of the epidemiologists as she spoke to someone from the airline company and confirmed that there was the potential, based on how this particular plane was built, for there to be air exchange between the cargo hold, where the luggage was, and where people sat in the plane. We had to know this, because if the lab findings suggested the possibility of anthrax, then we would need to recommend precautionary antibiotics to the passengers on the flight. Media interviews continued, along with continued testing on many samples from around the state, as we waited for updates from the lab about the white powder from the plane.

On Wednesday, the lab informed us that they had found the growth of a bacillus or rod-shaped bacteria of the same genus causing anthrax. There were many different bacteria in this category. If the bacteria were indeed the type that caused disease in humans *(Bacillus anthracis),* by the time we had definitively identified it in the lab, people would be at increased risk to develop serious illness from the exposure.

The Centers for Disease Control and Prevention (CDC) was working diligently to assemble and rapidly distribute recommendations for states as the reports of lab testing for white powder samples and real cases of anthrax in humans were reported. Information came to us as quickly as possible, and published in the *Morbidity and Mortality Weekly Report,* the CDC's weekly publication.[7] The CDC reported that for inhalation anthrax, although the exact incubation period was unclear, it was estimated to be between one and seven days, ranging up to 60 days.[7]

We knew immediately that the safest course to protect the public was to recommend precautionary antibiotics be given and taken until the final lab results were in. The rationale was although we felt that B. anthracis was not likely, despite the preliminary findings, (because there were so many forms of the bacteria, and they were commonly found in the environment), if it was anthrax and we waited the additional time to complete the culture testing, people could already be on their way to serious illness. Mortality from the inhalation form was very high; and described as "usually fatal" by CDC[8], so taking precautionary steps in the unlikely event this was real would be appropriate and protect the health of those on the plane.

We conferred with the CDC, because of the seriousness of our actions, and their national perspective in all this, and began to organize a clinic at the health department. Epidemiologists had contact information for all the passengers. The local hospital, our academic medical center, assisted in our efforts, as well as an infectious disease specialist and pharmacists. Sixty-six passengers, crew baggage handlers, and emergency responders were notified by phone and recommended to begin preventive antibiotics as a precautionary measure.[1,9]

We organized and held a clinic in the health department. The program for Children with Special Health Needs had a medical clinic area in our main building, with a waiting area, and exam rooms that were specially decorated to be friendly for the children they usually saw. We used clinic rooms decorated to put young patients at ease: the Jungle Room, the Farm Room, Up in the Air (decorated with planes and rockets), and Under the Sea (with an aquarium). Public health nurses, epidemiologists, and the infectious disease specialist came down to the health department to help. The lab notified us in the late afternoon; we organized during dinner time, and held the clinic from about 9 P.M. until well after midnight. Individuals were provided medical counseling and antibiotics, and instructions were given. One staff member patrolled the parking garage that was beneath the building as a "media bouncer" to protect the confidentiality of patients and not distract all of us from giving advice and preventive medication to all involved who needed it. Meanwhile another public information expert from my office prepared a media summary of what was happening.[9]

Law enforcement, the Vermont attorney general's office, the FBI and U.S. Attorney's office had all been making detailed inquiries throughout the incident, day, and evening, and we kept them apprised, along with the administration, of what steps we were taking and why. All of these events, if tests were positive for anthrax, had such dramatic ramifications for members of law enforcement that their interest was intense.

The clinic finished in the wee hours of the morning, and we went home tired but feeling like we had done everything possible to protect the passengers until the lab results confirmed or denied that it was anthrax. The only thing missing was the public notification. Our decision to not do this until after the clinic was complete was both because of the late hour and the necessity to act swiftly to set up and give advice and medication to a list of passengers, crew, and emergency workers. We didn't want there to be any delay or impediment from people seeking advice at the health department. Patient confidentiality was essential, but it was necessary to notify the public what was happening as well.

Early the next morning, we got a tip that that law enforcement officials, both state and federal, would likely be providing information about this situation at an 11 A.M. press conference Vermont's capital, in Montpelier, nearly an hour away from the health department. We were planning to issue a morning press release, but instead, decided on a press conference at our office in Burlington, at 10 A.M. Health officials needed to be speaking about health concerns. I spoke from a podium to a small room with television and newspaper reporters and told them that the bacteria growth of the rod-shaped bacteria meant that the substance could be anthrax and that we felt that this was possible but unlikely. The antibiotics were recommended as a precautionary measure while waiting for the definitive laboratory test results.[9]

Vermont had plenty of white powder scares, but no anthrax, and fortunately not even anything close to anthrax. The next day, there was a photo of the plane on the front-page along with a headline and front-page story, next to information about national and international anthrax investigations.[10] All local television stations carried the story. We began to get many more calls from concerned Vermonters, calls from local and national media. Epidemiologists, myself, and public information officers spoke nearly nonstop about the situation, while we waited for the lab results. Passengers on the plane, however, were remarkably calm. We were able to reach all those who were potentially impacted, and we were confident we had given medical advice and medication in sufficient quantity for the time being. Another front-page article on the same day carried the headline "Vermonters respond to threat with a guarded calm."[11]

It was an intense 72 hours. On Friday, the lab confirmed that the bacterium was not *Bacillus anthracis,* the bacteria that caused anthrax. All 66 people were contacted and told to discontinue antibiotics, and a press statement was issued. The final reports of this incident were carried on the evening news and newspapers the following day.[12,13] Newspaper articles that carried the reports that the tests for the white powder were negative also carried side-by-side reports of a *New York Post* staffer and New Jersey postal workers testing positive.[14,15]

White powder scares happened across our nation and in Vermont. The CDC reported that from October 3, 2001, until November 2, 2001, there were 21 cases of anthrax (16 confirmed and 5 suspected) of anthrax related to intentional bioterrorism acts. Reports of infected individuals came from the District of Columbia, Florida, New Jersey, and New York City.[16] The CDC reported that from September 11 to October 17, an estimated 7000 reports were made and more than 1000 tests of suspicious powders were conducted in health departments around the country.[16]

We were fortunate that our white powder was not anthrax. The plane left the airport and went back to its home base. Throughout this time, we worried about what we would do if it indeed was anthrax. If the tests had been positive for anthrax, the people on board, the crew, and emergency workers would have been protected.

Nationally, white powder was everywhere, some of it anthrax, but most of it not. The problem was that you couldn't tell which was which without testing. And the form of the disease caused by inhalation was rapidly progressive and often fatal. Such a climate, in the aftermath of September 11, 2001, had the ability to create public concern and panic. The most difficult challenge as a public health official, in addition to treating each situation as if it could be anthrax, was to be conscious of how health information was communicated and received. Our approach, to act swiftly and decisively, repeat important health messages to the public on a regular basis, didn't take the white powders away, but made sure the public would be protected should the worst occur and helped to keep the public calm during this time.

REFERENCES

1. Carney JK, Howland J, Erickson N. Bioterrorism: Public education using the internet. Abstract presented at 130th annual meeting APHA. November 2002. Philadelphia, PA.
2. Wright L. Scare grounds plane at Burlington airport. Leslie Wright. *Burlington Free Press.* October 17, 2001. P. 1A.
3. CDC. Ongoing investigation of anthrax–Florida, October 2001. *MMWR.* 2001;50:877.
4. CNN.com. Anthrax scares tax health system, law enforcement. October 18, 2001. Available at http://archives.cnn.com/2001/HEALTH/conditions/10/18/anthrax.impact/index.html. Accessed October 29, 2005.

5. Espo D, Associated Press. $1M reward offered: more anthrax found. *Burlington Free Press*. October 19, 2001. P. 1A.

6. Espos D, Associated Press. Anthrax links hunted. NY, DC cases show similarities. *Burlington Free Press*. October 17, 2001. P. 1A.

7. CDC. Update: Investigation of Anthrax Associated with Intentional Exposure and Interim Public Health Guidelines. *MMWR*. 2001;50: 889–893.

8. CDC. Emergency Preparedness and Response: Anthrax. Available at http://ww.bt.cdc.gov/agent/anthrax/faq. Accessed November 10, 2005.

9. Vermont Department of Health. Airline passengers get preventive medication. October 18, 2001. News release. Available at http://www.healthyvermonters.info/news.shtml. Accessed November 10, 2005.

10. Bazilchuk N. Vermont fliers treated as precaution–Cipro given in case powder was anthrax. *Burlington Free Press*. October 19, 2001. P. 1A.

11. Remsen N. Vermonters respond to threat with a guarded calm. *Burlington Free Press*. October 19, 2001. P. 1A.

12. Gram D, Associated Press. Powder found in luggage not anthrax. *Rutland Herald*. October 20, 2001. Available at http://www.rutlandherald.com. Accessed October 29, 2005.

13. Vermont Department of Health. Powder on Airliner Did Not Contain Anthrax. October 19, 2001. News release. Available at http://www.healthyvermonters.info/news.shtml. Accessed November 10, 2005.

14. Hallenbeck B. Tests clear powder found on Vt. plane. *Burlington Free Press*. October 20, 2001. P. 1A.

15. Gardiner S. Postal workers in New Jersey test positive. *Burlington Free Press*. October 20, 2001. P. 1A.

16. CDC. Update: investigation of bioterrorism-related anthrax and interim guidelines for clinical evaluation of persons with possible anthrax. *MMWR*. 2001;50:941–948.

20

The Stinky Tubing Saga

In the 1990s, there were many issues involving both health and agriculture. Our usual partners and colleagues had been doctors, nurses, and hospitals, but it seemed that we were seeing a shift in the nature of some of the food and environmental issues in public health. We worked hard to try and communicate on a regular basis with other state agencies that had potential health-related work, such as the environmental agency and the agriculture department. This communication came in the form of a meeting and handshake, commissioner to commissioner, and quarterly meetings with key staff, such as our environmental health director, state toxicologist, risk assessor, and epidemiologists. This was done to prevent situations in which one agency squared off with another in the press, and the public seeing and thinking that the government really didn't have its act together. Years earlier, one such public argument came over health statements about air pollution contaminants and their potential health effects—statements offered by an environmental agency employee, rather than a public health official. This damaged the credibility of both agencies, no matter who was right, and we felt that this was not the best way to practice public health, particularly with health issues that involved other public agencies. Despite our efforts to communicate more proactively on an ongoing basis, we had occasional surprises.

The problem that came to our attention one May involved malodorous tubing, "stinky" tubing that had been used to collect sap to produce maple syrup.[1] The odor, after evaluation by the best chemical and toxicological noses, was not totally characteristic of a single chemical or category. It was impossible to categorize with the smell test, to pinpoint exactly the nature of the stink. Some of the maple syrup producers had described the smell as medicinal, and the resulting syrup as bad tasting and not able to be sold. A syrup producer contacted the agriculture department to report the odor in the early spring; agriculture department staff investigated the situation and traced the odor to the plastic tubing that carried maple sap to collection buckets. The source of the tubing was further linked to a distributor in central Vermont and to a producer from Canada.[2]

The agriculture department worked with a food chemist at the University of Massachusetts to further study the tubing and staff at the agriculture department worked with the distributor to track down all the tubing. In May, a rural advocacy group made the issue public, and the health department became involved.[2] As many as 150 producers had possibly used the tubing, and it was estimated that the 250,000 feet of tubing could have impacted as much as

4200 gallons of syrup, less than 1% of the syrup produced each year[2]. It was also noted by the press that Vermont's maple industry generated more than $20 million each year[2]. At the request of the agriculture department, additional tests were done by the Massachusetts expert. The tests entailed running water through the stinking tubing at a high flow rate and analyzing what chemical compounds came out.[2]

While attorneys for health and agriculture worked to determine whether the known laws, regulations, or standards from the federal Food and Drug Administration for tubing used for food products had been followed, we were more concerned with any possible health effects from consuming syrup made from this tubing. Sap running through tubing from the trees, and then concentrated for syrup, could result in evaporation or concentration of contaminants, depending on their nature and chemical properties.[1] The agriculture department was trying to identify and find all such tubing that was being used, and we worked on the public health aspects.

Health department staff that were critical to answering such questions were experts in the lab, the state toxicologist, and risk assessment experts. Epidemiologists were also helpful, in the event we had to do any testing and controlled study. The Massachusetts expert working with the department of agriculture conducted tests designed to simulate syrup production, by running water through the tubing at a rapid flow rate.[3,4] We received a list of chemical compounds that had been detected when water was run through the stinky tubing in a simulated laboratory setting in Massachusetts. The immediate challenge was to figure out how we could determine if there was any risk to the public's health. We first had to determine if any of the compounds were potentially harmful to human health and try to prioritize and pick out the compounds that were most harmful to people: substances that caused cancer, or substances potentially harmful to the liver and kidneys, in humans or animals.

One compound on the list raised red flags. It was called 2,4,6- trichlorophenol (2,4,6-TCP) and was a fungicide that, as best we could tell, hadn't been produced in years, and had no current registration, or license, for use. The toxicological information found from the EPA suggested that this compound was a probable human carcinogen, and caused leukemia and lymphoma, a lymph gland tumor, in rats as well as liver tumors in mice.[5] There was no way that this compound should have been present in the tubing; it was not a normal component of plastic tubing. We didn't know how it got there, whether it migrated from contact with the plastic, or how the tubing became contaminated, but its presence in the Massachusetts scientist's work made it imperative to determine whether or not it was also in the syrup eaten by children and adults. With the help of the agriculture department, we needed to figure out whether or not any of the syrup made from the stinky tubing had been marketed and sold to the public and whether or not any harmful compounds found in simulated tests in the Massachusetts lab actually made it into the syrup that people were eating.

We also picked several chemical compounds that could serve as sentinel compounds, meaning that if these chemicals, that could cause the worst effects in humans or animals were present at very low levels, levels too low to be of concern to human health, it was unlikely that anything else really would be harmful. We didn't know if this was a problem or not—the scientist at the academic center had run water through the stinky tubing, and analyzed what came out. We didn't know if this meant that any of these chemical compounds were present or not in the syrup that people bought and ate, and we had to find out.

The other compounds we chose were Di-(2-ethylhexyl) phthalate (DEHP), acetophenone, and phenol.[1,5-7] Phenol was used in production of resins, synthetic fibers and many other products, and had a prominent odor. There was no evidence that it caused cancer in humans, but there was information about adverse effects on fetal growth in animals.[7] DEHP, a compound that makes plastic more flexible[6] was also a probable human carcinogen based on information from liver tumors in rats and mice.[5,6]

The presence of 2,4,6-TCP in the water from the stinky tubing and the fact that its health effects in animals were so serious (it was classified as a "probable human carcinogen"[5]) made it important to make this information public until we could quickly determine if this compound was in the syrup itself. This was not a small matter. The commissioner of agriculture was in the process of finding all the stinky tubing.[2] In an effort to alert consumers, we decided to notify the press about the situation. We informed the press that we were testing for compounds that were known to be harmful to animals. When reporters asked about how long it would take to get a definitive answer, I told them a week.[8] This was a major stretch and our laboratory would have to work at full tilt to get the answers we needed. Now we had to get the work done quickly.

Newspapers carried the initial story.[3,4] The issue became intensely public and news reports chronicled events over several days.[2-4,8,9] Some maple producers reacted angrily. As the agriculture department worked to recall the tubing that was still out there, the agriculture commissioner told the press that "we have contaminated tubing. We don't know if we have contaminated syrup."[9]

A senior manager told me I had better visit the lab—he usually didn't say this, but I knew it must be important. We sat down with one of the senior lab managers. The lab staff was thinking hard, but really didn't yet have an approach to testing for these four compounds. Agriculture officials would gather syrup samples, but lab staff had to come up with a methodology that would answer questions about potential health risks, and not gum up the chromatograph. It took about an hour, but we came up with a plan to get standards for the few compounds that were of concern, figure out the method, work closely with the other state labs as needed, and have all this done in less than a week. I was not sure when I entered the room whether this could happen, but as I left, I was confident that they had rallied, and would be talking with them frequently in the next few days.

The lab got the standards for the compounds we needed. During one of my visits, cans of maple syrup were lined up along the sides of the lab bench, as the technicians refined their testing methods. Agriculture officials collected syrup cans for us, using their knowledge of all the producers and who had this tubing. Forty-two samples were obtained, some from producers using the tubing and some from controls—producers who had used other tubing. There were also some samples from a single producer that had used the stinky tubing and some other tubing, some who had used it then switched to other tubing, some from syrup that had been marketed and some that had been held because its smell or taste were off. Working with the agriculture department staff, health department staff figured out that some of the syrup never marketed would represent the worst case scenario, and proceeded to develop a case-control type of study for maple syrup, looking at levels of the four compounds in syrup made with the stinky tubing and syrup that was not. The lab figured out how to perform the testing, with frequent cleaning of the equipment to ensure that the chromatograph still worked and was able to run nearly nonstop throughout the week.[1]

Public pressure was on for many reasons: producers who had come forward had had their syrup publicly noted—a concern to their future sales, the importance of the industry in Vermont, and the fact that the compound we were really concerned about caused cancer, at least in animals. The toxicologist and risk assessment expert were ready to make comparisons when tests were ready. They had exhaustively researched all available information about health effects of our sentinel compounds in humans and animals, studied all available standards and guidelines, and thought about safety factors to ensure risk to the public was limited. The two were prepared to look at both children and adults, and make assumptions about both for syrup consumption: children and adults ate four tablespoons of syrup each day for 365 days of the year for three years, the maximum time the tubing could possibly have been in use, and considered (even in Vermont), to represent maximum consumption and potential exposures to any contaminants.[1] They organized their information and assumptions, so that when the lab completed its testing, they could make the necessary calculations. For cancer-causing substances, the commonly used risk comparison was a level that was below a one in a million lifetime risk, over a 70-year lifetime, and staff worked to calculate any excess lifetime cancer risk. Protective factors were often built in for children, because they were growing rapidly, or on the assumption that they might be more sensitive to certain chemicals than adults. There was an expression that we always used: "You always err on the side to protect the public health," meaning if there were choices about how to make assumptions or calculations for a health risk, you always chose the one that was most protective of health. Besides cancer risk, a hazard index was used to quantify noncancer risks.[1]

The results looked at levels of the four compounds selected for testing, because they represented the ones with the worst possible potential effects on human health. Acetophenone was not found in any samples, and laboratory staff felt that because of its volatility, it likely boiled off during the process used to make syrup.[1] Phenol and DEHP were found in nearly all the samples tested in very, very low concentrations compared to the toxicological information. 2, 4, 6-TCP was found in 3 of 42 samples tested.[1] The lab confirmed that the compound was definitely the one we were concerned about and not a similar compound, and gave the information to the toxicologist and risk-assessment expert. Based on the information about cancer and noncancer risks, and the assumptions made for both children and adults, including body weight and levels of syrup consumption, the total potential excess lifetime cancer risk and the noncancer hazard index were calculated. Based on the testing information, assumptions used, scientific references, and resultant quantitative calculations, the total excess lifetime carcinogenic risks were far below the lifetime risk of one in a million, the comparison customarily used, and the non-cancer risks fell far below the hazard index of one, the reference used.[1]

We had to quickly get this information out to the public. The agriculture commissioner came to the health department, and we both jointly addressed the press in one of the health department conference rooms. We gave them the results of the findings and what they meant, trying to explain them in plain language. We didn't have much time beforehand, but I thought as I reviewed the results with our toxicologist and risk assessment expert how to translate this information and communicate it to the public. The extensive laboratory, toxicological, and scientific work that had gone on as staff sprinted through the week to test syrup and interpret results was detailed and complicated. Talking about "de minimis risk of one in a million," risk assessment methodologies, details of chromatography, and how much syrup children really ate and how many days they ate it, weren't really the concern, as we had always made assumptions most protective of health in our calculations, and also sent samples to another state lab and a Massachusetts lab to check our work.[10] The bottom line was whether or not it was okay to use the syrup.

We quickly decided to explain the findings by giving the syrup a "clean bill of health," and answered questions about how we did the testing and why we knew that. The front-page headline the next day read "Maple passes tubing test,"[10] and the article said that we had found no health risks, that the syrup had passed the tests, and accurately described what we had done and our conclusions. A similar article in another newspaper proclaimed "Health Department finds its Pure Maple."[11] A long week was over. The agriculture commissioner talked about certifying equipment to prevent similar problems in the future.[10] I was absolutely confident that the syrup indeed had a clean bill of health, and had the tests to prove it. The health department staff, in this circumstance, reacted promptly, thoroughly, and as a team. The lab showed a level of creativity that I had not seen before, and the exhaustive research by the toxicology and risk-assessment team gave me the information to do my job. The step of making our concerns public, when the decision to do testing in syrup had been made based on worrisome contaminants in tubing, was difficult, but necessary, and put pressure on us to come to a quick conclusion.

You never know what each day will bring in public health. There are times when you can only describe it as "every day is an adventure." Our work with agriculture officials was sometimes challenging and always interesting, but our teamwork was what served the public best. A public health laboratory able to respond to new and different situations, expert and capable individuals in toxicology and risk assessment, and the ability to respond quickly together, in a practical way when there is a serious health question, is essential to getting the job done. Although we never did find out exactly what made the tubing stink and how it really got there, we were indeed certain that there was no health risk to the public and were confident that our syrup had a clean bill of health.

REFERENCES

1. Vermont Department of Health. Maple Syrup Testing. Burlington, Vt: Vermont Department of Health, Burlington: 1996. Technical Report.
2. Good J, Liley B, Lisberg A. Syrup tubing tests delayed. Agriculture Commissioner regrets not reacting sooner. *The Burlington Free Press.* June 13, 1996; 1B.
3. Good J. Maple advisory issued. Suspect tubing raises concerns. *The Burlington Free Press.* June 13, 1996; 1A.
4. Derby D. State Says Bad Batch of Tubing May Taint Syrup. *Rutland Herald.* June 13, 1996; 1.
5. United States Environmental Protection Agency (EPA). 1996. Integrated Risk Information System (IRIS). National Center for Environmental Assessment. Cincinnati, OH. Available at http://www.epa.gov/iris/intro.htm. Accessed April 10, 2005.
6. Agency for Toxic Substances and Disease Registry. US Department of Health and Human Services. ToxFAQs for Di(2-ethylhexyl)phthalate (DEHP) 1993, 2002. Available at http://www.atsdr.cdc.gov/tfacts9.html. Accessed April 10, 2005.
7. Agency for Toxic Substances and Disease Registry. US Department of Health and Human Services. Public Health Statement for Phenol. Available at http://www.atsdr.cdc.gov/toxprofiles/phs115.html. Accessed April 10, 2005.
8. Derby D. Tubing Results Due in A Week. *Rutland Herald.* June 15, 1996; 15.
9. Good J. State hunts for tainted tubing. Letter asks producers to call, keep suspect tubing off market. *The Burlington Free Press.* June 14, 1996; 1B.
10. Maple passes tubing test. Officials find no health risks. Betsy Liley. *The Burlington Free Press.* June 22, 1996; 1A.
11. Derby D. Health Department Finds It's Pure Maple. *Rutland Herald.* June 22, 1996; 1.

21

Is There a Doctor in the County?

In the 1990s there was a growing focus of health policy discussions on access to health care. Policy makers talked about health insurance and ways to reform our health care system. In Vermont, there was a blue ribbon commission on health care, appointed by the governor, and later a health care authority was created and given broad responsibilities to present health care policy options to the general assembly. The public discussion on health care focused largely on health insurance and how we could make improvements in our current system or completely change it to provide health care for all our citizens.

I was involved in many aspects of the policy discussions, and served as a member of the blue ribbon commission, but my primary responsibility as health commissioner was the public's health. As the discussion and debate focused on access to health care, I often found it helpful to think about access to health care in the negative as well as the affirmative. What keeps people from accessing health care? What are the barriers? Are there ways to improve access that can address the barriers? I learned this lesson well when we worked towards and succeeded in improving access to prenatal care in Vermont. We addressed the existing financial barriers, as well as increased the number of practitioners. We worked on educating the public to improve the health of mothers and babies. We used simpler administrative methods and public health nurses to help women navigate the often confusing system. Thinking about what the barriers were and how we could lessen them was a concept that had a broader application to other public health issues, specifically access to health care.

What was it about health care that could improve health? If everyone had access to health insurance, wouldn't they go to their doctor, or other health practitioner, earlier, before they were very ill, possibly needing hospitalization? If there were insurance, wouldn't people access preventive care and prevent or detect early health conditions when they are more treatable? Screening for cervical cancer, breast cancer, or colon cancer; immunizations for children and adults; counseling to prevent or quit smoking, to not abuse alcohol, eat five fruits and vegetables a day, and get regular physical activity were all things that could potentially be improved though improved access, specifically financial access to health care. And, of course, the public health department had a critical role to play in making sure health improvements occurred, through linking special populations to services, such as providing guidelines for preventive care for children on Medicaid, providing screening for lead poisoning if needed, educating the public, and promoting health behaviors, all of which complemented the work of primary and preventive care in physician's offices. During the discussions about expanding access to health insurance, there were opportunities to improve public health even further, by linking our efforts to improve access to primary and preventive care to the insurance discussions.

But, Vermont was a rural state, and we wondered that even if everyone had an insurance card, would they all be able to get care? Would we even have enough doctors and other health professionals to achieve this? Other potential barriers included knowing when to go to the doctor, how to stay healthy with preventive care, and whether there was a doctor in the community. Although experts haggle about the numbers of doctors needed to adequately supply health care to our entire population, there was no argument that having enough primary care in rural areas was an ongoing challenge, but it was absolutely necessary if we were to improve health care access and, most importantly, improve health.

Recruiting and retaining an adequate supply of practitioners was difficult for many reasons. Medical training usually occurs in more urban areas, where there is ready access to diagnostic and therapeutic technology and specialists nearby. Physician groups and health systems may be larger, and "night-call" may be less frequent. In contrast, rural practices are often smaller, less dependent on nearby specialists and technology, and require more time on-call. Costs of medical training are high, and insurance costs contribute to ongoing expenses. Doctors in rural practice have to be independent and must be comfortable being generalists, particularly in more remote areas.

During the discussions about health insurance, we worried that we didn't have a mechanism or a system in place to make sure we had enough health professionals in all areas of the state. But how would we know if there was a doctor in the county? We had to find a way to size up our supply of primary care practitioners in all parts of the state, figure out whether we had enough, and target efforts to improve the supply where we were short. There were federal measures for comparison; while these didn't give a precise target, they provided a ballpark estimate of how many doctors were needed in a given population area. There were federal designations, designed to take into account populations, rural settings, and a few health status measures. We worked to apply for grants to take advantage of all of these, but it was still necessary to bring this national perspective home to Vermont. We really had no map, no data about where doctors were practicing, in what specialties, or in what Vermont location. To develop policies or programs to assure rural access, it was first necessary to know what was currently happening. The question was, how could we do this in a practical way with little state funding available for such initiatives?

We figured out a way to link our information needs to carry out our public health responsibility in the health care reform debate with information collected elsewhere. Professional licensure in Vermont was administered by the Vermont Secretary of State's Office, in the Office of Professional Regulation. It was here that professional licensing standards were set and enforced for public protection. The Board of Medical Practice, though quasi-independent, was administratively located with the other boards. Doctors in Vermont had to renew their medical license every two years in order to practice medicine. I thought that we should try to find out more about where doctors in Vermont were practicing, by connecting to this licensing process. We talked to the Board of Medical Practice, and they were willing to work with us.

We developed a survey to find out about the demographics of practicing physicians in Vermont: their age, gender, specialty, location, workload, and where they received their medical and residency training. The idea was that we would analyze the surveys and compare our results to national benchmarks to see if we had a physician shortage in parts of the state. Once we had this information, and a map, we could work with the University of Vermont College of Medicine, hospitals, and others to develop methods to recruit and retain primary care physicians. As physicians were licensed every two years, repeating this survey would give us a snapshot of how we were doing and over time allow us to measure our progress and target our efforts.[1]

In the first report, we found that we had severe shortages of physicians in 8 of 14 counties. Only 2 counties had an adequate physician-to-population ratio.[2] Although there was debate in the scientific literature about how accurate current benchmarks were, we reviewed the available literature and considered them a target[3,4] to help us frame some of our information in a way that we could more easily identify federally designated shortage and underserved areas. At the time, there were no more precise measures to incorporate trends in population demographics or details of community health status, but any benchmark we chose would have to be monitored over time, with formal surveys, such as the one done every two years, as well as the informal communication and working relationships with all the groups and organizations in Vermont equally committed to assuring access to primary and specialty care. Response rates were high and much information was gathered about where physicians received their education and post-graduate training, and about their collaboration with advanced practice nurses and physicians' assistants. We found out whether practices were accepting new patients, and about the age and gender distribution of primary care physicians, and in which areas of the state doctors were leaving or most likely to retire in the near future.[2]

This first step, documenting our supply and need, helped build a foundation for our efforts, working closely with the hospitals in Vermont, the University of Vermont College of Medicine, the legislature, primary care associations, and the federal government. Loan repayment, a recruitment center, curriculum changes, and the development of an Area Health Education Center program at the UVM College of Medicine (that reached across Vermont) all worked synergistically to improve our supply of primary care physicians in our most fragile areas. Over time, advanced practice nurses, physician assistants, and dentists were also surveyed. As of the year 2002, the statewide ratio of primary care physicians per 100,000 people had increased from 70 full-time equivalent physicians per 100,000 people in 1994 to 80 per 100,000 people, and improvement was seen in many counties. Although Vermont was making steady progress,[5] due to the programs, commitment, and collaborative work in place, assuring access to primary care in all parts of our rural state continues to be a challenge and a public health goal for the year 2010.[6]

Improving access to primary and preventative care is critical to improving the public's health. The age of the population, prevalence of acute and chronic health conditions, and other factors are important in the consideration of need for primary care professionals and the first practical step of knowing whether there was a doctor in the county helped us frame the issue and bring it to the attention of the public and policy makers. It was important to look, document, measure, and make this information relevant to the area that we cared about—Vermont. It was the first step in knowing whether our efforts in this important area would be successful.

REFERENCES

1. Carney JK, Moran-Green M, Thompson EB, Rosenstreich S. Vermont's Health Care Providers: A Comprehensive View. Abstract presented at American Public Health Association 122nd Annual Meeting. October 30-November 3, 1994. Washington, DC.
2. Vermont Department of Health. Vermont Health Care Provider Profiles. 1994 Physician Survey. Burlington, Vt: Vermont Department of Health.
3. ABT Associates, Inc. *Reexamination of the Adequacy of Physician Supply made in 1980 by the Graduate Medical Advisory Committee (GMENAC) for Selected Specialties–Final Report.* Springfield, Va: National Technical Information Service, US Department of Commerce; 1991. HRSA 240-89-0041.
4. Cooper RA. Perspectives on the physician workforce to the year 2020. *JAMA.* 1995;274:1534.
5. Vermont Department of Health. 2002 Physician Survey. Available at http://www.healthyvermonters.info/hs/phstat/provider/PHYSOZPP.pdf. Accessed November 10, 2005. Burlington, Vt: Vermont Department of Health.
6. Vermont Department of Health. *Healthy Vermonters 2010.* Burlington, Vt: Vermont Department of Health; 2000:5–7.

22

Regulating Nursing Homes: Community Health, Individual Health, and Public Resources in an Uneasy Balance

Patricia A. Nolan, MD, MPH

Fragile elders and severely disabled people often live in institutions that provide their homes, their room and board, and their medical, nursing, and social services. The residents of nursing homes, group homes, and assisted living facilities are vulnerable to poor care and financial and physical abuse because they are sick, demented, or disabled. The federal government regulates nursing homes, states regulate nursing homes, and so do some local governments. The Medicaid program pays for about one half of all nursing home care, more than $43 billion in 2001, and the amount rises each year. Two out of every three nursing home residents has at least part of their care paid for by this joint state-federal program.[1] Various public interests may be in conflict, complicating the issues of regulating and paying for nursing home care and protecting the vulnerable.

People rightly expect that nursing homes will provide high-quality care with kindness and respect and the public expects the government to assure this happens. When things go wrong from the residents' perspective, families and friends of residents expect the problems to be fixed, and those responsible identified and punished. The government's tools for punishing the errant nursing home–closures, fines, and withholding payments, for example–may compound the harms to residents. The current strategies promoted for improving the quality of health care include making information about quality more available to consumers and using root cause analysis and incentive payments for quality as tools.[2] Information about the quality of nursing home care is increasingly available, and some efforts at improving care with incentive payments for increased staffing or other tangible quality measures are underway. However, despite huge efforts to provide quality care and consumer information, nursing homes are particularly vulnerable to deteriorating quality of care. A case history from my experience in Rhode Island is instructive on what can go wrong.

In the early 1990s, a nursing home with strong community ties was failing. The community owners found a buyer who was more experienced in making deals than in operating nursing homes. The department of health opposed the reopening of the home because it was deemed unneeded, and the proposed renovations were too expensive. Our department also opposed the buyer's becoming a nursing home operator because of concerns about his financing and his lack of experience in health care. The Certificate of Need review found many problems with the proposals. The buyer made adjustments to satisfy the minimum requirements. When the US Department of Housing and Urban Development (HUD) approved the mortgage, the objections we had were moot: a higher authority effectively declared that the project was financially sound. The new owner had no history as a nursing home operator. Our ability to make a case that he was not a fit operator was severely limited by that lack of history. Ultimately he obtained a Certificate of Need, a nursing home license, and a HUD mortgage.

By the time the home reopened under its new owners in 1999, there was a poor relationship between the regulators and the facility. The first reinspection after licensing (2000) turned up several important deficiencies in care; the facility promptly corrected these deficiencies. This pattern was repeated in 2001 and 2002, but with different deficiencies. Our facilities regulation staff calls this pattern "yo-yo-ing" and considers it a sign that a facility needs scrutiny. After the 2002 inspection, we recommended financial penalties, but the facility corrected the problems and the fines were not imposed. However, we had a shortage of inspection staff and a number of other nursing facilities with significant problems involving patient care. Despite serious concerns, we received few complaints, and none that triggered special actions. This home did not continue to receive extra attention after it corrected the problems identified in late 2002.[3]

The same pattern occurred in 2003, but with repeated deficiencies, and resident care problems were significant. Residents with fragile skin were not being well managed. They were suffering skin breakdown and developing bed sores. These were not healing well because nursing care plans were not up to standard or not being properly and consistently carried out. Rumors of financial problems circulated, but the staff remained quite loyal. The state's ombudsman expressed great concern but did not press to move individual residents. In an effort to get the facility operator's attention, we recommended financial penalties to the Center for Medicare and Medicaid Services, which started the facility on the track for termination. The termination process gives the facility time to correct its deficiencies. Failure to make corrections results in termination of participation in the Medicaid and Medicare programs, which pay for a large majority of nursing home services. Closure or sale is the usual result.

The department of health was in an awkward position. Now we had a nursing home with a number of patient care problems and a history of being unable to sustain good nursing care for all its residents. If an inspector pointed to a nursing care problem, the staff would deal with it promptly, but the nursing management could not recognize developing problems or sustain improvements. While some residents were receiving poor care, many were pleased with the care and did not want the facility to close. A hold on admissions and readmissions was instituted to try to reduce stresses on the nursing staff, allowing it to get reorganized. Our regulatory action further exacerbated the financial problems of the facility.

The operator asked for an advance payment from Medicaid. This provided an opening for the health department to make very clear to the owner that turning around the situation required a long-term commitment. The department of health and the department of human services (DHS), our Medicaid agency, worked together closely, trying to determine the financial status of the home. We jointly informed the operator that the financial arrangements needed to be transparent *and* the nursing and dietary services had to be revamped. A clear message was delivered consistently: the facility must be in complete and full compliance by the end of April 2004, or there will be no further Medicare or Medicaid payments. Finally, in March 2004 the owner abruptly filed for bankruptcy protection and turned the facility over to a receiver.

As the receiver took over, media interest intensified. The question of whether the facility should close, displacing residents who were doing well in the facility, became front-page news. The receiver had a good track record of turning around failing facilities. Suddenly, a facility on track to be closed in early May was the subject of a concerted community effort to preserve its license. The administrator was discharged. A new nursing management team came in to try to turn the facility around. The union was trying to keep the facility going. The ombudsman worked with families to engage them in improving care. The governor publicly encouraged state agencies to try to get things resolved without closing the facility. He met with families, residents, and staff to cheer on the effort. DHS amended the Medicaid state plan to allow the nursing home to continue receiving payments after it was terminated from Medicare participation. In the end, the task proved impossible and the facility closed, requiring the resettlement of more than 100 people.

When the facility actually closed, it felt like a defeat. But once the home closed, the residents were resettled in other homes with no major problems. A good physical facility stood empty, waiting for a new owner.

However, the resulting media storm continued to build. An investigative series appeared in the *Providence Journal* weeks after the facility closed. These were stories about the ordeal of an individual resident whose poor care led the health department to place a hold on admissions. Her story of bed sores that worsened while the nursing home failed to get its act together was unfolded in a weeklong expose. The actions of the regulators (remember we had demanded improvements, imposed fines, stopped admissions, stopped readmissions, publicly condemned the facility, worked with the ombudsman to help families and residents, cut off state and federal payments and threatened to revoke its license) were judged insufficient. One colorful columnist called me immoral for not "doing something" about the poor care.[4] Public perception shifted from blaming the nursing home owner to blaming the regulators.

An investigation was commissioned by the governor and a series of hearings were held by other political leaders. In the next legislative session packages of bills were proposed by the governor and the department of health and DHS and by various legislators to increase financial scrutiny of nursing homes and care oversight, to increase public access to information about nursing homes, and to increase regulatory resources. At the end of the 2005 legislative session, a package of bills passed and was signed by the governor on July 5, 2005.[5] The new law clarified the powers and duties of the department of health, extended the authority for the state to examine nursing home finances, and strongly promoted public information. Key to change, the budget also provided additional staff resources for nursing home oversight. Some measures intended to increase collaboration among state agencies did not pass in the 2005 session.

How can we regulate nursing homes and protect individual residents while controlling costs? Can we prevent poor care by regulating nursing homes more stringently? It is not clear that we can. In this case, I believe the combination of the owner's financial dealings that diverted attention from resident care, a nursing home administrator who did not organize the facility to deliver good care, and a director of nursing who did not organize sustained nursing care systems contributed to a rapid downhill slide in the quality of care. Our system of regular inspections was able to point out these problems and document them, but did not have the power to achieve a change in direction. Other facilities with marginal operating capital and weak management have deteriorated and closed or changed ownership, often with much disruption in the lives of residents and their families.

Rhode Island has a stringent regulatory system: on average, homes receive four inspections a year. The federal nursing home regulations are detailed and stringent. The state mirrors them and adds a few regulations. The facilities regulation staff is well trained in how to inspect, how to document findings, and build a regulatory case. The surveyors are top-notch caring professional nurses, nursing home administrators, and other health care professionals. They are deeply concerned about the welfare of the residents of nursing homes. They are also trained that they are not the caregivers, and that they cannot substitute their judgment for that of the caregivers. Their job is to determine if proper care is given, and, if not, to require the facility to repair the problems.

Could we do more to protect the public's health if we concentrated on improving access to residential options for the frail elderly and the disabled? A number of lively experiments in long-term care alternatives have been developed in both the public sector (state Medicaid programs) and in the private sector (life care programs). The underlying premises are hard to test—Are home and community based options cost effective? Does quality of care and quality of life improve for most residents if more alternatives are offered? More home-like environments are highly desirable, but allowing "aging in place" is a challenge. Special arrangements can help meet one or two residents' skilled nursing needs, but as residents age and deteriorate, these assisted living facilities with insufficiently skilled staff, less stringent fire protection, and lower rates of reimbursement are quickly overwhelmed. The options for homes and community-based services are important, especially for improving quality of life. However, as an isolated strategy to improve long-term care, expanding alternative sources of care is unlikely to protect the severely incapacitated. It may siphon critical resources from the care of the most difficult nursing home residents.

The department of health responded to a different agenda than the media: we worked to document problems, to point out where changes were needed, and to hold the incompetent management of the facility accountable for fixing the problems. The media, and the general public, were very interested in how the state regulatory agency was going to fix the problems. Should the department change procedures to provide more direction and support to facilities on how to fix problems?

Improving communication with families and residents about the problems in a facility seemed like an easy step to take. Our inspectors are instructed to avoid giving advice on how to fix problems and to avoid taking direct action as problems are observed. Our interactions with the state's ombudsman are often very fruitful in helping individual residents and in placing residents when facilities are deteriorating or closing. However, in other instances, we did not meet each other's expectations, and residents and families were disappointed in the outcomes.

A particular customer service problem occurred over resident complaints. The department treated complaints as warning signs needing investigation. We triaged the complaints and scheduled investigations. We were not resolving the complaints for the complainants. In fact, we did not communicate with the complainants much at all. The public sees complaints as individual problems requiring immediate response. Families expect action. In other words, we treated complaints as evidence for regulatory actions. People wanted us to fix the individual resident's problems, rules or no rules. The department of health is changing its procedures to increase communication with the families and with the physician of record, hoping to meet family expectations. In addition, the agreements with the ombudsman have been revised to clarify expectations.

Caring for our vulnerable aged and disabled citizens is a growing challenge. Both regulatory and financing reforms are needed to meet the challenge. A lot can be learned from our failures!

REFERENCES

1. Government Accounting Office. *Medicaid Nursing Home Payments: States' Payment Rates Largely Unaffected by Recent Fiscal Pressures.* Washington, DC: GAO;2003. GAO-04-143.
2. See *Quality: Where is the Incentive?* A series of articles in *Health Affairs.* 22(2), March/April 2003; and *Patient Safety: Achieving a New Standard for Care,* developed by the Institute of Medicine and published by the National Academics Press, October, 2003.
3. Rhode Island Long-Term Care Coordinating Council, Task Force on Nursing Facility Closure. *Hillside Health Center: Doors Closed, Lessons Learned.* November, 2004.
4. Governor's press conference releasing the Hillside Report, Sept 20, 2004. www.ri.gov/GOVERNOR/?month=09&year=2004. Accessed December 3, 2005.
5. Governor's press release: "Carcien Signs Nursing Home Reform Legislation" July 5, 2005. www.ri.gov/GOVERNOR/?month=07year=2005. Accessed December 3, 2005.

Clorox and Cooling Towers

It was a Thursday, the first of August, usually a quiet time in the summer, a time when many people enjoy the Vermont summer. The epidemiology unit was contacted by a hospital in central Vermont to report a patient confirmed with Legionnaires' disease. The patient had symptoms of cough, trouble breathing, chills, head and muscle aches, and was sick enough to be admitted to the hospital. A test for the protein, or antigen, from the bacteria causing Legionnaires' disease in a urine sample was positive.[1]

According to the Centers for Disease Control and Prevention (CDC), there are anywhere from 8,000 to 18,000 people each year in the United States diagnosed with Legionnaires' disease.[2] Although the public hears about and remembers outbreaks, most of the cases occur in individuals called sporadic cases, and are not part of an outbreak. It is also reported that anywhere from 5% to 30% of people die as a result of their illness.[2] Symptoms include non-specific flulike symptoms such as fever, chills, and a cough that can be dry or produce phlegm. Many people with Legionnaires' disease have pneumonia when chest X-rays are taken. There are milder symptoms, without pneumonia; this is called Pontiac fever, and patients may recover on their own without antibiotic treatment.[2]

As there are many different kinds of pneumonia caused by many different microorganisms, specific tests, such as for a protein or antigen in a sample of urine, are done to make a specific diagnosis of Legionnaires' disease. Other tests to diagnose Legionnaires' disease involve testing the phlegm from someone with coughing symptoms or taking blood samples several weeks apart to see if there has been an increase in the antibody against the bacteria responsible for the disease.[2] People who are healthy may recover well, but people with chronic illnesses, such as heart or lung disease, or who smoke cigarettes or who have conditions that may weaken the immune system may contract pneumonia and have a more serious illness. Not only are such individuals more likely to catch the illness, but they are also more likely to die of it.[3]

Vermont had first hand knowledge of Legionnaires' disease in the late 1970s and 1980s, when there were two outbreaks of Legionnaires' disease in hospital patients and many deaths. It was a time when scientists and doctors were just learning about Legionnaires' disease, and Vermont had been heavily impacted.[4,5] Following the 1976 Philadelphia outbreak, 19 Vermont patients died in 1977. In 1980, 88 individuals became ill and 17 died from Legionnaires' disease in Vermont.[4,5]

Despite the long interval since these events, recollections of those outbreaks and the seriousness of them were still high, both among physicians who had been involved and the press. Legionnaires' disease was one of the diseases reportable to the department of health epidemiology unit, part of the disease surveillance, or early warning efforts to track, report, and stop as early as possible, outbreaks and epidemics of diseases. Each year, there were an average of seven sporadic cases reported to the health department,[6] most of them sporadic cases, meaning they were not related to any identified common source of exposure. One difficulty was that the scientific literature said cases were sporadic or isolated, but we sometimes wondered if that just meant that you couldn't track a source. In any event, the finding of a single case of Legionnaires' disease in Vermont meant the launching of an investigation; because if there were more cases to follow, we knew the situation could be serious or even fatal for people involved.

Since 1994, in Vermont, there had been 56 reported cases of Legionnaires' disease, and 11 of those people had died.[7] As Legionnaires' disease was one of the causes of pneumonia in the community, it was important to make sure physicians were thinking about it, as confirmation of the disease depended on doing the specific test for the disease. During an outbreak, it was critical to make sure that the public knew and understood symptoms that would direct them to medical attention, to make sure any and all cases were promptly identified.

Much had been learned about Legionnaires' disease since the 1970s. Although not spread person to person, disease outbreaks have been reported from contaminated water sources in a variety of settings, such as whirlpool spas, showers, cooling towers, other mists, but not home air conditioners. According to the CDC, the bacteria that causes Legionnaires' disease may be found in many types of water systems, but the conditions necessary for the bacteria to multiply and develop large numbers occurs in warm and stagnant water, with temperatures ranging from about 90°F to 105°F. To avoid the growth of bacteria, it is necessary for water systems to be properly designed and maintained.[2,3]

The patient confirmed with Legionnaires' disease had been an inmate at the Dale Women's Correction Facility in Waterbury, Vermont, for the previous year but had been released a short time before she was hospitalized. Because the incubation period for the disease is between 2 and 10 days, it wasn't possible to determine if her exposure was related to the correctional facility or came from the community.[1,3,6] A reported case of Legionnaires' disease gets high priority treatment from epidemiologists, not because it is spread from person to person, but because even though most cases cannot be linked to an outbreak, when outbreaks occur, they are serious and can be deadly. The same day this case was reported, an investigation was begun, and two epidemiology staff were sent to the Waterbury Complex, to learn more about the patient, to determine whether any other inmates, patients, or staff were sick. Epidemiology staff wanted to know if during the recent past weeks others had any respiratory symptoms. Another purpose of the visit was to provide clear and accurate health information about the situation and the reason for the investigation.[1,8]

Waterbury is right off the interstate highway between Burlington and Montpelier and close to recreation and tourist favorites. It was an old state government complex. In the late 1800s the Vermont State Hospital opened and

housed a significant population of individuals with mental illness, whose population decreased dramatically in the 1980s.[9] The Waterbury complex contained
the Vermont State Hospital and a large array of state government departments
and buildings: the Agency of Human Services, Department of Mental Health,
Agency of Natural Resources and related environmental agency departments,
Public Safety, the state police, the Vermont Department of Emergency
Management and the Emergency Operating Center, the corrections department,
and a state laboratory. Although other state departments were located in
Montpelier, and the health department was in Burlington, Waterbury and this
aging complex was home to many state departments and employees, as well as
being the home of the Vermont State Hospital.

The location of the multiple state government departments in this area had
implications for the investigation, because the epidemiology staff needed to
interview people from all the departments working in close proximity to the
Dale Correctional Facility. They met with administrative staff looking for respiratory illness in staff and patients at the state hospital. The epidemiology staff
reviewed files and interviewed staff with symptoms.[6,8] In addition, during their
interviews, they also noted complaints about water damage to ceilings and
water that had been dripping from pipes for the preceding few months.[1]

On the same day, epidemiologists were also told that a state employee who
worked in the same complex was in the hospital with respiratory symptoms.
This individual worked just across the street from the Dale building, where the
first ill person had resided.[1] Further discussions with the hospital personnel
found that there were three other patients living in a home in the village of
Waterbury who also had respiratory illness. Legionnaires' disease tests were
ordered for them all. Hospitals in the area were contacted about recent patient
hospitalizations with illnesses that fit symptoms for Legionnaires' disease.[1] A
press release was sent out that same day, on Thursday, talking about the single
confirmed case of Legionnaires' disease and the ongoing investigation.[6]

The investigation started with epidemiologists looking for serious respiratory illness, contacting hospitals, physicians, and going to the location where
the patient was living during the incubation period for the disease. As the disease must be specifically tested for, it was important to test individuals with respiratory illness, and be on the lookout for others hospitalized and not yet
diagnosed to see whether the one was an isolated case or just the tip of the ice-
berg. This active case-finding, as it was called, was essential—not just waiting for
illness, but aggressively looking for it.

Meanwhile, epidemiology staff, knowing how Legionnaires' disease could
occur in outbreaks, quickly talked with environmental health experts in the
health department's main office in Burlington. Although these environmental
health experts usually inspect restaurants and other food and lodging establishments, they were experts in diseases of a waterborne nature as well, and worked
closely with epidemiologists when a possible outbreak had a food or waterborne source.

The third major partners in the investigation were the public health nurses in
the closest district office to where the investigation was taking place, in Barre,
Vermont. Public health nurses, called "epidemiology designees" or "epi designees"
for short, were trained by epidemiologists and provided the local resources to help

when there was concern about an outbreak anywhere in the state. In quiet moments, they had other jobs, but could pivot and take on this critical role to rapidly expand resources during investigations or outbreaks.

The pace and activity of the investigation picked up, and the lab continued testing as cases were investigated. On Friday, health department staff went back to Waterbury to meet with staff in other buildings and received more reports of people sick who had worked or lived in Waterbury. A news release updated the public about the investigation.[8] A conference call was arranged with the CDC, who was routinely consulted for their national perspective and for their assistance in laboratory testing.[1] On Friday, August 2, a complete environmental or "sanitary survey" of the affected area was conducted by the environmental health staff. They looked at buildings, showers, where the drinking water comes from, and how high the water temperature gets. They looked for and inspected cooling towers. They looked on the roof for standing water and water leaks. They found that the south cooling tower across from the Dale building contained chemicals to kill algae but no residual chlorine.[1]

A second positive test was reported in a person who lived near the state office complex and regularly visited the complex. The same day, two days after the first case was reported, health department epidemiology staff were investigating many reports of respiratory disease, lab samples were being tested from patients, and environmental samples were taken from the cooling tower and in the Dale building, including the showers.[1] After the cooling tower samples were taken, it was chlorinated, and water temperatures in the agriculture lab and Dale building were raised for 24 hours to a high enough level to kill bacteria.[7] Samples were also taken from the home where the patient diagnosed with Legionnaires' disease had lived.[1]

During Sunday of the same weekend, health department environmental health staff continued to investigate for sources of Legionella bacteria. They found a second cooling tower in the Waterbury office complex, called the North tower, and tested and chlorinated it also. Inspectors drove through the town looking for other cooling towers. They even took samples from vegetable misters at a grocery store in town because the literature had cited such a source as responsible for an outbreak and because patients had shopped there.[1] Much of state government shuts down on the weekend, but I had spoken with the buildings commissioner and told him of the urgent need to work together to inspect, take samples, and clean and chlorinate when necessary. The state buildings department sent their staff to work side by side with the health department during the weekend.

Based on literature sources of previously reported outbreaks, not only were samples taken, but definitive actions taken while we waited for results, such as heating the water in the showers, chlorinating the cooling towers, so that if either proved to be the source, they would already be cleaned. From Thursday to Sunday, both epidemiology and environmental health staff worked to find and take care of any and all identifiable sources of Legionella bacteria in the area. Environmental health staff went door to door and found cooling towers in nearby businesses.[1] I drove around the area, within a 1-mile and 2-mile radius to make sure I was also immediately familiar with all the stores, businesses, houses, and state offices in the area. Because cooling towers had been the cause of so many other reported outbreaks, the ones in the area were further cleaned and disinfected. Other cooling towers in the area were tested, and owners were asked to disinfect them as a precaution.

Because of the report of Legionnaires' disease, the activity around the investigation, and the potential concern among local state employees, we wrote updates of the investigations and answered questions. Tourists called and asked whether the town was safe to visit and were reassured. I went to the town on numerous occasions for meetings and went to the radio station in town right in the middle of the outbreak to answer questions on the air and show my confidence in what actions health department staff had already taken. After talking with our epidemiologists, I also made the decision to give daily media information and updates, as proactively as possible, to try and get out timely, accurate information in a way that gave the facts, what people should expect, where to get more information, and who to call if you were sick. It was necessary during that time when we were actively searching for all cases to make sure people in the area, both the public and state employees, knew what symptoms to be on the lookout for and saw their doctor for testing if they had any of the symptoms. We also let physicians in the area know about the investigation, what types of tests should be done, and who to call with suspected cases or with questions. More than a dozen news releases were issued to provided updates about the investigation.

Daily press information required time each day to develop and answer any questions. Because the incubation period was anywhere usually from 2 to 10 days, if the source was in the complex, despite the fact that it had been cleaned and disinfected, we would expect to continue to see illness during the incubation period after exposure had occurred. We told people what to expect and why. Cases to date, numbers of negative tests (there were far more than positive tests), and symptoms that should prompt a call to their doctor were repeated in our daily written statements, our press releases, and on our Web site. We talked to the media, whether newspaper, television, or radio, on many days for several weeks.[4,5,10,11,12,13,14,15,16]

The communications effort was time well spent—an article in the newspaper talked about people at a local bar stopping to see the update on the TV, then going back to their conversations.[11] A state representative later told me that she had no calls from worried citizens in her area, and if they had been worried and nervous, she would have heard. State employees continued to do their work during this time of uncertainty. We continued to be accessible and provide regular updates.

The disease count increased—a third case occurred three days after the first reports, and we continued to monitor tests on patients and those from samples taken from environmental sources. On August 6, five days after the first reported case, there were three cases confirmed and four more suspected.[10] All were either state employees or lived or spent time in Waterbury. No one had died, but there were people hospitalized. At the same time, Great Britain was reporting its worst outbreak of Legionnaires' disease in a decade with 94 hospitalizations and a death. This provided another perspective on how potentially serious such situations were.[12]

The cases totaled 14 in Vermont by August 10.[13] Legionella bacteria were found in one of the cooling towers, though this wasn't enough to determine cause and effect, since the CDC had estimated that about 8 out of 10 cooling towers harbored the bacteria. By August 20, 18 people were diagnosed and one remained hospitalized–still no one had died. More than 120 tests had been negative so far.[17,18] The towers were suspected because of their close geographic proximity, their relation to previously reported epidemics, and the fact that so many people's illness could be explained by them through some type of outdoor air transmission. But that was not enough to implicate them as the cause.[13] At the end of the first week of August, a culture sample had been taken from the first hospitalized patient in the hopes that if positive, tests could be performed as to the specific type of Legionnaires' disease bacteria and link it to the tests of the cooling towers.[1]

Samples tested at the CDC from the south cooling tower were positive for Legionella pneumophila serogroup 1, type 1,2,3. Other samples were positive, but none for serogroup 1, one of the groups most commonly implicated in human illness. All the shower samples from the Dale building were negative at the health department lab. The samples taken from homes, the north cooling tower, and the supermarkets were also negative. Two cooling towers in the immediate area were tested, but none grew serogroup 1.[1]

Thirteen people were hospitalized and all recovered.[17] There were no deaths. When the epidemiology staff took detailed histories, looking for common exposures, such as jobs, homes, hobbies, and where they went grocery shopping, they found that seven individuals worked at the Waterbury state office complex, five lived in Waterbury, four worked and lived in Waterbury, one lived in Waterbury and worked nearby. One was a visitor to the state complex, two were visitors and residents, one was a patient at the state hospital and one was an inmate of the correctional facility.[1]

Nearly 200 lab specimens were tested in the lab during this time, with the vast majority testing negative.[1] In some cases, split samples were tested in the health department lab and also at the CDC, due to their expertise in testing for Legionnaires' disease. The health department laboratory, a small public health laboratory in comparison to CDC, could not perform all the typing needed to make a more precise match, and this was done at CDC.

Finally, the test from the phlegm from the first patient diagnosed tested positive for Legionella pneumophila, serogroup 1, subtype 1,2,3, from the laboratory at the CDC, the same type as the Legionella from the south cooling tower. The last person diagnosed with Legionnaires' disease got sick on August 10. This person would have been exposed on August 1 and 2 before the cooling tower was cleaned on August 3.[1,19] The outbreak had stopped.[16] Health department staff provided recommendations the state buildings department as well as the American Society of Heating, Refrigerating and Air-conditioning Engineers (ASHRAE) to reduce risk of Legionella in cooling towers. Later, health department staff reviewed plans for ongoing maintenance.[1,16]

The tracking and control of infectious diseases is a cornerstone of public health. Preventing epidemics and the spread of diseases is a core duty of public health departments. The successful performance of this duty relies on the ongoing surveillance, or early warning system, the clinical expertise and public health perspective of energetic epidemiologists, laboratory staff, environmental sanitarians, and public health nurses, along with the close collaboration of physicians, nurses, and hospitals. It further requires knowing the natural history of these diseases, the causes of outbreaks in other states and countries, and the ability to rapidly investigate potentially deadly situations on the suspicion of a few or even a single reported case.

Legionnaires' disease outbreaks can result in deaths and serious illness and have the potential to cause public concern, even alarm. The most important lessons from this outbreak investigation were the speed and skill with which department staff investigated and anticipated both the disease and related environmental factors, as well as the nearly constant communication throughout the outbreak that kept state employees and town residents calm and able to cooperate fully as the investigation progressed. Health department epidemiologists were capable and calm, providing leadership within the department and engendering public confidence. Communication, through daily press updates, gave the public the most current information, and gave us an opportunity to repeat symptoms, provide information about the disease, and tell people who to call and what to expect.

Because of the incubation period, we told the press that more cases were expected, and this helped as more cases were diagnosed and the tally was reported in our daily briefings. The outbreak was stopped—no further cases occurred after the incubation period of the disease following cleaning and disinfection of suspected cooling towers. Public health actions taken, based on rapid investigation and knowledge of other outbreaks, clear communication, and anticipating the potential harm from a single case, was critical to preventing more illness and protecting the public's health. This was public health in action.

REFERENCES

1. Vermont Department of Health. *Legionellosis Outbreak: Waterbury, Vermont, August, 2002.* Burlington, Vt: Vermont Department of Health; 2003.
2. Centers for Disease Control and Prevention. Legionellosis: Legionnaires' Disease (LD) and Pontiac Fever. Available at: http://www.cdc.gov.ncidod/dbmd/disease info/legionellosis_g.htm. Accessed October 29, 2005.
3. CDC. Legionnaires' disease. *MMWR.* 1997;46:28–34.
4. Legionnaires' Disease Found in Ex Inmate. Matt Sutkoski. The Burlington Free Press. August 2, 2002. P. 1B.
5. Sutkoski M. Doctors learned Legionnaires' disease lessons. *Burlington Free Press.* August 20, 2002. P. 1A.
6. Vermont Department of Health. Health officials investigate case of Legionnaires' disease. Burlington, Vt: Vermont Department of Health; August 1, 2002. News release. Available at http://www.healthyvermonters.info/news.shtml. Accessed November 11, 2005.
7. Vermont Department of Health. Legionniares' disease update, investigation uncovers additional cases. Burlington, Vt: Vermont Department of Health; August 5, 2002. News alert. Available at http://www.healthyvermonters.info/news.shtml. Accessed November 11, 2005.
8. Vermont Department of Health. Legionnaires' Update: No new cases Friday. Burlington, Vt: Vermont Department of Health; August 2, 2002. News release. Available at http://www.healthyvermonters.info/news.shtml. Accessed November 11, 2005.

9. Spaulding FP. Waterbury history. Available at: http://www.centralvt.com/towns/history/Hstwate.htm. Accessed October 29, 2005.

10. Sutkoski M. Legionnaires' mystery points to Waterbury. 3 cases confirmed, four suspected. *Burlington Free Press.* August 6, 2002. P. 1A.

11. Sutkoski M. Waterbury unfazed by Legionnaires'. *Burlington Free Press.* August 7, 2002. P. 1A.

12. Ross E. Disease spreads in Great Britain. One dead, 94 hospitalized in worst outbreak in ten years. *Burlington Free Press.* August 6, 2002. P. 4A.

13. Sutkoski M. Five more Legionnaires' cases surface. *Burlington Free Press.* August 10, 2002. P. 1B.

14. Larson K. Fifteenth case of disease confirmed. *Burlington Free Press.* August 13, 2002. P. 1B.

15. Mace D. Legionnaires' cases continue to roll in. *Rutland Herald.* August 13, 2002. Available at http://www.rutlandherald.com. Accessed October 29, 2005.

16. Sutkoski M. Cooling tower cited in outbreak. Legionnaires' made 16 ill. *Burlington Free Press.* September 7, 2002. P. 1B.

17. Vermont Department of Health. Legionnaires' Disease Update: Confirmed count now 18 cases. August 19, 2002. News release. Available at http://www.healthyvermonters.info/news.shtml. Accessed November 11, 2005.

18. Vermont Department of Health. Legionnaires' Disease Update: Investigators Focus on Cooling Towers. Burlington, VT: Vermont Department of Health. August 20, 2002. News release. Available at http://www.healthyvermonters.info/news.shtml. Accessed November 11, 2005.

19. Vermont Department of Health. Legionnaires' Disease Outbreak Traced to Dale Building Cooling Tower. September 5, 2002. News release. Available at http://www.healthyvermonters.info/news.shtml. Accessed November 11, 2005.

CHAPTER 24

Breaking Down Barriers to Health— Insuring the Children

There was a press conference scheduled at a local pediatrician's office. The announcement was for a new expanded insurance program to help pregnant women and young children. It was named Dr. Dynasaur, and pictured a friendly cartoon character, "Dr. Dynasaur," riding a tricycle (wearing a helmet of course) or wearing a stethoscope. The governor, the commissioner of social welfare (the department that housed the Medicaid program), myself, and the pediatrician talked about the reason for the program and what it would do. Vermont statistics in this area had shown troubling trends, the percentage of pregnant women receiving early prenatal care was too low, and the number receiving such care beginning much later was too high, a trend seen nationally as well. This problem was further complicated by too few physicians able to provide these services throughout our rural state. We had studied the literature and national recommendations and were working to try and remove some of the barriers to access faced by these women: finances (lack of health insurance); lack of transportation; lack of education about the value and importance of early prenatal care; administrative barriers such as long, complicated, confusing forms to enroll in government programs; and the lack of health professionals.

In Vermont, steps were taken to remedy this problem in a comprehensive way. One of the biggest hurdles was the financial one, and expanding state-funded health insurance for pregnant women and children was a critical step. Thus, the creation of the Dr. Dynasaur program. This by itself wouldn't absolutely guarantee that access to prenatal care climbed rapidly; we also had to make sure the other barriers were addressed as well. A nearly 20-page application for insurance was reduced to two sides of one page to enroll in the Women Infants and Children's program (WIC) and Medicaid or Dr. Dynasaur. A media campaign, promoting the importance of early prenatal care and providing help in accessing health care was created. It was formed from a public-private partnership and coalition and starred a public health nurse, Vermont's trusted health professional, giving a message about the importance of prenatal care, and included a toll-free number to call to "Help Your Baby, Help Yourself." It was called the helpline, for short. Callers talked to a friendly voice and were helped with finding a doctor, finding out what programs were available, and getting an appointment.[1]

During one legislative session I was testifying about my budget and the funds needed for these activities. The public health nurses had told me a story about a woman who called the helpline. She was eight months pregnant, with no prenatal care or insurance. A public health nurse found her a doctor and got her an appointment, and met her at the doctor's with the short application form, and yes, the outcome for mother and baby was positive. The committee, who usually had at least two members who were either really asleep or just pretending, woke up and listened as I told this story. They asked questions. We had tremendous support, and our outcomes measurably improved.

The Dr. Dynasaur program was designed to remove the financial barrier to health care by expanding eligibility to health insurance.[1] It was named and promoted this way to make it recognizable and easier to call and enroll. From many of the stories we had heard, and from the literature in prenatal care, it was obvious that many government programs were difficult to understand and the extensive paperwork was difficult to fill out. Confusing enrollment forms and procedures were limiting access to health care. Two departments worked together to simplify the forms and to remove the bureaucratic barriers. A few years prior, public health nurses had also redirected their efforts to prioritize their visits to women of highest medical and social risks. Pregnant teens were at especially high risk, and a program in the Agency of Human Services, our umbrella agency, worked to help them. Reimbursement to physicians providing prenatal and delivery services was increased, and the legislature gave funds to the health department to provide grants to communities to increase the availability of comprehensive prenatal care services.[1]

Health outcome statistics supported the effect of this comprehensive approach, one that was designed to remove a myriad of possible barriers to care. The percentages of pregnant women who received early prenatal care increased, and the proportion receiving care late decreased; this held true for all women and also specifically for teens. Infant mortality also improved significantly during this time. Investments by the state and public-private partnerships, crafted in a comprehensive way, provided measurable improvements in health.[1] Focus, policy commitment, and emphasis on prevention were essential to the success of the efforts. We realized that a comprehensive effort that included financing of health insurance, simplifying forms, educating women, reaching out to link at-risk women with needed care, promoting the program, and including the legislature and private sector in our efforts was an important approach that resulted in improvements in birth outcomes for Vermont children. Comprehensive public health approaches, designed to systematically improve knowledge as well as remove financial barriers, and administrative hurdles, were also later used in other areas such as preventing childhood lead poisoning, reducing smoking, preventing deaths from breast cancer, and improving access to primary and preventive health care.

Health care reform efforts in Vermont, like efforts at the national level in the early 1990s, were both complex and controversial, particularly since the state was struggling to regain its financial footing from a difficult financial recession.[2] A government agency was created, called the Vermont Health Care authority. It had to deliver two plans to the Vermont legislature: a single-payer plan and a multiple-regulated payer plan. Although debate and discussion was vigorous, a comprehensive plan was not adopted at the time, nor was such a plan adopted at the national level.

In Vermont, however, there was still extensive support and commitment by the administration and the legislature to make further progress to improve access to health care by expanding eligibility to health insurance. In 1989, Dr. Dynasaur had been created as a state-funded program for women and children through age 6 who had no health insurance and were unable to qualify for the state's Medicaid program.[3] Children were covered up to 225% of the federal poverty level (FPL) and pregnant women up to 200%. A few years later, in 1992, this coverage was integrated into the state Medicaid program and expanded.[3]

In the 1995–1996 legislative session, there was tremendous discussion and debate as the legislative committees wrestled with the means to also increase health care access for adults, along with the financing to sustain this. Raising the price of tobacco products was a means to provide funds, and also to prevent young children from starting to smoke, a health issue that had grown in severity as well. Act 14 (H159) passed by the legislature and signed by the governor, had as its purpose, "to finance health care benefits for uninsured or underinsured low-income Vermonters. To the extent permitted by appropriations, the revenues generated by this act will finance the existing Medicaid program and will increase the number of low-income Vermonters with health benefits coverage, integrate certain publicly funded beneficiaries into mainstream medical care, bring Medicaid beneficiaries into managed care plans, extend pharmaceutical benefits to low-income elderly and disabled individuals, increase residential care, increase home and community-based Medicaid waiver services, and enhance access to health care benefits paid under the Medicaid program by increasing reimbursement levels for physicians and other providers."[4] This was a tremendous task and responsibility. The act established the Vermont health access trust fund in the state treasury for this purpose, raised the price of cigarettes and other tobacco products, and created a legislative oversight committee. In addition to funds appropriated for health insurance for adults, increased reimbursement rates were budgeted for physicians and dentists, and money was budgeted for the health department to fund the loan repayment program for the recruitment of primary care providers. The federal government (Health Care Financing Administration) approved a waiver in July 1995 to facilitate administrative efforts to further develop the program.[5] In 1998, Dr. Dynasaur was further expanded; it covered children though age 17 in families with incomes up to 300% of the FPL. (In 2002, for children, income guidelines allowed earnings up to $45,216 for a family of three.)[3]

The goals of Dr. Dynasaur were first to promote access to prenatal care for pregnant women and give young children health services, particularly emphasizing preventive care. The larger goal, the one that was sometimes controversial, was to ensure universal access to health care for all Vermont children. This gradually occurred as the income eligibility for Dr. Dynasaur expanded and alongside with private insurance, provided coverage for essentially all Vermont children.[3] The coverage for children eligible for Dr. Dynasaur was as comprehensive as Medicaid and included routine checkups and needed laboratory tests, childhood immunizations, limited dental services, and other services.[3]

When this was being first implemented, it created difficulty for physicians in some areas of the state, as reimbursement for services for children now eligible for this program were low. In areas where physicians saw a high proportion of children in their rural practice who were enrolled, maintaining the practice became challenging. Despite these difficulties, health providers continued to work closely with state agencies, and their support contributed greatly to the success of these programs and the subsequent improvements seen in the outcomes for children's health.

For adults, a variety of programs were offered from the Agency of Human Services through its Office of Health Access, including the Vermont Health Access Plan.[5,6] Increasing the percentage of people with health insurance was a public health goal of *Healthy Vermonters 2010,* Vermont's priorities for improving public health.[7] The use of measurable goals and objectives supported and facilitated the close cooperation of multiple departments in the Agency of Human Services. The administration strongly supported the development and implementation of this approach.

Somewhere in the discussion about health reform, there also seemed to be an opportunity for public health, but there was also a danger. At first there was the simplistic notion that improving access to health care would be all that we needed to improve health. We had to respond quickly to disprove this idea. We provided examples of the core duties of public health, including our role of working closely with health professionals, and gave examples such as the prevention of epidemics, protecting health through the environment, promoting health behaviors (such as reducing smoking), monitoring the health of the population, and linking special populations with services, such as the diligent work that had been done to deliver services to Vermont children with special health care needs. The opportunities for education and discussion with legislative committees during this time challenged our staff to communicate the roles and responsibilities of public health, in any discussion of health care reform, no matter what shape the health care delivery system took. Explaining with examples the relationships between health care and public health in improving health outcomes was critical. We used the *Healthy Vermonters* approach of measurable outcomes, as often as we could, to explain what was required to improve health, using public health issues as examples.

Improving access to health care in order to improve health outcomes also required enough primary care providers in all areas of our rural state, something that was an ongoing challenge. The first profiles that showed numbers and types of physicians, and where they were located was presented in a visual way through a Vermont map. This map showed legislators exactly where small offices, reimbursement rates, and high debt levels were impediments to recruiting and keeping health professionals. The legislature understood why this situation was so important to correct and funded the growing collaborative work between the health department, the University of Vermont College of Medicine, and Vermont hospitals all over the state, as the university developed Area Health Education Centers throughout Vermont. Primary care provider trends were tracked and publicized, and a process to help address the high costs of education through loan repayment programs was begun.

Started in 1995, the Vermont Health Access Program (VHAP) was expanded until, as of 2003, adults at or below 150% of the federal poverty level (which translated to an annual household income of just over $33, 000 for a family of five) were covered.[6] According to the Vermont Behavioral Risk Factor Surveillance System, 88.4% of Vermonters aged 18–64 reported having health insurance in 2000, and 88% reported having health insurance in 2003, as compared to 82.2% reported for the United States in 2002. Our target for the year 2010 was 100%. In addition, for people over 18, nearly 87% had an ongoing source of primary care in 2003, and contrasted to 79% for the rest of the United States.[8]

In Vermont, what was remarkable was the determination and persistence in finding ways to insure all Vermont children and many adults. Despite the national debate and momentum and the analogous efforts here, the successful efforts to improve access were more pragmatic and incremental, but determined to achieve goals. There were many opinions as to the way Vermont should proceed, but the important fact was that steps were taken to continue to make improvements in children's health by making sure they had health insurance. We learned from our earlier efforts to improve prenatal care that providing health insurance was a necessary step, but we knew there had to be other efforts in place as well to improve health outcomes. Health planning took a broader approach to health, and it was recognized that health included health care and much more. Although prevention is the best investment that can be made in health, and many services have been shown to be cost-effective,[9] barriers to access remain.

Reaching our 2010 goals for public health include removing barriers to health, improving access to health care, increasing knowledge, expanding transportation, having enough health professionals, increasing coverage of clinical preventive services, and creating partnerships between health care and public health at every step of the way. To prevent some of the conditions that we will continue to see in the near future, such as diabetes, heart disease, and cancer— all becoming even more urgent as our population ages—will also require a focus on communities, the environment, habits and behaviors, and economic and social factors, including health literacy. Vermont's efforts to improve health through increasing access to health care required partnerships, sustained leadership and commitment, and the willingness to be pragmatic and persistent.

REFERENCES

1. Carney JK, Berry P, Thompson E, Brozicevic MM. Improving access to prenatal care in Vermont. *Am J Public Health*. 1996;86(6):880–881.
2. Carr J. Vermont's Fiscal Fitness. Available at http://www.vermontguides.com/2001/1jan/jeffcarr.htm. Accessed March 28, 2005.
3. Office of Health Access, Vermont Agency of Human Services. Vermont's Dr. Dynasaur Health Insurance Program. Waterbury, Vt: Vermont Agency of Human Services; 2002. Available at: http://www.ovha.state.vt.us/docs/HISTORYDRD.PDF. Accessed January 4, 2005.
4. Acts of the 1995-1996 Vermont Legislature. No. 14 (H159) An act relating to financing of health care. Available at: http://www.leg.state.vt.us/DOCS/1996/Act014.HTM. Accessed March 17, 2005.

5. Office of Health Access, Vermont Agency of Human Services. Vermont Health Access Plan: Key Milestones. Waterbury, Vt: Vermont Agency of Human Services 2002. Available at http://www.ovha.state.vt.us/docs/1115milestones.pdf. Acccessed April 8, 2005.

6. Office of Health Access, Vermont Agency of Human Services. Vermont Health Access Plan (VHAP). Income Guidelines. 2003 Available at: http://www.path. state.vt.us/programs_pages/healthcare/vhap.htm. Accessed April 8, 2005.

7. Vermont Department of Health. *Healthy Vermonters 2010.* Burlington, Vt: Vermont Department of Health; 2000:6–7.

8. Vermont Department of Health. Behavioral Risk Factor Surveillance System. *Healthy Vermonter* 2010: Objectives and Vermont Summary of BRFSS Data. Available at: http://www.healthyvermonters.info/hs/brfss/ BRFSSobjective.htm. Accessed April 8, 2005.

9. Satcher D, Hull FL. The weight of an ounce. *JAMA.* 1995;273: 1149–1150.

CHAPTER 25

Knowledge is Power—Preventing
Breast Cancer Deaths

The Center for Disease Control and Prevention's *Morbidity and Mortality Weekly Report* size and appearance have changed, but the content has always been timely and relevant for those in public health. Formerly, it was a small size, black and white, just a little too large to fit in your back pants pocket for leisure reading, but just the right size to be carried and hidden easily for reading during tedious meetings. I read it every, every week, usually right when it arrived, by mail, and later electronically, to see what new conditions were being reported elsewhere, to see how we compared to other states and nations, and as my way of keeping our work and data in context. The clear descriptions of outbreak investigations and the insightful editorial comments were most helpful whether dealing with infectious diseases, trends in chronic conditions, or emerging health threats.

One afternoon between phone calls, meetings, and paperwork, I sat at my desk and read an article from the *Morbidity and Mortality Weekly Report* about the national perspective on breast cancer deaths.[1] What immediately caught my attention was the black-and-white map of the United States, shaded according to whether the death rates were higher or lower. Death rates in northern states were higher, and I studied the map and saw that Vermont was printed black, in the highest death rate category.

It was a rare quiet moment, where I had a minute or two to think before speaking to anyone or answering a call. I thought to myself "What are we going to do about this?" and then read the article carefully. Death rates that were high could be from more women getting breast cancer, or from those getting the disease not getting the best possible care, whether it was not getting screened for early detection or not receiving state-of-the-art treatment in a timely way. It was not possible from the article to distinguish between the two, and we did not have the data at the time to tell whether the amount of breast cancer in people newly diagnosed breast cancer, the incidence rate, was higher than other places in the country, or whether our death rate was high because of the difficulty people had in the rural parts of our state getting access to timely and appropriate health care. I read the rest of the article carefully, looking for hints of what approach we might take and what might be our next step.

There was no real practical way to actually "prevent" breast cancer through primary prevention, as most risk factors cited were largely uncontrollable. However there was a figure in the literature that stated that breast cancer death rates could be decreased by an estimated 30% if women received mammograms at recommended intervals.[2,3,4] If we couldn't prevent breast cancer, and if we couldn't tell if our high rate of deaths was from more cancer or from lack of access to the best possible treatment, we could still lower death rates by nearly a third if women received mammograms at recommended intervals to detect breast cancer earlier at a more treatable stage. This meant that women would not only have to get a mammogram once, but would have to receive them regularly, at the recommended intervals. Though it was not an easy task, it was something we could possibly achieve.

This issue followed on the heels of a crisis in access to prenatal care and a growing interest in providing more universal access to health care in Vermont. As momentum for this issue increased there was also a small but influential legislative voice who said efforts to promote breast cancer screening should wait and be tied to our ability to provide health insurance for all of our citizens. Although not a loud public tension, we hesitated only momentarily before deciding that the urgency of the issue made it essential for us to move ahead.

At the same time, there was much interest and enthusiasm in Vermont around cancer, with the formation of a cancer coalition, the publishing of a simple and elegant five year cancer plan,[5] and the release of *Healthy Vermonters 2000*,[6] which listed cancer as a priority area. There was also a focus on early detection of breast cancer at the national level.

We had initiated our cancer prevention and control efforts with a federal grant, as state funds were difficult to come by, especially for new initiatives. State budgets were approved every year, and the biggest driver of the next year's budget was the current year's budget. One of our management goals was to have data drive public health policy to the extent possible, and as we began to focus more and more on measurable health outcomes as a framework to measure our progress in public health, special surveys, in addition to the usual Behavior Risk Factor Surveys, were done to determine screening rates and barriers to women getting mammograms at the recommended intervals.[7] As expected, breast cancer screening rates in Vermont were far below national and Vermont goals. The biggest barrier, however, was lack of awareness, or women not knowing that mammograms were needed. After lack of awareness, the other reasons for not getting a mammogram were procrastination, a physician not recommending it, not having any symptoms, and cost. Although a common perception at the time was that cost was the primary reason that women did not get mammograms and clinical breast exams as recommended, and that providing health insurance would remedy this situation, the reality was that lack of knowledge about the benefits of screening was the immediate barrier.[7]

A statewide media campaign was started to encourage women 40 and older to have regular mammograms. The campaign included posters, television and radio ads, and a toll-free phone number to get further information about early detection of breast cancer and where mammography facilities were located. The campaign itself was a public-private partnership between the health department, the University of Vermont Cancer Center, the state medical society, and the largest health insurance company in Vermont. Community action meetings were sponsored by the health department in various parts of the state to raise

awareness and promote community momentum, and worksite educational programs, reduced-cost screening programs, and community education meetings
were some of the results.[7]

Other activities supported our efforts. A law was passed by the legislature
that required third-party insurance coverage for annual mammograms for
women aged 50 and older, and younger women as advised by their physician.[8]
An extensive worksite education campaign targeting working women was developed and implemented by nurses and allied health workers in partnership with
the University of Vermont, Vermont hospitals, and home health agencies.
Public education efforts occurred both in the media and through grassroot
efforts in communities, and were carried out by trusted public health and
health care professionals, along with many other groups, organizations, and
individuals.

After extensive efforts to raise awareness and educate Vermont women about
the importance of early detection in our fight against breast cancer, we conducted another survey to look again at the barriers identified to screening and
whether or not our work was having any impact. We concluded that despite the
national attention to this issue as well, the efforts in Vermont had resulted in
increases in screening rates for breast cancer, and most importantly, a decline in
the lack of awareness barrier that prevented many Vermont women from receiving mammograms.[7]

As national surveys[2] showed that both cost and fear of radiation had been
cited as barriers to getting regular mammograms, or even a single one, and
since we were aggressively promoting their use, at the same time we also conducted a special statewide survey (by the health department radiological health
staff) to inspect all mammography X-ray units in Vermont, using methodology
from the National Evaluation of X-ray Trends (NEXT) to look at the quality
and dose from mammograms performed in Vermont. Image scores were found
to be acceptable with lower average doses seen than were noted in the national
surveys. This work was done to ensure that at the same time we were promoting
mammograms for early detection of breast cancer to help lower Vermont's high
death rate and improve women's health, we were also protecting health by
ensuring the quality and safety of the facilities used.[9]

As educational efforts continued and more women understood that early
detection of breast cancer, when there were no symptoms, could be lifesaving,
discrepancies in screening rates among women with different educational levels
and income became apparent. Our educational efforts, though valuable, didn't
address all the barriers. Screening rates were increasing–from 1993 to 1997,
more than 63% of Vermont women over 50 had a mammogram and clinical
breast exam in the past two years. But in 1997, less than 50% of women with
annual incomes below $15,000 were screened as compared to nearly 80% of
women with incomes over $75,000.[10] There now was clearly a disparity in
screening rates among those women with limited income and education, pointing our campaign against breast cancer in a new direction.

Again, with the help of federal grants, the Ladies First program was begun in
1995. It was called "Ladies First" because the name was chosen by Vermont
women themselves. It was a health screening program for women that paid for

services, annual mammograms, clinical breast exams, and other screening, and provided services close to home.[11] Before starting the program, we wondered what would happen if a woman were diagnosed with breast cancer through Ladies First but had no insurance? After some calculations, we estimated that if it were to happen, the numbers would be small. After phone discussions with hospitals, an informal understanding was reached that somehow we would handle it if it happened. No papers were ever written or signed, but it was enough assurance, based on our ongoing relationships with hospitals in Vermont, and we proceeded.

Ladies First was announced at a press conference, where the program was explained and women were given a toll-free number, and told to call "Kate," the actual name of the person who originally had the job of answering the phone and helping women enroll. Kate helped women determine if they were eligible, helped them enroll, and helped find a location convenient to home. In a 5-year period, more than 9000 screenings were performed, more than 3500 women were enrolled, more than 700 health professionals around the state were enrolled, and all of the state's mammography facilities were participating. Most of the cancers detected had been in early stages.[11]

In a creative and comprehensive social marketing strategy, health department staff made sure Ladies First was well publicized. In a quiet effort called "Operation Ladies Room," the easily recognizable tear-off messages with the toll free number were put in over 3000 ladies rooms in locations around Vermont.[12] Cancer survivors told their stories in the press, in weekly newspapers and flyers, and in monthly magazines, describing how they had breast cancer detected early and survived. Ladies First also targeted women with special needs, such as hearing impairment and the needs of women in wheelchairs.[13]

The percentage of Vermont women who had mammograms as recommended, in the past two years, increased to more than 75% by the year 2000,[14] surpassing the *Healthy Vermonters 2010* 2010 target. In addition, breast cancer deaths had fallen since 1990. From 1995 to 1999, 36% of breast cancers were detected by mammography as compared to 2% from 1974 to 1984.[15] And although differences in screening rates were still being seen, progress was steady, with now 60% of women over 50 with limited incomes and 88% of women with higher incomes receiving screening.[15] The story is far from over, but the efforts to educate women and remove barriers to access were succeeding.

In my epidemiology training in public health school, I was taught that the use of epidemiology to understand problems that you didn't yet fully understand was like peeling the skin from an onion, layers were removed, and you were left with more layers, and over time, as you were able to use the data to peel away more and more layers, you got to the onion itself. However, there is rarely enough time or data, to be able to study the problem to the degree that you would like. Sometimes you can peel another layer or two from the onion skin, then it is time to act. There is never enough time, and problems are much too pressing to sit in our epidemiologic kitchen and wait to see the entire onion. It is not an excuse for abrupt or careless decisions, or not trying to use all available data to best understand the problem at hand; it is just the reality of practicing public health in the real world.

In public health practice, what you never seem to have enough of is time. There is always a public urgency to problems, sometimes pressure to act quickly, a public outcry, or most often a public health issue, no matter how you uncovered it, that just *has* to be remedied, with waiting viewed as an unacceptable option. Sometimes public health action was driven by national attention to an issue, sometimes a crisis occurred, and sometimes the moment of decision came from seeing a piece of data, a chart, or a map. And, the moment when you became aware of a problem, despite not being able to anticipate every dollar you would need to fully finish the job or despite not every person agreeing with your approach, you knew something must be done, and quickly.

Although health departments and the public see this most clearly for infectious diseases, there is no less urgency for chronic conditions. We found out that Vermont had a high breast cancer death rate, and decided to do something about it. Some of the steps were immediate, some required getting more data, but the decision to act was made and steps were taken, based on the potential to reduce deaths by improving access to screening and early detection. Three years later, we found that after trying to educate Vermont women and raise awareness about the importance and efficacy of screening, and remove a knowledge barrier, we found the discrepancies in screening rates based on income and education that led to the creation of a program to address it—Ladies First. But, if the educational steps had not been taken first, progress would not have been seen so fast because it was this barrier that was nearly overwhelming.

For breast cancer, knowledge is power, and one of the most important things that we did was to help give Vermont women the knowledge to improve their own health. We started this at a time when we had no cancer registry and did not yet have as much information as we needed to reduce deaths from breast cancer. But we took what information and science we had at hand and applied it in a systematic way and measured the results to see if what we did worked. The knowledge gained resulted in more women being screened and programs being created in a way that women would use them. Though the issue is far from over, death rates have fallen and screening rates are up. Progress is being made.

REFERENCES

1. CDC. Progress in Chronic Disease Prevention. Chronic Disease Reports: Deaths from Breast Cancer among women—United States, 1986. *MMWR.* 1989;38:565–569.
2. CDC. Use of Mammography—United States, 1990. *MMWR.* 1990; 39:621, 627–630.
3. Shapiro S, Venet W, Strax P, Venet L. Periodic Screening for Breast Cancer: the Health Insurance Plan Project and its Sequelae, 1963–1986. Baltimore, Maryland: The Johns Hopkins University Press; 1988:1–214.
4. Eddy DM. Screening for breast cancer. *Ann Intern Med.* 1989;111: 389–99.
5. Vermont Coalition for Cancer Prevention and Control. *Vermont Plan for Cancer Prevention and Control: 1990–1995.* Burlington, Vt: Vermont Department of Health; 1989.

6. Vermont Department of Health. *Healthy Vermonters 2000.* Burlington, Vt: Vermont Department of Health; 1992.

7. Carney JK, Ewing JF, Finley CA. Progress in breast cancer screening. *J Public Health Management Practice.* 1996:57–63.

8. Acts of the 1991–1992 Vermont legislature. Act 40 (H160) Insurance coverage of mammograms. Available at http://www.leg.state.vt.us. Accessed November 12, 2005.

9. Carney JK, McCandless RN, Clemmons PE. A statewide survey of Vermont Mammography X-ray facilities. Abstract presented at the American Public Health Association annual meeting. Washington, D.C., November 1992.

10. Vermont Department of Health. *Cancer in Vermont. A report of the 1994–1996 cancer incidence data from the Vermont Cancer Registry.* Burlington, Vt: Vermont Department of Health; 2000:11. Available at http://www.healthyvermonters.info/hs/epi/cdepi/cancerregistry/CancerInVT.pdf. Accessed March 31, 2005.

11. Vermont Department of Health. Breast cancer survivor Pauline Couture of Westfield tells her story in new Ladies First "Every Woman Matters" campaign. Burlington, Vt: Vermont Department of Health; 2000. News release. Available at http://www.healthyvermonters.info/news.shtml. Accessed March 31, 2005.

12. Walsh M. Program urges cancer screening: over 1000 women enroll in first year. *Burlington Free Press.* October 1, 1996; 1A.

13. CDC. State programs in action. Vermont women with special needs have access to vital cancer screenings. Available at: http://www.cdc.gov/ nccdphp/pc_factsheet/pe_cancer.htm. Accessed March 31, 2005.

14. Vermont Department of Health. *Behavioral Risk Factor Surveillance System (BRFSS): Healthy Vermonter 2010 Objectives and Vermont Summary of BRFSS Data.* Burlington, Vt: Vermont Department of Health. Available at http://www.healthyvermonters.info/hs/brfs/BRFSSobjective.htm. Accessed May 3, 2005.

15. Vermont Department of Health. Cancer in Vermont. A report of the 1995–1999 cancer incidence data from the Vermont Cancer Registry. Burlington, Vt: Vermont Department of Health; 2003; 10. Available at http://www.healthyvermonters.info/hs/pubs/2003/2003CancerInVT.pdf. Accessed March 31, 2005.

26

The Great Tobacco Wars: Part 1— Changing Our Culture Around Tobacco Use

There were 400 middle school children marching up the street with banners, noise, and the enthusiasm of a crowd this large. They marched up the front steps to the statehouse carrying a huge banner painted with the words "If you Smoke, You'll Choke and Croak."[1] Many students held smaller posters. These were the Vermont Kids Against Tobacco, or VKATs, taking part in their annual rally at Montpelier High School and the march to the statehouse. I was watching them from a second-floor window in the governor's ceremonial office area in the statehouse. The long line of young children, carrying banners that were hand painted, and interspersed among the crowd, created an interesting picture from my upstairs perch. Others nearby noticed the small parade's approach, and each year, the rally and statehouse march was captured by the press.

Once there, VKATs met with the governor in the house chamber, where they presented the results of one of their activities, Operation Storefront, a nonscientific survey done in their local communities to raise awareness about some particular aspect of tobacco prevention and control, to bring a critical gap in enforcement of current laws to the attention of legislators, and to raise awareness of a new issue that needed legislative attention. The health department started the program with 10 schools in 1995 and expanding to 56 schools by 2005.[2] Their rally was an annual event that was hard to ignore. On this particular day, they met with statehouse leaders and presented their results from their survey of 171 stores around the state: 15% had illegal self-service displays, and 27% placed tobacco near candy.[3] The type of peer leadership was not only effective among the young people themselves, but it was obvious that it had an impact on political representatives from both parties. The publicity associated with it provided another opportunity to get the word out about the effects of smoking on health, and why we needed a public health approach to prevent young people from smoking. An editorial in the Burlington newspaper a few days later called the activity "A Healthy Rebellion,"[3] and wrote about the "research, enthusiasm, and conviction" these young people showed. Through their creativity, Vermont Kids Against Tobacco helped promote a positive health message, most importantly to their peers, but also to their parents, policy makers, and the public. They did nonscientific surveys, showing real findings from their own communities, summarized them, and presented them to state policy makers. This particular year, there was a proposal to increase the price of cigarettes. Other years, a variety of legislation was being considered.

Such strategies were used in tobacco prevention and control, prior to the receipt of larger funds from the tobacco master settlement agreement. Inexpensive, grass root efforts based on science and practical thinking were at the heart of these modest programs. The thinking was that kids could more effectively influence other kids than we could, coming from our position in government and closer to the age of their parents. These groups grew and expanded around the state, one part of an effort to change our culture around tobacco use.

During this time, strategy for legislation was built on the premise that specific, carefully chosen policy initiatives could help raise awareness about smoking and create a foundation and framework for programs. The Vermont Coalition for Cancer Prevention and Control, in its first cancer plan[4] called for the consideration of legislation that promotes clean indoor air in public places, increases the state excise tax on tobacco products, prohibits the sale of tobacco products in vending machines, and other tobacco-reduction strategies. Such a coalition, funded by a federal grant, provided a framework and experience in the health department's work with coalitions, and much attention and interest on the part of legislators, the administration, and members of the coalition focused on policy changes through legislation.

Healthy Vermonters 2000,[5] and later *Healthy Vermonters 2010,*[6] our blueprint for improving public health, had tobacco as a priority area for public health efforts. A coalition called the Coalition for Clean Indoor Air helped with legislative efforts to promote and secure passage of Vermont's Comprehensive Clean Indoor Air law, through the work of its individual members. The coalition was informal, and comprised state agencies, legislators, citizens, health care professionals and organizations, nonprofit agencies, and many others. Department of health staff provided administrative support, but the group was loosely organized and momentum came from individual groups participating. Efforts were coordinated, but there was no independent budget, lobbyist, or layers of organizational bureaucracy that slowed the group. Individual groups and organizations were free to promote their own organization's interest, but efforts focused on a common goal—to reduce smoking.

The result was a group that was informal, loosely organized, and very hard to stop. The department of health provided clear articulation of the public health impact of smoking, had the support of the administration in its prevention efforts, and testified along with large numbers of other groups and organizations when such bills were considered. Additional funding requests in the forms of requests to the legislature was not allowed (the unwritten budget rules prohibited this), and one of the immense challenges, in addition to opposition by the tobacco industry, was to be able to make progress in tobacco prevention and control with sparse funding. What the coalition strategy accomplished, by making all of our priorities harmonious, was to make the entire group and its member organizations a very loud choir, supported by many legislators of different parties. In addition, the very loose organization made the organization nimble, difficult to track, and defend against. *Healthy Vermonters 2000,* in the priority area of tobacco, called for a reduction in youth smoking, adult smoking, smoking by pregnant women, increasing the percent of primary care providers who assist with tobacco use cessation, and to enact a comprehensive clean indoor air act.[5] The fact that legislators of all parties were ongoing active participants of the coalition efforts was a key component to ongoing working relationships in the legislature. We were very conscious of what was allowed and not allowed in our role as government officials. The coalition had similar requirements, as they were not an independent organization. There were trade-offs to such arrangements. An organization attached to a government department receiving grants had to abide by such rules, and such an organization experiences some loss of complete autonomy. But independent coalitions had to become financially self-sufficient, which created a different challenge. Such trade-offs were sometimes discussed, but the informal, focused, and more nimble model was highly effective for many years.

Tobacco-related legislation was common, supported by different administrations, and many legislators. In 1991, a youth access act prohibited sales to people younger than 18, established licenses and established penalties for illegal sales.[7] The passage of Vermont's clean indoor air act was a time of intense legislative focus on tobacco. The bill was supported by the coalition. H159 was introduced into the House of Representatives in January, when the session started, with a total of 98 sponsors, an incredible legislative coalition for public health. The lead sponsor was an incredibly energetic and knowledgeable advocate for tobacco prevention and control. The premise of the bill was the determination by the Environmental Protection Agency (EPA) that environmental tobacco smoke was a "group A" carcinogen, along with dioxin, benzene, radon, and asbestos.[8] The bill cited the studies showing a risk of lung cancer among nonsmokers, health effects in children such as respiratory infections and decreased lung function, and worsening of asthma. The purpose of the act was to "protect public health by reducing exposure to environmental tobacco smoke."[8]

There were numerous hearings, and coalition members from pediatricians to representatives from malls in two parts of the state came out to support the bill. One hearing had more than 20 witnesses advocating for health. The original bill contained a broad inclusion of public places and exceptions for designated smoking areas that were "physically separated and effectively segregated and separately ventilated." Public places included any commercial establishments, public transportation, health facilities, and so on, and exempted entire rooms or halls used for private social functions. Fines were detailed as enforcement provisions. The bill, after being somehow being called into and stuck in the house appropriations committee for a day, passed the House, and contained a detailed list of places of public access, and included restaurants, bars, and cabarets. During subsequent discussion in the Senate, controversy increased around the inclusion of restaurants, and testimony was given by business groups, restaurant owners, hotels, the chamber of commerce, as well as health advocates, coalition members, and tobacco interests. The Senate compromise, after intense discussions in the health and welfare committee, kept the detailed list of places of public access (including restaurants), called for the prohibition of lighted tobacco products in any form "in the common areas of all enclosed indoor places of public access and publicly owned buildings and offices,"[8] but the amendment included a section that gave restaurants, bars, cabarets, hotels, or motels two additional years to comply with the law. It also only allowed, after 2 years, businesses issued a cabaret license, the license that defined a bar, as designated smoking areas. If a cabaret was part of a larger facility, it could be a designated smoking area if separately enclosed (not separately ventilated) and separately licensed as a cabaret. The enforcement called for the proprietor or an employee to ask a person to extinguish a lighted tobacco product, and if the person refused, to ask the person to leave the premises. In addition, the bill stated that the statewide law did not supercede a municipal ordinance at least as strict.[8]

The bill passed, with Senate amendment, and was signed into law. It was cited as the nation's toughest law for clean indoor air[9] and was well publicized locally and nationally,[10] because restaurants were included. However the spokesman for the Tobacco Institute called it a "tough law on paper, but there are no enforcement mechanisms or fines."[10] Initially, critics had cited the cost of enforcement of such laws as barriers, and indeed it seemed the legislative process had stripped the enforcement provisions from the bill. The bill relied on self-policing by owners or proprietors of public places. But actually, since the bill was placed in Title 18, the home of the public health laws, it fell under the general enforcement abilities cited in those sections and given to the health commissioner and local boards of health. They included the ability, after always first seeking and exhausting efforts to seek voluntary compliance, to issue health orders, other enforcement measures, and bring civil court actions, by going to superior court where civil penalties up to $10,000 per day could be sought, and criminal fines up to $5000 for each violation.[11]

What we learned between the time the original law went into effect and the end of the 2-year phase-in period was that strong educational efforts, mailings to impacted businesses, public brochures, and a toll-free number were effective at educating people about the law. About 450 warning letters were sent in response to complaints, but no enforcement actions had been necessary initially. Appropriate legal authority for public health and educational efforts made the law practical to implement.[12] However, as expected, numbers of cabarets continued to increase, and over the subsequent years, the need to tighten the law became apparent, as cabarets increased from 84 to more than 400 in a period of several years.[7] This loophole was finally closed in 2005.[13]

Why did this law pass and why was it important? It passed because of broad support. Nearly two thirds of the members of Vermont's House of Representatives were initial sponsors of the bill. Educational efforts to enlist legislative support took much time, but resulted in a large number of initial sponsors. Both the focus on health by the department and the coalition members, along with the federal report on the effects of environmental tobacco smoke, were all important in the timing of the efforts. Broad public support enabled the passage of a critical law at a critical time to help Vermont's prevention efforts against tobacco use. The benefit of such laws, in addition to the direct benefit of reducing exposure to environmental tobacco smoke, was to reinforce the message that most people didn't smoke, contributing to efforts to change the culture around tobacco use. From a public health perspective, this was an important step, one that was part of a foundation of laws and policies that reinforced messages that promoted health.

Several other critical bills passed during this time, prior to funding from the master tobacco settlement agreement. A bill passed in less than three months that prohibited tobacco use on school grounds and at school functions.[14] There were only three hearings needed, in education committees on both sides, and it was an opportunity to spend time in the education committees to talk about public health. The urgency of the health issue, as smoking rates were at their highest level, made more uniform policy for schools a legislative priority. As smoking rates in grades 8 through 12 peaked in the mid 1990s, efforts became increasingly focused on comprehensive ways to prevent young children from starting to smoke. Efforts were made to increase the price of tobacco products to fund increased access to health care, another critical policy discussion during this same time. This effort provided opportunities to talk about the impact of raising the price of cigarettes and other tobacco products on preventing young people from starting to smoke.

Efforts to pass laws that took away the authority of cities and towns to pass tobacco ordinances stricter than state laws were unsuccessful. Such ordinances created momentum to generate stronger laws when needed and allowed communities to pass such ordinances, something that needed to be preserved; such local control was good for public health, and the debate, discussion, and controversy they provoked was often an important step to counter and impact local health issues. They were sometimes also a first step in a later statewide policy change.

A law restricting minors' access to tobacco products was intensely debated and enacted into law during the 1997–1998 legislative sessions.[15] The bill was designed to toughen the enforcement provisions of illegal sales to minors. Vermont Kids Against Tobacco had been working on this issue, and the Operation Storefront effort showed directly, from the surveys done by children, that 81% of the stores surveyed had self-service tobacco displays, 57% had them next[7] to the candy, and 44% had them displayed below three feet tall. These facts (as well as a perception that it was easy for youth to buy cigarettes illegally) led to some vigorous legislative discussion. Nationally, this was also a point of focus, and the legislative findings cited the fact that over half a billion packs of cigarettes are sold illegally each year to children under the age of 18 years.[15]

The bill prohibited vending machines, with few exceptions, and banned self-service displays, but exempted cigarettes in unopened cartons and smokeless tobacco in unopened multipack containers, along with cigars and pipe tobacco in a humidor on a sales counter in plain view.

The testimony, held in the house health and welfare committee was intense as exceptions for cigars and smokeless tobacco were attempted. Humidors, containing cigars, had to sit on the counter, negating attempts to have freestanding places. During one hearing I envisioned a humidor the size of a refrigerator sitting in the middle of the limited floor space of a small store, and we argued against it. Discussions of costs, placement of products, and impact on small stores were heard, but in the end, after some compromises, the law for enforcement of illegal sales was strengthened, cigarette packs were put behind the counter, and there were some exemptions for cigars and smokeless tobacco.[15]

We were all working to change our culture around tobacco use. There was always the need to manage our public resources efficiently and promote public health, using strategies to do so with limited resources. It was also when we were trying to increase access to health care through expansion of health insurance. Raising the price of tobacco yielded funds that were designed to help get more people access to health care, and this price increase would help us prevent children from starting to smoke, no matter where the funds were targeted. Resources were always limited, which was why we were a broad coalition of stakeholders; all were focused on improving health outcomes. Our priorities became focused on one thing—to reduce the effects of tobacco. At one point, the executive director of the cancer society came to visit me, as funds were meager, and offered to work together. I remember sitting at the table in my office and discussing our mutual priorities. That kind of conversation set the tone for the time; our willingness to help each other pooled many more resources than even a moderately funded tobacco program. Each organization brought its own resources, energy, commitment, and focus to the efforts, all with the same goal, to impact public health by reducing smoking: reducing the impact of environmental tobacco smoke, reducing illegal sales, and preventing children from starting to smoke, with the cumulative effect being to build a stronger and stronger foundation to support health. It was fast, loose, and often appeared that no one was in charge, a strategy key to the coalition success, but we each knew what we needed to do in our own roles, and were intent on accomplishing it. The grassroots efforts of the Vermont Kids Against Tobacco (VKATs) cannot be underestimated. While we were all working so hard to act at the policy level, they kept it (and us) down to earth. By the time the Master Settlement Agreement was in the wind, we were all ready, our foundation was in place, and smoking rates were taking a turn for the better, especially among young children in Vermont.

REFERENCES

1. Rathke L. Burlington Free Press Youths stage rally against smoking: 400 students march on Montpelier. *Burlington Free Press.* February 8, 2001. P. 1B.
2. Vermont Department of Health Tobacco Program. Available at: http://www. healthyvermonters.info/hi/tobacco/tobacco.shtml#two. Accessed March 24, 2005.
3. A Healthy Rebellion. Editorial. *Burlington Free Press.* February 10, 2001. P. 10A.
4. Vermont Coalition on Cancer Prevention and Control. *Vermont Plan for Cancer Prevention and Control.* Burlington, Vt: Vermont Department of Health; 1989.
5. Vermont Department of Health. *Healthy Vermonters 2000.* Burlington, Vt: Vermont Department of Health; 1992.
6. Vermont Department of Health. *Healthy Vermonters 2010.* Burlington, Vt: Vermont Department of Health; 2000.
7. Vermont Department of Health. *Vermont Best Practices to Cut Smoking Rates in Half by 2010.* Burlington, Vt: Vermont Department of Health; 2000. Available at http://www.healthyvermonters.info. Accessed March 24, 2005.
8. Acts of the 1993–1994 Vermont Legislature. Act. No. 46 (H.159). An Act Relating to Clean Indoor Air—Environmental Tobacco Smoke. Available at http://www.leg.state.vt.us. Accessed March 28, 2005.

9. Liley B. No butts about it: Public smoking ends. Nation's toughest law takes effect Thursday. *Burlington Free Press.* June 29, 1993. P. 1A.
10. Larrabee J. Vermont law sweeps smokers under the rug. *USA Today.* May 17, 1993. P. 3A
11. Vermont Statutes, Title 18 VSA Chapter 3, Sections 124–131.
12. Carney JK, Hamrell MC, Wargo WE. No Butts about it: Public smoking ends in Vermont. *Am J Public Health.* 1997;87:860–861.
13. Acts of the 2005–2006 Vermont Legislature. Act No. 34 (H.241). Prohibition of Smoking in All Public Places. Available at http://www.leg.state.vt.us. Accessed November 11, 2005.
14. Acts of the 1995–1996 Vermont Legislature. Act No. 52 (S.72). An Act Relating to Prohibiting Tobacco Use on School Grounds and School-sponsored Events. Available at http://www.leg.state.vt.us. Accessed March 28, 2005.
15. Acts of the 1997-1998 Vermont Legislature. Act No. 58 (S. 156). An Act to Restrict Minors' Access to Tobacco Products. Available at http://www.leg.state. vt.us. Accessed March 28, 2005.

27

The Great Tobacco Wars: Part 2— How We Nearly Lost Our Footing

If the Great Tobacco Wars in Vermont, Part 1, told our tale of how we collectively worked to change the culture around tobacco in Vermont, Part 2 is how we nearly lost our collective footing during our disagreements over how to spend the funds the Master Settlement Agreement brought into the state.

Because of a well-crafted section that defined public health hazards and risks in Vermont law (the attorney who originally wrote it couldn't possibly have imagined how useful it was for just about any public health issue that came along) and the strategy of the Vermont attorney general's office, my name was on Vermont's lawsuit against the tobacco industry, along with the attorney general's.[1] Fortunately, in November 1998, the Vermont Attorney General announced a settlement, called the Master Settlement Agreement (MSA) that would bring Vermont nearly $30 million per year into perpetuity.[2] Although the MSA contained some other provisions designed to protect public health, many public health experts felt that spending the money on science-based, comprehensive programs to reduce tobacco use would be the primary positive potential impact if the money was well spent. A tobacco task force was created by the legislature with the governor's support and instructed to bring recommendations back to the legislature the following January. A tobacco litigation fund had been established where all money coming into the state from the settlement would be deposited as well.

The Centers for Disease Control and Prevention (CDC) in August 1999 had published a well-timed document, called Best Practices for Comprehensive Tobacco Control Programs.[3] In it was the scientific basis for comprehensive tobacco prevention and control programs, based on the experiences of Massachusetts and California, two states that had well-developed and well-funded programs prior to most other states and prior to the Master Settlement Agreement. In the document, the CDC recommended for each state a range of funding for program elements such as community programs, chronic disease programs, school programs, enforcement, statewide programs, countermarketing, cessation programs, surveillance, evaluation, administration and management. The target for Vermont, according to the CDC, was between $7.9 to $15.9 million per year, which gave a per capita funding range of $13.42 to $27.06. It also included chronic disease programs in its total, defined as programs to reduce the burden of tobacco-related diseases at a funding level of $2.78 to $4.16 million per year.[3]

While we marveled at the skill with which the CDC prepared the document to help states secure funding from the MSA, we noticed that the inclusion of the chronic disease programs (we already had funding for a cancer registry) and funding levels were at both an absolute and per capita rate that we could only dream of. I thought it was unlikely, if not impossible, that such levels of funding would be supported, but we were determined to make a run at the best-funded, most comprehensive program that we could. The health department budget for tobacco was small in the mid-1990s and mainly came from federal and other grants. But in the late 1990s funding increased from federal and foundation sources, and the CDC portion increased to states, in preparation for health department roles in establishing comprehensive programs with settlement funds, allowing the staffing and infrastructure to be built and ready to go.

The Tobacco Task Force met over the summer and fall. I was a member, and it was chaired by a senator and representative and included the attorney general, education department commissioner, two other legislators, a low-income advocate, a public health advocate, and two experts from the University of Vermont College of Medicine, one a smoking prevention expert and the other a smoking cessation expert. The task force had an elegant strategy to support the use of settlement funds and a public strategy designed to engage people in the dialog and gather support through this process. Public hearings would be held and the ads said "How should we spend 30 million dollars?" an eye catching phase. The "$1/_3$, $1/_3$, $1/_3$" proposed division of money, one third for a comprehensive tobacco program, one third for support of other health programs, and one third into a permanent tobacco control trust fund, was simple and easy to understand. The creation of a new independent board to administer the tobacco program by enlisting members of the public and private sector was being promoted. I argued against the creation of a new board at one meeting, but it was clear that I was not in the majority, and could only register my objection in the minority view section of the report. Through the summer, the task force had discussions and presentations by local and national experts. Public meetings were scheduled throughout the state in October to get input on how the state's $800 million should be spent.

Initial budget discussions occurred in the administration during the summer months, leading up to the governor's budget presented to the legislature in early January, and I did my best homework to gain the support of those I worked for. Access to health care was another top priority in public health, and a top priority of the administration, and it became clear that at least some of the funds would be directed to continued efforts to expand access to health care. From a public health perspective, much of this made sense; if you increased the ability of adults to have financial access to health care, it would be easier to connect this with smoking cessation efforts. On the other hand, health care was expensive, for adults, and large expansions would be more costly than tobacco prevention and cessation programs. It was not an either/or, it was a matter of degree, and whether or not we could successfully argue for a sizable tobacco program in the governor's budget and be buttressed in the legislative process. We worked during the budget process, using the unwritten rules in which you argued your best case on the inside, to try and take advantage of this new funding for public health.

Tobacco was in the news all summer long. Talk of the settlement, the task force, and public health antismoking activities, some linked to alcohol and drug prevention in communities, were all ongoing. Ads that had been successfully aired in other states were aired in Vermont.[4] Public health nurses and outreach staff surveyed nearly 3000 Vermonters all over the state. People at farmer's markets, fairs, clinics, grocery stores, laundromats, and other locations were surveyed about tobacco issues during the summer and results were released in September.[4] Vermonters, when asked, overestimated the percentage of smokers for children and adults, and most Vermonters were concerned about tobacco use in their communities. Although the information was qualitative, many ages were surveyed, and people were surveyed all over the state.[4]

Public hearings of the Tobacco Task Force scheduled to be held in October were well publicized. The *Burlington Free Press* called me about them and I highlighted the hearings importance as well as the statistics. When asked about the need for a new board and couldn't the health department administer the funds, I said that we could. The editorial publicizing the six forums was called "Clearing the Haze" and talked about the unique opportunity to reduce our number one public health problem, and printed a schedule of the hearings. The editorial went on to say that the unique opportunity to reduce smoking wouldn't happen if money was spent to cover health care needs unrelated to tobacco or if "the money is wasted to create a new antismoking bureaucracy" and that the health department was "capable of overseeing the money."[5]

And on we went: "$\frac{1}{3}$, $\frac{1}{3}$, $\frac{1}{3}$." and a new independent board, versus likely less money for the program and administration by an already existing health department. The disagreements were tricky; on the one hand we had to articulate our disagreement with the creation of a new board, and on the other, there was no way we would get $10 million for a Vermont tobacco program, and we had to be careful that such areas of disagreement didn't undermine public and legislative support for addressing the issue. So, our strategy throughout was to use our areas of disagreement to focus on the areas of agreement, that we needed to reduce smoking, and take advantage of the opportunity for more publicity. We all agreed on needing to address the most important preventable public health issue in Vermont, and even controversial or competing portions of the proposal gave public opportunities to reiterate the reason reducing tobacco use was so important for public health.

I had used much energy to gain support of the administration I worked for and laid out an approach that would help us in our efforts to reduce the impact of tobacco on health. The administration was highly supportive, but in the real world of competing priorities, efforts were also being made at the same time to continue to expand and fund health care, for both children and adults. In contrast to a categorical approach, the implications of this were that we would link our smoking cessation efforts to health care. We already had strong relationships with physicians, nurses, and hospitals. People who smoked who would gain access health care, would also hear the strong advice, and be offered means to stop smoking. Free-standing cessation methods were also needed, but achieving a high rate of access to health care, for adults as well as children, was a benefit for health, including tobacco control. Of course, the devil was always in the details, and the internal haggling to get a share of tobacco funds, expressly for prevention, control, and comprehensive programs, was all part of the budget process.

In October, in the midst of the public hearings, at a part of his weekly press conference, the governor and I announced a $10 per capita proposal to cut smoking rates in half over the next 10 years, which became instantly controversial[6] and was a surprise to the task force. Under this proposal, more money would go to health care to improve health care access for Vermonters with limited incomes, and the tobacco program would be funded at a much higher level than currently, but short of the CDC minimums. The subsequent public meetings provided much opportunity for public discussion about tobacco, including controversial areas. Soon after, the attorney general announced details of the new settlement money now available to Vermont.[7] It was a very exciting (and interesting) time in tobacco prevention and control.

The road to bigger and better tobacco prevention and control programs was not a straight or smooth one. It was characterized more by zigzags and bumps (and occasional bruises) as we did our best to work with our allies who had been so instrumental in previous years. The work of the Tobacco Task Force report was just the beginning of an exciting but intensely competitive effort to create, with this new money, an effective tobacco control and prevention program that would be comprehensive and sustained. This time, however, the competition was not against the industry.

We had also decided to create a Vermont document about how the health department would further public health efforts, using a comprehensive public health approach, that would show where we had come from, where we were, what steps had already been taken, and how we would reach our year 2010 goal. During the Tobacco Task Force deliberations, the discussion of a new independent board came with the discussion of the development of a future plan for tobacco prevention and control. It seemed that this would be slower than it needed to be, and we really had all the science and Vermont data and working relationships to get started sooner. We worked on this throughout the fall, and produced a 28-page document, based on the CDC approach, called *Vermont Best Practices to cut smoking rates in half by 2010*.[8]

Reducing smoking by 50% over a decade was ambitious but achievable, and a goal of cutting smoking in half in 10 years was easy to understand and focused on results we wanted to achieve. The document laid out the progress to be made in all areas of a comprehensive program: from community programs to programs in schools, from laws and policy to enforcement. The document said what we needed to do, using a public health approach that built on all of our many existing connections and relationships. It wasn't a document talking about money; it talked about progress, actions, and results. The message was that if we followed this plan, we would see smoking reduced, and here's how it would happen.

While the task force members talked about a future plan that would be developed, we put ours on the table, consistent with CDC, the best available science. It was practical and ambitious, but with achievable goals. And besides, smoking was already declining, so the data (speaking for itself), even without our advocacy, would suggest building on something that was already working.

The Tobacco Task Force report, released mid-November, was a comprehensive document, called *Blueprint for a Tobacco-Free Vermont, the Final Report of the Tobacco Task Force,*[9] and it detailed in an excellent way both the science behind the need for comprehensive programs and funding recommendations. As smoking rates declined, and as money coming in that was tied to these rates would also decrease, there could easily be an unintended disincentive to put all energy possible to reduce smoking, and it was felt that investing in a Tobacco Trust Fund would help prepare the state for the days when funds were reduced because less people were smoking.

The press conference to release the report was held in a large and ornate statehouse committee room. The task force members were there, as were children attending, who sat in front of the podium. The two task force chairs and the attorney general talked about the final report and the findings and the recommendations and opened the event to questions. Since I had been a minority voice against the creation of a new independent board, not surprisingly, the press asked me several questions, looking for controversy. I had decided, throughout, that it was absolutely essential, to highlight the importance of smoking as our most important preventable public health issue and our areas of agreement. Although I stated my concerns about a new organizational structure, I quickly moved to all the areas of agreement and opportunities to impact public health. It proved to be an opportunity to speak strongly, over and over, about the importance of reducing smoking.

The debate moved to the legislature in January. The legislative lines were drawn. There were two companion bills, one in the Senate and one in the House, that put into law the task force report.[10] The House health and welfare committee took up their bill right away in January, when the legislature returned. The bill outlined a new administrative structure—an independent board, with detailed composition and funding that had all the powers of a state agency and would oversee all funds and aspects of tobacco prevention and control. Our rationale for not supporting the creation of a new independent board to administer all aspects of the program included concerns that it would be too slow, as it would take time to develop and create those relationships and partnerships that were necessary for a comprehensive public health approach to reducing smoking. It had taken the health department years to develop these relationshps. Also, we worried that with this much money at stake, anything but getting results at breakneck speed would leave the program and funds to be picked off for nonhealth priorities. Tobacco was the leading "real killer" of the population.[11] The way in which the health department was administering its meager funds was already getting results through the use of a comprehensive public health and grassroots approach that involved many strong and existing day-to-day relationships.

At the end of January, the governor and I announced at his weekly press conference the latest results of our Youth Risk Behavior Survey, showing a drop in smoking rates in Vermont eighth through twelvth graders, with the sharpest decline being seen in the younger students, where prevention efforts in legislation, enforcement against illegal sales, raising the price of tobacco products, and community efforts, had been focused. We released the tobacco statistics and included them in our *Vermont Best Practices* document. Our goal was to cut smoking in half by the year 2010 by building on the progress we were already seeing. We put our plan on the table to cut smoking in half and outlined the elements and next steps. Newspaper articles carried the news of our progress the next day as well as our plan outlined in *Vermont Best Practices to cut smoking rates in half by 2010.*[12]

In our view, results were critical, as the competition for what was a very large amount of money coming into the state was already intense and would likely increase. However, the majority of task force members, and some members of the key health committees disagreed, and it was clear from the first committee meeting (there were more than 20 committee meetings on both the House and Senate side over these issues) that the bill was going to be rapidly passed out of the committee. It did.

Fortunately, for us, the bill traveled across the hall on the third floor of the statehouse, to the House government operations committee, the committee that looked at new departments, government restructuring, and how the government ran. They asked a lot of questions. It was in this committee that after much testimony and committee discussion, the accountability for results shifted from a new independent board to a shared responsibility between the health department and a Tobacco Prevention and Treatment Board that would be situated in the Attorney general's office. The committee discussed that despite the source of funds, the accountability rested with the legislature, and the committee made substantive changes to the bill. There was extensive testimony and debate with the appropriation committee as well, as there were differences in amounts of money going to public health and health care in each one, and the bill that passed the House contained a shared responsibility for the program, and the board now became situated, after a floor amendment, in the state treasurer's office.[10]

The language was still too cumbersome, but the bill's accountability for public health had dramatically improved since the task force report and House bill. The discussion picked up again on the Senate side, and the final legislative language regarding money and also board and department responsibilities was written into the appropriations act, called the "Big Bill," where it was guaranteed to pass, as the Big Bill funded all the money of state government for the year.[13]

The final bill was ultimately a compromise, with more than $6 million going to tobacco prevention and control, including funds for the state departments of health, education (who worked to increase the number of science-based programs in school curricula) and the department of liquor control (that performed the enforcement operations to prevent illegal sales). A tobacco trust fund and the Tobacco Litigation Settlement fund had already been established and a Vermont Tobacco Evaluation and Review Board was established and situated in the office of the Secretary of the Agency of Human Services, the same umbrella agency that included the Department of Health. The roles in the areas of community grants, countermarketing, independent evaluation, enforcement, and other activities were defined and timelines established. The board composition and the process for board members and the creation of a conflict of interest policy were spelled out. The board had its responsibilities, the departments of health, education, and liquor control had theirs, and the partnership defined. Although it would require a little different way of connecting our work, it was a good compromise, with checks and balances, and most importantly, a strong commitment to a comprehensive and sustained program to reduce smoking.

The session was intense, and I thought long and hard about tobacco, and whether what we were proposing was really best, both in the short term and long term. I was a minority voice, and with the strong support of the people I worked with, continued to articulate the reasons for our objections to the creation of a new tobacco superstructure. Our goal was not to have a bigger department or budget, but to reduce smoking. I had plenty of time to consider and reconsider my rationale as we participated in hearing after hearing. Although the final bill was a compromise (putting public health funds in the health department and creating a new evaluation and review board), it would ultimately greatly benefit the public.

Public health, in the form of the department of health, had staff that had shown tremendous energy, creativity, and efficiency in their efforts, putting science into practice to reduce smoking. We worked in an administration that was strongly supportive of public health and health care. The new tobacco evaluation and review board worked in partnership with public health, had a critical review and evaluation function, and the potential to provide an independent assessment of progress and recommendations for funding. The evaluation and review board could provide shelter in the event that a controversial countermarketing campaign was needed–something that had created attention and subsequent attacks on funding in other states.

Their most important function was the independent review and recommendation for the annual program budget to the governor, joint fiscal committee of the legislature, and the House and Senate appropriations committees each year by October 1, well in advance of the governor's January budget address and the legislative deliberations that occurred during the winter. The greatest future danger, was not in the program content and direction, where there might be only minor differences, as the health department had a long track record of using the best available science and working with nearby experts (using an informally created Scientific Advisory Panel) to help get the scientific information on the table. The greatest danger was what would happen in future years with the money used to sustain the comprehensive efforts. In the appropriations process, the greatest driver of the next budget is the previous year's budget, and although the legislature makes some modifications, the governor's budget is usually the basis for major decisions. Such a structure, in which the health department, the state's public health agency, and the tobacco evaluation and review board, who had a complementary and independent role, provided a "check and balance" that while not guaranteeing funding of the program at the same level into perpetuity, would give it the best chance of continued focus, despite future changing administrations and competing public health needs.

What to do when you have more money than you have ever had? You must use your resources in a way that will get the best possible results as quickly as possible. It is how you spend the funds that is critical. It is important to have a plan on the table, based on the best available science, to have community partners in place, and be ready to move forward. It took a little time to develop a rhythm for the use of these new funds–an administrative rhythm that made good decisions in each program area—but it happened. Countermarketing campaigns were developed and implemented, based on the notion that "8 out of 10" Vermont kids don't smoke. Youth groups empowered themselves in a larger youth movement. Toll-free quit lines were developed, funded, and evaluated. Hospitals and doctors and the University of Vermont helped train physicians, and provide community support, as well as help people to quit. Community grant criteria were developed and communities funded.[14] The price of tobacco products went up, a major deterrent to youth smoking. Science-based curricula were put into place in more and more middle schools, aimed at children just considering the deadly habit. And, most importantly, smoking declined among adults (in a small way) and steadily among Vermont's youngest citizens. The bottom line was that kids were smoking less.[15] Was smoking solved as a public health issue? No way, not yet, but we were well on our way.

As of 2005, collaborative work continued[16] and Vermont remained one of 10 states who have committed substantial funding for tobacco prevention programs and ranked number 11 in both FY 2004 and FY2005.[17] Most important, however, is that far fewer Vermont kids are smoking.

REFERENCES

1. State of Vermont Chittenden County, SS. State of Vermont Plaintiff Vs. Philip Morris, Incorporated; RJ Reynolds Tobacco, Nabisco Holding Corp., RJR Nabisco, Inc. American Tobacco Corp, Brown and Williamson Tobacco Corp; Liggett and Myers, Inc. Lorillard Tobacco Co Inc, United States Tobacco Co, BAT Industries, PLC, British American Tobacco Company; The council for Tobacco Research-USA, Inc, and the Tobacco Institute, Inc. Defendants Chittenden County Superior Court Docket No. 744-97. Available at http://www.stic.nev.edu/vt/complaintdoc. Accessed March 28, 2005.
2. State of Vermont, Office of the Attorney General, Vermont Attorney General Announces Tobacco Settlement. November 20, 1998. Montpelier, Vt: 1998. News release. Available at http://www.atg.state.vt.us. Accessed March 28, 2005.
3. Centers for Disease Control and Prevention. *Best Practices for Comprehensive Tobacco Control Programs.* 1999. Atlanta, Ga: US Department of Health and Human Services; 1999:79.
4. Remsen N. Poll: Fewer smoke than people think. *Burlington Free Press.* September 30, 1999. 1A.
5. Editorial. Clearing the Haze. *Burlington Free Press.* September 21, 1999. P. 9A.
6. Blowing Smoke. Editorial. Rutland Herald. October 8, 1999; 8.
7. State of Vermont, Office of the Attorney General. Attorney General William H. Sorrell Confirms Final Approval of Tobacco Settlement; $9.8 Million to Flow to Vermont Now, with $26.3 Million Starting January 2000. November 12, 1999. News release. Available at http://www.atg.state.vt.us. Accessed March 28, 2005.
8. Vermont Department of Health. *Vermont Best Practices to cut smoking rates in half by 2010.* Burlington, Vt: Vermont Department of Health; January 2000. Available at www.healthyvermonters.info/hi/tobacco/pubs/tobacco2000.shtml. Accessed March 28, 2005.
9. Vermont Tobacco Task Force. *Blueprint for a Tobacco-Free Vermont: Final Report of the Tobacco Task Force.* Montpelier, Vt: 1999. Available at http://www.leg.state.vt.us/tobacco/finalreport.pdf. Accessed March 28, 2005.

10. Bills and Acts of the Vermont Legislature, 1999–2000. H.310 and S.243. Available at http://www/leg.state.vt.us. Accessed March 28, 2005.
11. McGinnis JM. Actual causes of death in the United States. *JAMA*. 1993; 270–2212.
12. Gram D. Associated Press. High schoolers smoking less, state reports. *Burlington Free Press*. January 23, 2000. P. 6B.
13. Bills and Acts of the 1999–2000 Vermont Legislature. Act 152 (H842). Appropriations for state government. Available at http://www/leg.state. vt.us. Accessed March 28, 2005.
14. Vermont Department of Health Tobacco Control Program. Available at http://www.healthyvermonters.info/hi/tobacco/tobacco.shtml. Accessed March 24, 2005.
15. Vermont Departments of Health and Education. Youth Behavior Risk Factor Survey. Montpelier, Vt: Vermont Department of Health and Education; 2003. Available at www.healthyvermonters.info/pubs.shtml. Accessed March 28, 2005.
16. Vermont Department of Health, Vermont Department of Education, Vermont Department of Liquor Control, Vermont Tobacco Evaluation and Review Board. Vermont Tobacco Control Work Plan 2004–2005. Available at http://www. ahs.state.vt.us/TobaccoBoard/RFP's/workplan0405.pdf. Accessed November 10, 2005.
17. Campaign for Tobacco-Free Kids. FY2005 ranking of state funding for tobacco prevention. Available at http://www.tobaccofreekids.org/reports/settlements/ Accessed on October 26, 2005.

28

Rabies—Preventing Public Fatigue About a Fatal Illness

Health officials from Vermont and New Hampshire[1] investigated and managed animal rabies and human exposures on both sides of the river. On one occasion, a cat bit its owner, was then shot by the owner, and the animal was tested at the health department lab. Because the cat's brain wasn't intact, it was impossible to determine for sure whether or not the animal was rabid, as brain tissue is used in a dead animal to test for the rabies virus. Such an inconclusive result, with the whole story of events, prompted precautionary measures that assumed that the cat could be rabid and steps were taken to prevent human rabies in exposed individuals.[1]

The story had started in a household in New Hampshire where there were nearly a dozen dogs and a litter of puppies, more than a dozen cats, mice, hamsters, and gerbils. Because the cats had been kept indoors, the owners didn't vaccinate them because they didn't think they could contract rabies in that way. A cat had been found dead in the basement, and people became suspicious about the possibility of rabies. Another family was involved from Vermont because one of the cats had been given to them.

Officials from both states worked together and with the families involved to make sure exposed people were referred to physicians for preventive shots against rabies, and other animals evaluated by veterinarians to make sure the situation didn't get worse. Public health officials in both states reminded the public about the importance of pet vaccination against rabies, even for indoor cats, as well as large barn animals. They told the public through newspaper interviews about how the rabies animal epidemic was spreading and what people could do to protect themselves and their families.[1]

Such stories were unfortunately not rare. Two years earlier, the Centers for Disease Control and Prevention (CDC) had reported an unrelated situation in New Hampshire in which the New Hampshire public health lab had diagnosed rabies in a kitten bought in a New Hampshire pet store and more than 650 people had to receive postexposure prophylaxis (rabies shots) as a result.[2]

Rabies is a fatal illness in animals and humans,[3] with only a rare human survivor reported after clinical symptoms and illness set in.[4] On the East Coast, raccoon rabies has traveled north, posing a real risk of harm to unvaccinated animals and potential exposure of humans to the fatal virus. In February 1992, the fox strain of rabies was confirmed in foxes in the northwestern part of

Vermont and in June 1994, raccoon rabies was first documented in southwestern Vermont. Since then hundreds of cases of animal rabies have been reported.[5]

In the early 1990s, when raccoon rabies was moving up the East Coast, there was preparation for the animal epidemic, or epizootic, and much discussion and planning about how to prevent its impact on animals and people in Vermont. In 1991, the governor issued an executive order[6] creating the Vermont Rabies Task Force. The order highlighted the fact that raccoon rabies was reported 100 miles south of Vermont and fox rabies was in upstate New York, and that there was "fear that infected animals would reach Vermont when Lake Champlain froze over."[6] A task force was created because the responsibilities were divided among different state and federal agencies, and a coordinated approach was needed. I was a cochair, along with the commissioner of agriculture, to be helped also by the commissioner of the department of fish and wildlife, who employed the state game wardens. The task force included the commissioner of the department of public safety, and private sector representatives as well. The order required us to develop strategies and an action plan to deal with this within 90 days. This executive order, issued by the governor, gave a strong public message that this was an imminent public health priority. Its composition and direction gave government departments the message to cooperate, and quickly. The order also instructed the group to be a source of information to the public.

The task force met, was highly productive, and issued its report on time. One of the recommendations was to fund a position for a public health veterinarian, in the health department, in anticipation of the tremendous resources and credibility needed to protect public health. The state had a state veterinarian, located in the department of agriculture, but the risks of rabies included the potential for human exposure and illness, and the issues were related to both human and animal health. This recommendation, and the hiring of a public health veterinarian in the department of health, was a step that was instrumental in our sustained approach to preventing rabies in humans and animals.

The public health strategies subsequently used included clarifying and updating the current law, educating the public, and finding ways to ensure vaccination of domestic pets. During the following session of the legislature, the authority of the commissioner of agriculture was clarified and strengthened, required vaccination of domestic pets including, dogs, cats, and ferrets, as well as wolf hybrids, and the licensing of dogs and wolf hybrids.[7] In the discussions about the need to vaccinate cats (it was felt that exposure of cats to raccoons was possible due to their sharing of some habits and environments), and require them to be licensed, some pet owners testified as to the difficulty of cats having to wear collars, and the impracticality of their being required to be licensed, so the bill was a compromise in this area. In addition to many other provisions, the law set aside a mechanism for the town clerks, who were responsible for pet licensing in the towns, to have a one dollar fee collected to go to the departments of fish and wildlife, agriculture, and health, to add a modest amount of resources, as the game wardens now had a new and difficult responsibility as did officials at the other departments. These extra duties and funding would be needed, we estimated, for at least the next decade.

Federal agencies were also extremely helpful, and one of the important steps taken early on was to establish a toll-free hotline, with the word "rabies" in the number, to give the public access to information, and connect people with health department experts, if there was a human exposure, or if testing of animals was needed at the public health laboratory.

Public education was the centerpiece of the strategy, and Vermont's public health veterinarian was a credible and tireless spokesman. Messages to appreciate wildlife from a distance, not to touch or feed wild animals, to make sure pets are vaccinated and kept up to date, and other advice were repeated at first, and each time a new animal was tested positive for rabies. Although we all announced when raccoon rabies hit Vermont, to reinforce the seriousness and reiterate the public messages, it really was the ongoing, day-to-day, familiar voice of Vermont's public health veterinarian, that kept the issue in the news, statewide and locally, in print and on television, with different angles, but always with the same advice to protect the public.

The CDC reported that in 1995 40% of the raccoons tested were positive for rabies, and in addition to more than 100 rabid raccoons, there were 31 foxes, 38 skunks, 2 woodchucks, 1 pig, 1 beaver, and a cat.[5] Vermont's public health veterinarian noted that there had been 829 confirmed animals with rabies in Vermont from 1992–2000, including cats, dogs, cows, bats, and horses.[8]

Rabies was in the news, in usual and unusual circumstances. A rabid raccoon entered a home through a cat door and chased the family cat around.[9] In another report, a cat was drooling with paralysis in its hind legs.[8] A rabid gray fox, a rabid woodchuck, and a rabid bat resulted in rabies information written in another news report,[10] along with the hotline number. Two donkeys in Rutland County,[11] confirmed with rabies, provided an opportunity to reinforce advice about rabies and the importance of immunizing pets. Each rabid animal reported prompted the same public advice: vaccinate your pet, avoid wild animals, and call the hotline—the same advice, over and over, at each and every public opportunity.

When Vermont joined research efforts to use the oral rabies vaccine to keep raccoon rabies from spreading across the Vermont/Canadian border in 1997,[12] it was important to craft public messages that didn't create a false impression that this would eliminate the need for public caution and pet vaccination, as we had been recommending. Public meetings held before the first bait drop served to further educate the public in the affected areas and answer public questions and concerns. Public education efforts and news reports continued,[13–16] and the health department updated it Web site and public information materials on an ongoing basis.

Sometimes in public health it is difficult to keep public attention high through the press when an issue, even a serious and fatal issue, goes on for years. Ongoing educational efforts to encourage certain actions and behaviors, such as vaccinating pets, even when the disease is nearly always fatal, like rabies, become challenging after initial efforts are made and time has passed. Getting the press's attention and overcoming "public fatigue" from hearing the same advice over and over, was a real danger. If people were no longer interested in hearing the message, they may not be listening to the advice. The rabies epizootic, or animal epidemic, was not a sprint, it was a marathon, and experts predicted that it would last for a decade, or more. Rabies cases in humans (none) and animals (hundreds) were required to be reported to the health department through the usual disease surveillance system that tracked measles, hepatitis, and AIDS. Finding ways to overcome public and media fatigue were difficult, but press releases, using every reported animal, particularly ones occurring less frequently, such as horses, donkeys, and cats, gave a new opportunity, because they weren't the (by now) usual rabid fox, skunk, bat, or raccoon that was creating havoc in a community. It was essential to have a capable and credible spokesman in public health, and we were indeed fortunate to have our public health veterinarian who was tireless in his efforts to protect the public, despite the nearly continuous work needed. Rabies bait-drop research trials provided additional opportunities for public education, and it was a challenge to make sure Vermonters didn't let down their guard. In Vermont, since the animal epidemic began, there had been hundreds of animals with rabies, and no person had gotten rabies. We intended to keep it that way.

REFERENCES

1. Cronin E, Montany G. Dozens of pets euthanized due to rabies scare. *Caledonian-Record*. April 22, 1997. Available at: http://www.caledoniarecord.com. Accessed March 2, 2005.
2. CDC. Mass treatment of humans exposed to rabies—New Hampshire 1994. *MMWR*. 1995;44:484–486.
3. Vermont Department of Health. Rabies in Vermont. Available at: http://www.healthyvermonters.info/hs/epi/idepi/rabies/rabies.shtml. Accessed March 2, 2005.
4. CDC. Recovery of a patient from clinical rabies—Wisconsin, 2004. *MMWR*. 2004;53:1171.
5. CDC. Update: Raccoon rabies epizootic—United States, 1996. *MMWR*. 1997;45(51&52);1117–1120.
6. State of Vermont. Executive Order (No. 14-91). Rabies Task Force 1991. Vermont. Statutes, Title 3 Executive Orders/Chapter 18, Health/No.18-5. Rabies Task Force (No. 14-91). Available at http://198.187.128.12/mbPrint/11e7311.htm. Accessed March 3, 2005.
7. Acts of the 1993–1994 legislative session. Act 213 (S115). Domestic Pet Control. 1994. Available at: http://www.leg.state.vt.us. Accessed March 3, 2005.
8. Smith RF. First domestic rabies reported in cat. *Rutland Herald.* June 3, 2000. Available at: http://www.rutlandherald.com. Accessed March 2, 2005.
9. Smith RF. Pet owners warned after rabies turns up. *Rutland Herald.* May 10, 2002. Available at: http://www.rutlandherald.com. Accessed March 2, 2005.
10. Rabies cases on the rise. *Times Argus.* August 28, 2001. Available at: http://www.rutlandherald.com. Accessed March 2, 2005.
11. Dritschilo G. First case of rabid donkeys recorded in Vermont. *Rutland Herald.* February 15, 2002. Available at: http://www.rutlandherald.com. Accessed March 2, 2005.

12. Vermont Department of Health. Rabies Bait Drop fact sheet. Available at: http://www.healthyvermonters.info. Accessed June 17, 2005.
13. Associated Press. Anti-rabies bait drop begins Monday. *Rutland Herald.* August 4, 2001. Available at: http://www.rutlandherald.com. Accessed March 2, 2005.
14. Smallheer S. Dairy farm tackles rabies scare. *Rutland Herald.* February 2, 2002. Available at: http://www.rutlandherald.com. Accessed March 2, 2005.
15. Dritschilo G. Rabies cases rise sharply in county. *Rutland Herald.* April 3, 2002. Available at: http://www.rutlandherald.com. Accessed March 2, 2005.
16. Vermont briefs: Rabid cow. *Rutland Herald.* July 31, 2002. Available at: http://www.rutlandherald.com. Accessed March 2, 2005.

CHAPTER

29

Bug Spray and Birdbaths— West Nile Virus

We received many letters each day, and Vermont citizens often called and sent emails. Sometimes the notes and calls were critical, other times just concerned and asking for information. Sometimes people wrote or called in reaction to a media report or to bring a health issue to our attention. I read letters carefully, because it was one small but important way to measure how what we were doing was being received by the people we were trying to help, the public.

During the time when we were drafting Vermont's prevention plan for West Nile virus, we received much feedback, particularly about the use of pesticides. We considered the spraying of pesticides as a "last resort" and tried to emphasize the use of public education and surveillance as our primary approach. An editorial in the *Burlington Free Press* expressed a similar sentiment that "Vermont should not rush to spray pesticides in response to the relatively small health threat posed by the West Nile Virus."[1]

In late August 1999,[2] two patients with encephalitis were reported to the New York City Department of Health. Active surveillance and further investigation revealed more patients, with a number of patients being identified from a small area in Queens. At the same time, New York City noted an increase in dying birds, particularly crows, along with the zoo deaths of captive flamingos and a pheasant. By the end of September, 17 confirmed and 20 probable cases involving humans had been identified and reported from New York City and nearby counties. Four deaths were reported in people older than 68. Citywide pesticide applications were begun, telephone hot lines rang off the hook, public information materials and mosquito repellent were widely distributed.[2] An analysis of the genetic viral material from zoo birds, human brain, dead bird and mosquitoes showed them to be all alike and although the virus was thought to be the St Louis Encephalitis virus (SLE), it was subsequently identified as a similar but distinct virus, West Nile virus.[2,3] Because mosquitoes were so common and deaths had occurred, publicity about the initial reports from the Centers for Disease Control and Prevention (CDC) pushed the issue rapidly to the top of the priority list for public health. The epidemic in New York City had 61 human cases and seven deaths, along with high death rates among horses, crows, and zoo birds.[4]

West Nile virus was first isolated in the West Nile province of Uganda in 1937,[2,5] with human epidemics reported in South Africa, Israel, southern France, southeastern Romania, and south-central Russia. It had been noted in temperate regions of Europe in recent years, with the most serious potential complication being encephalitis, a fatal inflammation of the brain seen in both humans and horses. It could also kill domestic and wild birds.[6]

At the health department, we gathered all available information from the CDC and met to establish short-term steps such as keeping track and trying to anticipate what the CDC would recommend, noting which aspects would be difficult to implement in Vermont. One advantage that we already had was a strong communication, both formal and informal, with physicians, nurses, and hospitals in Vermont to allow reporting of human illness, and these health professionals served as a vehicle for information to patients. If we made sure that physicians and nurses had all the information right away, they were always a tremendous help in our efforts to identify illness and address health concerns from patients and the public.

Much of the fall was spent monitoring the situation, and the return of cool weather bought some time for planning. In January 2000, the CDC released guidelines for surveillance, prevention, and control of West Nile virus (WNV).[4] They called for increased surveillance, including bird monitoring (particularly of dead crows), mosquito surveillance, looking for the distribution of mosquitoes and their larvae, increased veterinary surveillance in horses, alerting of physicians and other health-care professionals with general information about what was known, and for health workers to report viral encephalitis to health departments. Ensuring adequate laboratory capacity for specialized testing in regional laboratories and reference laboratories was also recommended. Prevention and control measures included mosquito control by local programs to reduce larvae. Public education about the disease, how it is transmitted, and ways to prevent exposure through mosquitoes were recommended and became our top priority. In the case of West Nile virus, CDC emphasized the importance of sharing accurate data among local, state, and federal public health agencies, and those concerned with agriculture and wildlife.[4]

Planning efforts began to evolve in Vermont and it was clear that to develop and implement a successful prevention strategy, there would need to be strong relationships with other agencies, especially the Department of Agriculture. A task force was convened to develop a plan for the state of Vermont. Members included commissioners of health and agriculture, the state epidemiologist, state public health veterinarian, state entomologist, the state agricultural veterinarian, epidemiologists from the health department and representatives from the public health laboratory, public information staff, and from the Pesticide Advisory Council, a group that gave thorough review and advice to the commissioner of agriculture on the use of pesticides.

Vermont's plan emphasized the areas recommended by CDC, making it specific to Vermont. It strongly emphasized public education about WNV and how it is spread, included information about the need to eliminate mosquito breeding habitats, and personal measures that could prevent or greatly reduce the risk of exposure to West Nile virus. Pesticides would be used only as a last resort. Surveillance activities—our early warning system—included dead bird surveillance systems, and it was important for state and federal agencies to be closely involved in this effort.[5]

Public education encouraged people to report dead birds. Efforts included refrigerator magnets and flyers with a cartoon bird lying on its back, feet in the air, above the caption "Have you seen a dead bird?" with a toll-free number and the phone number of the local health department district office. Mosquito surveillance was proposed to provide better information on the types of mosquitoes and where they were found, to map and identify the distribution and habits of mosquitoes that were vectors of WNV, to allow targeted use of larvicides. Information was summarized for physicians in an issue of the Disease Control Bulletin, a newsletter that had been published by the health department for years to summarize health issues and update physicians and hospitals around the state, to raise awareness, and prompt calls to the health department. Horse surveillance was recommended by providing information to veterinarians and horse owners across the state. Surveillance and public education efforts increased as time went on.

Not only did this plan identify who would be responsible and do what, its development and implementation created even stronger working relationships between the departments of health and agriculture, critical to a successful program. How many times have citizens been critical of government agencies acting in different directions? We learned that if another state agency gave conflicting advice, it hurt us too, because most people saw the collection of state agencies and departments as "the state" or "the government" and loss of credibility in one department had the potential to hurt the credibility of another. It was in our best interest to work closely with other state departments. Over time, we found that the quarterly meetings between key staff at the two departments worked much more effectively than formal signed Memorandums of Agreement and paper pledges to work together.

In our overall response to WNV, public education strategies were paramount, and information came both from the health and agriculture departments. Health department staff worked hard to fully engage agriculture experts as partners in our planning and implementation efforts, and it showed up in the media. One report of the response to West Nile virus showed a health department epidemiologist being interviewed; another report featured the agriculture department's state entomologist, our mosquito expert, and the message to the public was entirely consistent. Such consistent messages not only reiterated essential health information, it gave the public confidence that the issue was being addressed.

The agriculture department had a fact sheet[7] explaining about *Bacillus thuringiensis israelensis* (Bti), a naturally occurring soil bacterium that can kill mosquito larvae. The health department fact sheet[8] gave background about West Nile virus, explained that people get WNV usually from the bite of an infected mosquito, and that mosquitoes are infected when they feed on an infected bird, and that most mosquitoes are not infected with WNV. Points of emphasis were that most people infected have no symptoms, about 20% have a mild illness, and a small percentage, less than 1%, can develop encephalitis or meningitis, particularly seen in older individuals.[8]

The health department gave advice about how individuals could protect themselves and their families, and included times when mosquitoes are most active, and guidance or the appropriate use of insect repellents for adults and children.[8] Suggestions regarding ways to reduce mosquitoes around homes were practical: emptying trash cans or other containers that held water, particularly old tires; changing water in birdbaths every three or four days; and being conscious of standing pools of water and ways to reduce them. A toll-free number was included and educational materials were included on the health department Web page.

Media alerts were frequently issued and questions from print, television, and radio reporters provided opportunities to reiterate health information and common-sense recommendations. When bird surveillance was initiated, press reports talked about how WNV was transmitted, and that crows were particularly susceptible. Birds were being sent to the National Wildlife Health Center in Wisconsin for testing. At the time, the state epidemiologist characterized the risk to the public as "very, very low" but emphasized that the state had monitoring systems in place and wasn't going to sit and wait.[9] Both health and agriculture officials were quoted. Another article announced that mosquitoes would be tested for WNV.[10]

In October 2000 a hermit thrush tested positive for WNV and the news release emphasized that spraying was not recommended.[11] To date, more than 550 dead birds had been reported, 213 were sent for testing, and 153 of them tested negative.[11] Just before the news that a bird had tested positive, the state epidemiologist had told the press that WNV was already likely in Vermont, based on the fact that it had been seen in two New York counties that bordered Vermont.[12] He reiterated steps the public could take at home and talked about the state's ongoing efforts. When the first bird tested positive, health officials explained that "it was only a matter of time" and how it had been expected. Because of the time of year, with cooler weather making mosquitoes sluggish, there was no reason to consider spraying.[13]

The following summer, the paper described a college student working as a virus field agent for the health department and how she trapped mosquitoes with a trap that used light and dry ice, and recorded each mosquito's position with a global positioning system.[14] Surveillance and public education activities continued, and the CDC also updated states and the public on a regular basis. The local paper published a front-page headline when a horse and two birds were infected in a northern county.[15] It was the first horse infected and the news went statewide,[16] but the response from health and agriculture departments was the same—the horse was the first case in horses, but not surprising, according to the state veterinarian and the state epidemiologist, who clearly said "We have been looking for the WNV, we have expected it, and now we are finding it and we are prepared to deal with that."[16] When the first probable human case of WNV happened in September 2002, it was not unexpected. The individual, identified only by gender and county of residence, was released from the hospital, and the health department epidemiologist emphasized that most people with WNV have no symptoms, repeating ways to avoid mosquito bites and how to reduce mosquito populations near homes.[17]

And on it went. It was a busy summer and fall, one that had seen blue-green algae and Legionnaire's Disease, as well a regular news releases and media coverage about West Nile virus. Each bird, horse, and finally human case provided another opportunity to remind Vermont residents what practical steps they could take to protect themselves and their families, and to put risks and the disease into perspective.

The issue of spraying to reduce mosquito populations, either from the ground or from airplanes, had prompted public comments in the draft state plan from the health and agriculture departments, and pleas to use common sense and a realistic perspective on health risks, as they were balanced with risks to people and environment. The use of larvicides, an important part of the planning efforts, was not so controversial and it was essential to provide clear communication about what was and was not being considered, while repeating the same practiced health advice, over and over again. "Change the water in the birdbath regularly," not "get rid of the birdbath" was an example of the type of information given. These efforts to remind individuals and families about how to reduce risks from mosquito bites (most of which did not carry West Nile virus) went a long way toward putting in place the public education, surveillance, and contingency planning that was needed. Much of the public education could be described as "consciousness raising" about mosquitoes and their habits, reporting dead birds, and where to get more information, delivered by capable epidemiologists from the health department and experts from the department of agriculture, both giving similar advice from different perspectives. It was a conscious strategy to publicize frequent reports about dead birds, testing results, annual statistics, and human illness.

West Nile virus activity increased in the United States with four states seeing activity in 1999 and 44 in 2002. Increases were seen in horses, birds, mosquitoes, and humans. WNV was first documented in Vermont in October 2000, in a dead hermit thrush found in southern Vermont. Two years later, WNV activity encompassed the vast majority of Vermont counties. More than 100 dead birds, five horses, and 11 mosquito pools had tested positive and Vermont's first human case was diagnosed in 2002.[5]

In August 2004, two birds from the state's largest county tested positive for West Nile virus, though no human cases were found. In 2003, 116 birds from nearly all Vermont counties were found to have the virus, as well as four horses and three humans.[18] Public health efforts continue.

An epidemiologist, a regular spokesperson on this issue, said that the health department expected to find West Nile in birds every year.[18] She reiterated again the message that was so successful in communicating this issue to Vermonters—that we heard about it, we planned with the department of agriculture, we have been monitoring it through surveillance, and when we saw it, we were prepared. The proactive and sustained partnership with the Vermont Department of Agriculture, and the calm and prepared tone, always with repeating common-sense advice to the public was an example of a proactive public health response to a serious issue. There were deaths in New York City as the initial momentum around West Nile virus began. Developing a plan with concrete priorities and using proactive communication with credible spokespeople not only ensured that Vermont was prepared to deal with West Nile virus, but did so in a way that it put health risks in perspective and advocated practical, common-sense measures.

We planned, anticipated, monitored, collected, counted, acted, communicated, and were ready. When West Nile virus was found in Vermont, it was expected. There was no panic, 100,000 calls to the toll-free number, or media frenzy, just many, many opportunities to repeat health advice to the public, and do our job.

REFERENCES

1. A matter of choice. *Burlington Free Press.* Editorial. May 31, 2001; 6A.
2. CDC. Outbreak of West Nile-Like Viral Encephalitis–New York, 1999. *MMWR.* 1999;48:845–849.
3. CDC. Update: West Nile Virus Encephalitis, New York, 1999. *MMWR.* 1999;48:944–946.
4. CDC. Guidelines for Surveillance, Prevention, and Control of West Nile Virus Infection–United States. *MMWR.* 2000;49:25–8.
5. Vermont Department of Agriculture and Vermont Department of Health. The State of Vermont West Nile Virus Surveillance and Response Plan. Final Working Plan, August 2001 (revised July 2003).
6. CDC. West Nile Virus. Background: Virus History and Distribution. Available at: http://www.cdc.gov/ncidod/dvbid/westnile/background. htm. Accessed April 11, 2005.
7. Vermont Department of Agriculture. West Nile Virus: Controlling Mosquito Larvae with *Bacillus thuringiensis israelensis (Bti).* Vermont Department of Agriculture. Montpelier, Vermont.
8. Vermont Department of Health. West Nile Virus. Burlington, Vt: Vermont Department of Health. May 2003. Fact sheet.
9. Associated Press. State to watch for dead birds. *Rutland Herald.* April 26, 2000. Available at: http://www.rutlandherald.com. Accessed April 12, 2005.
10. Barna E. State to test mosquitoes for virus. *Rutland Herald.* August 8, 2000. Available at: http://www.rutlandherald.com. Accessed April 12, 2005.
11. Vermont Department of Health. Hermit thrush test positive for West Nile virus in Putney. No spraying planned. Burlington, Vt: Vermont Department of Health. October 13, 2000. News release.
12. Associated Press. West Nile virus likely in Vermont. *Rutland Herald.* August 4, 2000. Available at: http://www.rutlandherald.com. Accessed April 12, 2005.
13. Sneyd, R. West Nile virus shows up in Putney. *Rutland Herald.* October 14, 2000. Available at: http://www.rutlandherald.com. Accessed April 12, 2005.
14. O'Connor, K. GMC student tracks deadly virus. *Rutland Herald.* August 27, 2001. Available at: http://www.rutlandherald.com. Accessed April 12, 2005.
15. Hallenbeck T. West Nile virus infects horse, birds in Franklin County. *Burlington Free Press.* August 23, 2002. P. 1A.
16. Associated Press. Horse, two birds test positive for West Nile. *Rutland Herald.* August 22, 2002. Available at: http://www.rutlandherald.com. Accessed April 12, 2005.
17. Vermont Department of Health. State health officials announce probable human case of West Nile virus. Burlington, Vt: Vermont Department of Health. September 10, 2002. News release. Available at http://www.healthyvermonters. info. Accessed April 14, 2005.
18. First West Nile of year found. *Rutland Herald.* August 27, 2004. Available at http://www.rutlandherald.com. Accessed on April 12, 2005.

30

Investigating Cancer Clusters— Stepping Out from Behind the Podium

We all drove in the car to Rutland, down Route 7–it took about an hour and a half–for a community meeting about cancer concerns in the town elementary school. With me were our toxicologist and environmental epidemiologist, two individuals who had done much of the background work leading up to the meeting. As we entered the large room, with folding chairs, I remembered a television segment in which I had seen one of my staff talking to a group about cancer questions. What I remembered most was seeing him behind the podium, and the image of a barrier between him and the sometimes hostile and questioning audience. I decided at that moment to skip the podium, and to step out directly in front of the audience, very close and quite vulnerable to the people attending. The room was filled with about 40 people from the community–parents, teachers, and others, who were very concerned and questioning the health of the school, and what we were doing about it. There were reporters from the newspaper and one television station.[1]

I explained to the audience that I did not feel that the cancer cases reported were connected and that we weren't dealing with a cluster. I talked a little about the guidance that we used from the Centers for Disease Control and Prevention and the National Cancer Institute, and how we came to that conclusion. Cancers of different types had been reported from school employees in the age ranges that they were usually found.[1] For example, lung cancer, prostate cancer, and colon cancers were all found. Five staff members had been diagnosed with cancer several years prior, and one additional person more recently, prompting a renewed concern for the health of the school and the community.[1]

I told the audience that it would worry us more if the cancers were all the same type, if we were seeing even a small number of usually rare tumors, or if the cancers had been seen in people younger or older than the usual age range in which the type of cancer usually occurred. I talked about how cancer is not one disease but many different diseases, and that it is more common as people get older, and that some risk factors we knew and some we didn't.

I related how we had reviewed school records, and had taken an unannounced walk-around tour of the school looking at the physical facility, school grounds, and nearby neighborhoods.[1] A history of the area noted that it had been previously used for agricultural purposes.[1] There were many questions from the audience and my approach was to simply try and answer them the best that I could, and honestly. Some questions were straightforward and some mathematical. Someone raised concerns that some soil on the playground may have come from a landfill. We had gotten agreement from the state environmental agency to test soil samples from the playground.[1]

The chairwoman of the Healthy School and Neighborhood Review Committee said that there were a handful of thyroid cancer cases in the surrounding community. I had not heard that previously and said I would look into it. I explained about what we do with our cancer registry, started in 1994. One man asked about comparing cancer cases in the school to the number of people working there. I responded that I didn't think it would be helpful.[1] A question was raised about studying school graduates. The questions went on for an hour or so, and I did the best I could to answer all questions, as did our toxicologist and epidemiologist, but our conclusion that the cancer cases didn't represent a cluster remained.[1] The audience, though very concerned, was not angry. We stayed until all questions were asked and people were leaving. Tests that were promised were subsequently completed.

The newspaper reported that questions about this school had arisen several years earlier when five longtime employees, four teachers and a retired nurse, were diagnosed with different types of cancer.[2] The school hired a contractor and began testing air, water, and soil. News reports told about the different types of cancer found: lung cancer in a longtime smoker, breast cancer, acute myelogenous leukemia, and others.[2]

At the time, the principal wrote a letter to parents that school officials would take steps to make sure the school was safe. Private companies were hired to perform sampling. The department of health had reviewed the information obtained. A nearby landfill was also investigated, as was air, soil, and drinking water. The principal updated the town select board about the history of the concerns and investigation, and the fact that tests found no link between the school environment and the illnesses,[3] but a sixth person diagnosed with cancer years later prompted a renewed level of concern and activity.[3] The health department, the Centers for Disease Control and Prevention, and the Agency for Toxic Substances Disease Registry, as well as the Vermont state Agency of Natural Resources Air Pollution Division, were all contacted by the school.[2] Several weeks later, a community group was organized to identify environmental factors related to the six cancer cases.[4] The group was called the Healthy School and Neighborhood Review Committee and it conducted an informal survey in the area of the school, which found that some nearby residents had been "diagnosed with cancers, tumors, and autoimmune illness."[4] A review of land history and use, geology, groundwater, the water supply system, oil storage tanks, chemical use, and asbestos had been conducted by a private company and a further review of land records was planned. The committee also planned to review state activities and recommendations to ensure things were done correctly, and served as a link to help the school board and school officials.[4]

The first meeting of this group occurred during a snowstorm[5] to discuss the response to date of the six cancer cases in four years at the elementary school, all among staff. Fourteen committee members divided into eight subcommittees to look at "water, air, soil, power, the school building, surveys and health testing, communications and grants, and consultant review."[5] Radon tests were planned and possible grant applications were discussed. News reports indicated that parents were concerned about their children's health and wanted a thorough evaluation of the school and news of a future health department team unannounced walk-though was discussed.[5]

I worked with our health department staff, listening to the history of the concerns and investigation and reviewing all that had been done. We decided, with permission, to verify definitively the reports of types of cancers and ages of persons involved. The environmental epidemiologist used available registry data to confirm reports and to look at cancer rates in the area, though the geographic area and numbers were small. After review of all the information collected to date, and review of literature, from national experts, we concluded that the cancer cases among the school staff were unrelated, and not a cluster. That was the conclusion that I presented at the public meeting.[1] The follow-up tests from the questions at the public meeting on water, soil, and air did not indicate potential health hazards, however the chair of the neighborhood committee still wanted continuous air testing. A letter sent from the assistant United States surgeon general to the school assured that the review of the environmental tests was not remarkable.[6] But still some members of the group wanted a more comprehensive report and the chair wanted to recruit an environmental engineer to review the data. Despite the call for further testing and analysis, the school was opened on time.[6]

Addressing the questions of cancer clusters is complex and not easy. Literature on this subject reinforces that, except in a handful of mostly occupational settings, many such investigations have had a low yield of meaningful results. Questions of cancer clusters often come from the public—a concerned citizen or a school official trying to answer questions from concerned parents. Many resources and guidelines are available to public health agencies,[7,8,9] however, despite many investigations, one review of more than 20 years of more than 100 cancer cluster investigations at the CDC showed no clear cause for associations found.[10] Some authorities recommend a four-step approach, but emphasize that agencies must be flexible.[9] In Vermont, we had developed information about monitoring cancer that was available to health professionals and the public.[11]

The immediate concern for some of these cancer cluster questions is that if there is more than a single person with cancer, even different types in older individuals, then there must be an environmental reason and an investigation should be launched. The latency of exposure to carcinogens and the subsequent development of cancer make this difficult to study. The assumption that cancer is all the same disease, the gaps in our scientific and epidemiologic knowledge, and the uncertainty around all of this, make it difficult to give negative answers in a public climate fraught with concern over serious diseases.

In reality, when we saw the data, there seemed to be little to suggest that this was out of the ordinary compared to what could be expected in a population of these ages—different types of cancer in adults, all in the age range where such cancers occurred. We would have been immediately concerned if there were several cancers of the same type, particularly a rare cancer, or if there were cancers that usually occurred in older people seen in the wrong age group. Although this was not the case here, federal agencies had been called, contractors hired, tests performed, and committees organized and the investigation had been ongoing, renewed when another diagnosis was made, making this difficult to manage and even more difficult to communicate.

We decided that the best approach was to meet the local school officials and concerned citizens where they were, accept the investigation as it was proceeding, and go visit. They had already made decisions to do testing, but it was all based on an assumption that there was a cancer cluster—and there was no talking them out of it. We had to work with the committee formed and do our best to give accurate information to concerned parents and citizens. It was essential to go visit—all of us, walk around, review information on paper and in person. Consultants were no substitute for public health officials at the school. The purpose of the visit was to look around the area, but more importantly, to try and speak face to face with the parents, teachers, and community residents who were concerned and had been so for a long time. I took key staff, the department experts, to discuss concerns and findings. Finally, after drawing our conclusions, we needed to spend time at a community meeting, where without a podium we could stand in front of the crowd to explain what we thought, why we thought it, and answer what questions we were asked. Was all the testing needed for scientific purposes? Probably not, but it was clear that, given where the community was in its thinking and concern, it was necessary. Any test that could have reasonably been linked to any cancer, including asbestos and radon, was already being tested for. After the test results were unremarkable and our findings were in, was everyone satisfied? No, not immediately, because a momentum of concern had developed that would take time to go away.

Much of what has been written as guidelines for the investigation of cancer clusters is helpful, but the most important thing that I learned is how important it is to be flexible in your approach. People are concerned, frankly scared, when there is a question of cancer where they live or where their children go to school. These concerns cannot be dismissed and must be dealt with directly, sometimes face to face, no matter how difficult it is to do, and despite the fact that you may not have a precise answer to every single question. Giving out specific information about what we do know about types and causes of cancer won't take away concerns, but can help give a perspective. This situation had gone on for several years, had newspaper and television coverage, and it is likely that not all concerns have been allayed. But the best way to deal with such situations is to size them up, get all the data you can, and be direct in your approach to communicate what you know and what you don't know. Stepping out from behind the podium, literally and figuratively, was important to our communicating with the community and best dealing with this situation.

REFERENCES

1. Renzi A. Cancer cases among school staff unrelated, health chief says. *Rutland Herald.* May 9, 2001. P. B1.
2. O'Connor K. School responds to new cancer case. *Rutland Herald.* February 13, 2001. Available at: http://www.rutlandherald.com. Accessed February 25, 2005.
3. Renzi A. More tests find no cancer connection at town school. *Rutland Herald.* February 27, 2001. Available at: http://www.rutlandherald.com. Accessed February 25, 2005.

4. Renzi A. Neighbors probing "cluster" of cancer. *Rutland Herald*. March 18, 2001. Available at: http://www.rutlandherald.com. Accessed February 25, 2005.
5. Renzi A. Group addresses cancer cases at town school. *Rutland Herald*. March 23, 2001. Available at: http://www.rutlandherald.com. Accessed February 25, 2005.
6. Curtis B. Rutland town school tests come back clean. *Rutland Herald*. August 22, 2001. Available at: http://www.rutlandherald.com. Accessed February 25, 2005.
7. Centers for Disease Control and Prevention, National Center for Environmental Health. Cancer Cluster Frequently Asked Questions. Available at: http://www.cdc.gov/nceh/clusters/faq.htm. Accessed February 25, 2005.
8. National Cancer Institute. Cancer clusters. Available at: http://www. cis.nci.nih.gov/fact/3_58.htm. Accessed February 25, 2005.
9. Guidelines for Investigating Clusters of Health Events. *MMWR*. 1990;39(RR-11):1–16.
10. Caldwell GG. Twenty-two years of cancer cluster investigations at the Centers for Disease Control. *Am J Epidemiology*, 1990;132:S43–S47.
11. Vermont Department of Health. Monitoring Cancer in Vermont. Burlington, Vt: Vermont Department of Health. Available at: http://www. healthyvermonters. info/hs/epi/cdepei/cancer/monitorcancer.shtml. Accessed on February 25, 2005.

CHAPTER 31

Timing Is Everything— Tattooing and Body Piercing

The hearing was, to describe it simply, colorful. In one of the larger hearing rooms in the Statehouse, the legislative committee sat behind great wooden tables, while a small parade of heavily tattooed individuals entered the room and testified to support the regulation of tattoo artists. One by one, they sat at the table, arms covered with a variety of colorful and artistic designs as the committee listened attentively and asked questions. At one point I gave testimony—not to promote tattoos, but to make them safer, as long as people were going to get them. The committee, following testimony and discussion, passed out the bill that would require registration of tattoo artists.

In Vermont, as tattoos gained popularity, in the mid-1990s, we were approached by tattoo artists who wanted to be allowed to perform their art in the state. We looked up the current law, which allowed tattoos to be performed only by medical doctors who specialized in them. I had never heard of this type of medical specialty, so the law effectively made tattooing illegal. In addition, there were potential public health concerns about use of unsterile needles or improper infection control measures, potential risks for blood-borne diseases such as hepatitis B or C, and potentially HIV infection.[1,2] We reviewed the scientific literature to see what had been reported about the risk of infections and found a few citations for outbreaks of hepatitis.[2] Bacterial infections and allergies to dyes used in the tattoo process were other potential health risks. So, we reasoned, if more people were now actually getting tattoos, and it was for all practical purposes not allowed under the law, then the potential risks from underground practices that had no government oversight or other protection required, could cause potential public health risks.

The potential risk warranted changing the law and I discussed this possibility with administration staff, who concurred. We talked about the option of the health department regulating this, but as most professional licensing and regulation was situated in the Office of Professional Regulation, in the Secretary of State's Office in Vermont, we decided it could be best done there, with standards and regulations connected in some way to public health. A bill was drafted with several sponsors and introduced into the House of Representatives, where it went to the House Committee on General, Housing and Military Affairs.[3]

I had never spent much time with this committee, and the only thing that I remembered was that its chair was not a strong supporter of our antismoking efforts. But, after an initial conversation, we sat down in the Statehouse cafeteria one morning and over coffee I explained the health concerns. He said that his committee would take up the bill, and they did.

Testimony was provided by the secretary of state's office, the tattoo artists themselves, and me. My emphasis was simply on potential health risks, and the public health rationale that we wanted to prevent potential problems rather than wait to see if such infections materialized, as more people were getting tattoos. I explained the difficulty in potentially linking reported diseases with tattooing, and also the more general public health principal that, given what we know, we should try to prevent problems before they occurred and that we had worked out a way between the Secretary of State's office and the Department of Health to try and do this. I told them that it was important to make tattooing legal and regulated; otherwise, we couldn't be sure it would be as safe as possible. The tattoo artists wanted to be able to legally run their shops. We all tried to answer the committee's questions. The Office of Professional Regulation would register tattoo artists and the Secretary of State would have advisor appointees to counsel them regarding the regulation on such matters. The director of the Office of Professional Regulation would adopt rules for infection control procedures and public health practices, after consultation with the health commissioner, to protect the public from infectious diseases. The Commissioner of Health also had the responsibility to recommend sanitary standards for the tattooing facilities. So the net effect was to provide a coordinated effort within those agencies to better protect the public.

The bill went to the House Ways and Means Committee regarding the fees involved and went on to pass the House and Senate, and was signed into law.[3] There were three hearings, little controversy, and no press attention. The process to take public health information and make it easy to use by tattooists was tedious, but there was little controversy or activity on the bill until sometime later, when body piercing became a question.

Several years later, the House of Representatives passed a bill that would prohibit people under 18 from getting body piercing or tattoos. The bill now included body piercing as a regulated profession in the state. In the previous law, minors had been able to get a tattoo with parental consent.[3,4]

The Office of Professional Regulation in the Secretary of State's Office, each year, sent a large bill to the Government Operations Committees and sometimes to the Health and Welfare Committees to update, amend, or add new regulation to its extensive responsibilities in this area. Since the original bill had passed, the increase in body piercing, and potential for similar risks as tattooing, including both blood-transmitted and bacterial infections, brought the issue again to the legislature.

Our epidemiology field chief testified for the health department about the public health aspects and potential risks associated with body piercing.[4] Despite the views of the Government Operations Committee, however, concerns arose from other representatives about the rights of minors. The bill was postponed and the issue was not resolved until the following year. During the winter, when the legislature resumed its activities, the Senate delayed acting on the large professional regulation bill because of the tattoo and body piercing issue, specifically the section regarding whether and under what circumstances minors could have their bodies pierced or tattooed. The Senate version of the bill that passed the House the previous session allowed minors to get pierced or a tattooed, only with parental permission. A conference committee was organized, including members of the House and senate to work out the differences, but then action was delayed.[5]

What was happening related to a controversial bill that would require parental notification for minors to obtain an abortion. That bill had passed the Republican-controlled House in late 2001, by a vote of 78 to 55,[6] and was sitting in the Health and Welfare Committee of the Democrat-controlled Senate. The questions that had caused delays resulted from the juxtaposition in timing of the bills in opposite chambers of the legislature, controlled by different parties and dealing with issues that were controversial. Perception of potential inconsistency in positions requiring parental consent for tattoos versus abortions caused a flurry of media reports, and the entire professional regulation bill stalled for the moment.[7]

A House–Senate conference committee for the tattoo and body piercing segment included the provision for parental notification, and the bill went to a second conference committee. A move to again restrict minors from having tattoos or body piercing stalled the bill again.[7,8] The usually innocuous bill that regulated a long list of professions through the Secretary of State's office was now stalled because of debate over the possible link between parental consent for tattoos and body piercing and parental consent for abortions. Some Senators vigorously opposed the suggestion of a link between the two, but the perceived controversy, called by one reporter "uncomfortable comparisons,"[9] had the effect of stalling the large professional regulation bill and the section needed, from a public health perspective, to regulate those performing body piercing as well as tattooists.

Our role, except for testimony by health department staff on the potential public health risks related to body piercing, was minimal, except that while the health department epidemiologist was testifying on the body piercing bill, I was busy working to help with a massive overhaul of how medical practice and physicians were regulated, a bill that had come about due to a public consensus that the Board of Medical Practice needed strengthening and tighter accountability by moving it to the Department of health, and changing its composition and standards of practice to better protect the public. This bill represented a huge change in how physicians were regulated, following much publicity around some tragic events that occurred to patients. I had spent much of the legislative session working extensively with legislative committees, the Board of Medical Practice, and the medical society to craft legislation that was tough but fair and would achieve the goal of better protecting the public. This bill became entangled in the entire professional regulation debate and controversy, and it was only in the middle of May, very late in the legislative session, that an agreement was finally reached on the body piercing bill and the medical regulation bill passed as well.

The Senate finally agreed to take up a House-passed bill that revamped how Vermont regulated doctors and moved accountability to the Department of Health. The House dropped the requirement that minors be required to get parental permission or be banned from getting a tattoo or their body pierced, the section discussing minors simply was deleted,[9] and the large professional regulation bill moved as well.

Although we were innocent bystanders, when the timing and controversy erupted, there was much at stake, and I saw firsthand what can happen when there is a controversy relating to bills under debate and discussion, particularly near the end of the legislative session, and the unintended consequences that can happen. In the end, tattoos and body piercing were both regulated by the Office of Professional Regulation in the Secretary of State's office, along with many other professions, and the Board of Medical Practice and its responsibilities moved to the Department of Health. Sometimes timing is everything, and despite your best efforts, controversies erupt and bills stall. But even in those moments, you just have to weather the unintended storms.

REFERENCES

1. Ko YC, Ho MS, Chiang TA, Chang SJ, Chang PY. et al. Tattoos as a risk of hepatitis C virus infection. *J Med Virol.* 1992;38:288–91.
2. Limentani AE, Elliott LM, Noah ND, Lamborn JK. An outbreak of hepatitis B from tattooing. *Lancet.* 1979;14:86–8.
3. Acts of the 1995–1996 Vermont legislature. Act 79. An Act relating to tattooists. H178. Available at http://www.leg.state.vt.us. Accessed April 3, 2005.
4. Schmaler T. House voted to bar teens from getting pierced, tattooed. *Rutland Herald.* May 23, 2001. Available at: http://www.rutlandherald.com. Accessed April 8, 2005.
5. Mace D. Tattoo provision stalls House bill regulating professions. *Rutland Herald.* January 10, 2002. Available at: http://www.rutlandherald.com. Accessed April 8, 2005.
6. Vermont Legislative Session 2001–2002. H218. Available at http://www.leg.state.vt.us. Accessed April 3, 2005.
7. Mace D. Body piercing legislation has parties divided. *Rutland Herald.* March 27, 2002. Available at: http://www.rutlandherald.com. Accessed April 8, 2005.
8. Sneyd R. Senate kills body piercing bill. *Rutland Herald.* April 3, 2002. Available at: http://www.rutlandherald.com. Accessed April 8, 2005.
9. Mace D. Agreement reached on body piercing bill. *Rutland Herald.* May 17, 2002. Available at: http://www.rutlandherald.com. Accessed April 8, 2005.

CHAPTER 32

Calling in Extra Help— Diarrhea on a Dairy Farm

A *US News and World Report* article in late November 1997 showed a picture of a sick calf lying down and the story contained a bold cover title: "Outbreak: Danger in the Food Supply." The article continued: "First, a calf on this Vermont farm got sick. Then the cows started dying. Then the people fell ill. Soon, federal scientists were hunting down a virulent new microbe."[1]

An outbreak of Salmonella Typhimurium DT 104 was reported in the spring on a dairy farm in a northern Vermont county, less than an hour from the Canadian border. Cattle on a dairy farm developed bloody diarrhea and several died.[1,2,3] A calf had become ill, and despite treatment by the owner and their Veterinarian, it had died the same evening.[1] More animals became ill with bloody diarrhea and despite treatment with the usual hydration and antibiotics had died. The local veterinarian sent samples to the Cornell University veterinary lab and later to the USDA lab in Ames, Iowa.[1]

Results of cultures showed Salmonella Typhimurium that was resistant to a list of antibiotics: ampicillin, chloramphenicol, streptomycin, sulfonamides, and tetracycline. The type was determined to be type 104 or DT104.[1,2] Less than a week later, a young child had also become ill, a week after the cattle developed diarrhea, and Salmonella Typhimurium was also identified.[1,3] More animals became ill, more family members developed diarrhea and one was hospitalized.[3] Both the Centers for Disease Control and Prevention (CDC) and the United States Department of Agriculture (USDA) were asked to help state agencies of health and agriculture with the investigation of the outbreak and to make recommendations to prevent further illness.[4]

At the time, Salmonella Typhimurium DT 104 had already been found in sheep, pigs, goats, cats, dogs, mice, and other domestic and wild animals.[1,2] The Vermont state epidemiologist's call to the CDC resulted in an investigator, known as an Epidemic Intelligence (EIS) Officer, being sent to Vermont. The CDC had a limited number of available investigators, but they were sent when there was something of potentially national significance, something that might help better understand an emerging infectious disease.[1]

The CDC visited the farm in late May.[1,3] At the same time, CDC was also investigating outbreaks of DT104 in California and Washington State[1] and the Vermont investigation was part of a national effort.[4] The farm agreed to work with both state and federal agencies throughout this time.

State and federal officials interviewed family members and gathered specimens to be analyzed for DT104.[1,3] Specimens were obtained from family members, animals (including family pets), and environmental samples from feeds, milk tanks, and drinking water to be tested for DT104. Nine people had diarrhea, and five of the ill individuals were confirmed with DT104.[1,3] On the farm, twenty-two of the nearly 150 cattle had become ill and thirteen died.[1] Three of the six dogs had cultures that were positive, but were not ill.[1] Samples from the milk tank filters tested positive for DT 104.[1,3]

The farm, despite the severe impact of this illness on both the animals and some family members, was very cooperative with the health and agriculture departments in Vermont, as well as the two Federal agencies. In addition to helping prevent similar illness among farm animals on that farm, on other Vermont farms, and among humans, it was important to better understand how such infections occur, to try and prevent similar situations in other locations throughout the United States. Although this drug-resistant form of Salmonella had been noted in the United Kingdom, there were limited reports of this in the U.S. to date, and limited experience and guidelines for prevention. The first reported outbreak in the U.S. was among school children in Nebraska, although a definite source had not been determined.[5]

When the data from the cultures, interviews, and other information was analyzed, it was found that drinking raw (unpasteurized) milk and caring for sick animals were risks for human illness in humans.[1,3,6] Animals who became ill were often young and being kept in the calving pen was a risk for animal illness.[6] Although the exact source of the infection could not be determined,[6] the investigators noted that this was the first DT104 outbreak in the U.S. where animal to human transmission was found.[3] Investigators had some hypotheses about how the bacteria got there, such as by birds or wildlife, or on footwear, but were not certain as to the precise reason and way the outbreak started.[6] However, based on the investigation, recommendations were made to avoid drinking raw (unpasteurized) milk, to wash hands after handling animals, and to avoid eating in the barn area,[1,3,6] and to continue to track S. Typhimiurium DT 104 closely through disease surveillance in both animals and humans.[2,3]

Awareness was also raised, through the news media, with further details given about the investigation and recommendations from the state agriculture commissioner to farmers.[7,8] A related editorial reinforced key recommendations and tried to put risks in perspective.[9] An article written in the health department Disease Control Bulletin, a well-read publication that was widely distributed to health professionals and hospitals summarized the outbreak and recommendations.[2]

At the time of this outbreak, there was little known about these outbreaks and ways to prevent them in the U.S., despite the fact that such disease in animals and humans had been reported in the U.K. years earlier. The CDC later reported that S. Typhimurium was the most commonly isolated Salmonella serotype in the U.S. in 1999, accounting for nearly a quarter of all Salmonella cases reported.[10] CDC further estimated that multidrug resistance was common, being seen in nearly 46%. Outbreaks investigated revealed association with eating and drinking unpasteurized dairy products[11,12] and contact with pets.[10] More recently multidrug-resistant Salmonella Typhimurium has been associated with rodents bought in pet stores.[13]

One of the great challenges in public health is to try to stay ahead of infectious diseases. A national focus from the CDC on emerging infectious diseases led to an increased awareness among public health professionals about many different categories of these infections. Similar work was done over many years in Vermont to bring such infections as campylobacteriosis, salmonelllosis, E.coli O157:H7, yersiniosis, and many others to the attention of health professionals and the public.[14] The first step in dealing with these infections was to raise awareness, such that efforts would shift to detecting them early, and ultimately trying to prevent them.

Although the working relationships with physicians, nurses, and hospitals were excellent and comfortable, the shift in the nature of these infections made relationships with other government agencies and individuals essential. A task force had been created to look at health and agriculture issues and a public health veterinarian, located in the health department, who started work in the health department in anticipation of the rabies animal epidemic, provided valuable expertise from a public health perspective. In this outbreak, communication from a local veterinarian to public health officials helped with the initial investigation of this situation. But health and agriculture issues always had implications and ramifications for the agriculture industry. Agriculture officials in Vermont had the responsibility to both promote and regulate the industry, a delicate balance, always with potential for conflict. In this case, they worked with us side-by-side, and the prompt work to identify the situation, link local veterinarians to public health, and the cooperation of the farm family, despite the potential for negative publicity were helpful in doing all that was possible in a short period of time to understand and control the outbreak.

Decisions to involve federal agencies, whether health or agriculture, were made immediately, because in this context, there were implications beyond Vermont, and knowledge obtained could be potentially beneficial to others in Vermont, and other states. However, such involvement of federal agencies may also come with a price. The outbreak was the cover story for an issue of *U.S. News and World Report.* Although Vermont was aggressive in investigating this new virulent form of Salmonella at a time when little was understood throughout the county, there was the potential to provide a false negative impression of Vermont agriculture, analogous to avoidance of restaurants when an outbreak hits the news. Is this a reason to be less aggressive? Of course not, but calling in the CDC was a very big deal and calling in two Federal agencies, to work with two state agencies almost never happened. Decisions to do so are made both quickly and carefully. The CDC's expertise was needed here and the cooperation of the farm in a national farm study of this illness could help other farmers prevent this same situation.

The rapid investigation and control of infectious diseases is one of the core responsibilities of public health, but it has become more complicated with emerging infectious diseases, sometimes seen in new and different settings. These investigations sometime require partnerships with agencies not usually seen as public health entities. National experts remind us of the emergence, reemergence, and persistence of microbial threats to public health[15] and task forces struggle with efforts to not just respond, but to be proactive in comprehensive approaches for these complex issues.[16] No state wants to be famous for cattle with drug-resistant organisms, any more than a restaurant wants to be known for having had a disease outbreak occur from eating there. But despite the fact that the story in U.S. News was really highlighting the difficulty with preventing food-borne illness, it was also an example of a very cooperative farm and public health doing its job, wherever it was happening, when the stakes were high, the disease serious and not well understood, all in an effort to try and prevent illness from happening again.

REFERENCES

1. Spake A. O is for Outbreak. *US News and World Report* November 24, 1997; 70-84.
2. Salmonella Typhimurium DT 104. Vermont Department of Health. Disease Control Bulletin. September 1998. Available at http://www.healthyvermonters. info/dcb/091998.shtml Accessed March, 29, 2005.
3. Friedman CR, Brady RC, Celotti MJ, Schoenfeld SE, Johnson RH, Galbraith PD, Carney JK, Robbins K, Slutsker L. An outbreak of multidrug-resistant Salmonella serotype Typhimurium definitive type 104 (DT104) infections in humans and cattle in Vermont. In: Program and abstracts of the International Conference on Emerging Infectious Diseases; March 8-11, 1998; Atlanta, Ga.
4. Vermont Department of Health. May 28, 1997, News Alert.
5. CDC. Multidrug-Resistant Salmonella Serotype Typhimurium–United States, 1996. MMWR 1997; 46:308-310.
6. United States Animal Health Association 1997 Committee Report of the Committee on Food Safety. Available at http://www.usaha.org/reports/ food97.html. Accessed July 29, 2004.
7. Hemingway S. State seeks federal salmonella study. Fairfax outbreak is still a puzzle. *The Burlington Free Press.* November 20, 1997; 1A.
8. Hemingway S. Salmonella spurs state to urge farm precautions. *The Burlington Free Press.* November 21, 1997; 1A.
9. Keeping food safe.Editorial. *The Burlington Free Press.* November 24, 1997; 6A.
10. CDC. Outbreaks of Multidrug-Resistant Salmonella Typhimurium Associated with Veterinary Facilities: Idaho, Minnesota, and Washington, 1999. MMWR, 2001 (50): 701-704.
11. Billar, RG, Macek MD, Simons, S, et al. Investigation of Multidrug-Resistant Salmonella Serotype Typhimurium DT 104 Infections Linked to Raw-Milk Cheese in Washington State. JAMA 1999. 281: 1811-1816.
12. Fey, PD, Safranek TJ, Rupp M et al. Ceftriaxone-resistant salmonella infection acquired by a child from cattle. NEJM 2000; 342: 1242-1249.
13. CDC. Outbreak of Multidrug-Resistant Salmonella Typhimurium Associated with Rodents Purchased from Retail Pet Stores–United States. MMWR 2005; 54(17): 429-433.
14. Foodborne Disease Surveillance. Vermont Department of Health. Disease Control Bulletin. December 2001. Available at http://www.healthvermonters. info/dcb/122001/shtml. Accessed November 28, 2005.
15. Institute of Medicine. Microbial Threats to Health. Emergence, Detection, and Response. 2003. National Academies Press, Washington DC. Pp1-18.
16. Institute of Medicine. The Emergence of Zoonotic Diseases. Understanding the Impact on Animal and Human Health. Workshop Summary. 2002. The National Academies Press, Washington, DC.

33

Restoring Public Confidence— Strengthening the Board of Medical Practice

Late in 2001, a reporter from the *Burlington Free Press* wrote a series of articles[1] that told horrifying stories about medical errors by Vermont physicians licensed by the Board of Medical practice, and the lack of information about physicians available to the public. These high-profile medical misadventures and their reporting helped create a public momentum for change in how physicians were regulated in Vermont. I was totally immersed in these changes and saw first hand the skills and talents of legislators from many political backgrounds working together to strengthen this important board and improve the public's health.

In Vermont, hospitals were licensed by the Department of Health, and emergency workers were licensed or certified by the same department, but the majority of professionals, including health professionals such as nurses, dentists, and cosmetologists and many others were regulated through the Office of Professional Regulation under the Secretary of State, an elected official. The regulation of physicians had been a special circumstance; they were regulated by the Board of Medical Practice that was administratively attached to the Secretary of State's office, but was really quite independent. This arrangement had to be renewed every two years during the legislative session, but provided a level of autonomy and independence for physician regulation that was unlike other professions.

There had been some attempts to change this, but it remained until late 2001, when a wave of news articles raised questions about the board and the availability of information to the public, with even many professionals agreeing that more information was available in choosing a plumber or a car.[1] During January 2002, it was clear that there could be a change. Newspaper accounts of the board's actions, or lack of action, had created public unrest to the degree that this would become an issue for the legislature.

The Vermont Medical Society approached the governor with the notion that this board might perform better under the direct oversight of the Department of Health. That would place the ultimate responsibility with an appointee, the health commissioner, and make the governor ultimately responsible for public protection in this area. The idea caught on and a bill was introduced. It was clear in January that this was now a priority for my work during the session. I worked with the current board members, who supported this change, their executive director, the medical society, and many others to quickly understand all the issues from the past, how other states disciplined doctors and made information available to the public, and all the nuances and issues in the current law.

The legislative committee that took up this task was the Government Operations Committee in the House. This committee had responsibilities to deal with what its name said—government operations—and looked at department restructuring, programs, and any proposals that impacted the workings of government. It wasn't usually a high-profile committee but had many seasoned legislators on the committee. What was also notable was the geographic and political spectrum the committee covered—rural to urban and conservative to progressive—a recipe that had the potential to make consensus challenging. I had spent time previously with this committee and respected the chairman and committee members for many reasons: their ability to dissect and understand the complex relationships of one part to another part of government, the serious way in which they approached their responsibility, and the demeanor of the committee as it did its work.

I had the opportunity to testify on this bill, H755, many times, and tried to talk about key areas of the law that might need modifying as they changed the form and oversight of the medical board. There was testimony from patients and consumers, current members of the board, physicians, the Secretary of State's office, and others. Because the highly publicized cases involving doctors had been so public, there was more often than not a reporter in the room and the entire course of the legislation was accompanied by many newspaper articles.[1-7]

During my initial testimony I outlined several changes that the bill would accomplish, and why they were desirable: changing the responsibility for oversight of the board to the department of health, where it would become the health commissioner's ultimate responsibility; adding three more public members, necessary to ensure more public input into a process that was still largely comprised of professionals; changing the standard of care to which physicians could be held, which became the most controversial of all the provisions; and making a database of demographic, educational, and previous disciplinary events available to the public.[2,3]

Members of the board were behind the changes and agreeable to becoming part of the Department of Health. Despite the fact that resources would be stretched, the new database had to be accomplished within current resources—adding a requirement for additional funding would have added another hurdle, the appropriations committee. The medical society did not agree with the proposed change in the standard of unprofessional conduct. However, the language in the current law had required care must be a "gross" or "repeated failure" to meet standards of practice[3] for the board to be able to take action, meaning that you had to wait until a physician did something pretty bad or made multiple mistakes for the board to be able to take any disciplinary action. I thought that the board needed better tools to be able to do its job and a public health approach would be to change the standard to allow the board to act when there was a failure to meet the standard that was less severe. That would let it intervene at an earlier time, before a serious mishap had occurred, a patient was harmed, or multiple mistakes had been made. Physicians feared additional malpractice suits.[4]

I watched as the House committee worked together, and passed this complex bill out of committee. This one provision, changing the standard of care to a much simpler level, enabling the board to act on a single failure of a physician, was controversial—some lawmakers felt we would become a haven for malpractice suits, some physicians and the medical society felt the bill had gone too far the other direction in response to all the controversy. This standard ended up being taken up by the House Judiciary Committee, a committee largely composed of attorneys who felt they were more expert in these matters than the House Government Operations Committee had been, a committee that more nearly reflected the composition of our citizen legislature. The full house gave preliminary approval on a vote 136–1,[4] but it was clear that this matter wasn't finished yet.

The Judiciary Committee heard testimony on the issue and decided to submit its version of the standard of care for a vote during the full House debate of the final bill. I sat in the gallery on the day of the House floor debate, in one of two rows of seats in the back of the House chamber. Sometimes I was there for moral support to the committee; sometimes a note or two could be passed during the heat of the arguments. The floor debate on this provision of the bill, despite the fact that the rest of the bill was agreed upon, was intense. The House Judiciary Committee members made their arguments about why their provision was superior to the House Government Operations one: doctors would not leave the state and malpractice cases would not increase. Never flinching, the House Government Operations Committee members, one at a time, Republicans, Democrats, and Progressives, rose to be recognized by the House speaker and spoke to the issue, passionately and in plain English. They needed no legal training to articulate their rationale to the entire House of Representatives that their standard would be best for the public, and would not be used to needlessly punish doctors. One of the individuals and families of the highly publicized cases was also sitting near me in the gallery, watching the debate. During the floor battle the amendment of the House Judiciary Committee was defeated by a vote of 81–56,[5] and the bill moved to the Senate. A newspaper editorial called the committee members "Doctors of Lawmaking."[6] Although time was running short before the end of the session, we were optimistic that the Senate would pass the bill and it would reach the governor's desk this year.

The momentum carried though to the Senate, but once again the provision related to the definition of unprofessional conduct, or the standard of care to which physicians were held, was controversial. It became clear that some modification of the bill might have to occur for it to successfully sail through the Senate. It was ultimately decided to adopt a more stringent standard than was previously held, but more like the one currently used by the Board of Nursing, a board that had high credibility in Vermont. Bills that are passed with different language in the Senate than the House must have a conference committee, with representatives from both sides, to reconcile which changes will remain in the bill that goes to the governor's desk. The standard was reconciled,[7] all other provisions remained and the bill was signed by the governor to become law in July of that year.[8] There was agreement that the bill would do a better job protecting the public, restore the credibility of the Board of Medical Practice, and make more information available to consumers than in the past.[9]

I saw something with my intense involvement in the bill's development and passage that I had not seen in quite this way before. Although there were definite times when I was on the opposite side of my professional peers, because of my responsibility as health commissioner, we still got the job done, with no loss of respect between us. The Medical Board members agreed to make changes as well, making the task workable. They had been under fire, but took a high-road approach to the issue, because of their dedication to their work. I felt that the bill would give them better tools to do their job, and they had the support of a larger department, the Department of Health, that could provide resources and advice, as well as accountability.

I also felt a deep respect for the members of the House Government Operations Committee. Politics were never a part of their discussion, as they took testimony, weighed options, sought council from experts and people they trusted, and came up with a bill that was the right remedy for the current situation. Then, when it would have been far easier and expeditious to modify parts of the bill to get it through faster, they had the courage of their conviction and argued successfully against a committee of individuals more formally trained and versed in the nuances of the law. I was proud to watch what they did that year, and even prouder to have been part of it. It was how a law should be passed and within a few short months there was an increase in accessibility of the board,[10,11] and the information available to the public. Vermont has always prided itself on high-quality health care and the quality of the medical professionals here. Now public confidence was restored, and if there was a physician who was not meeting the standard of care of his or her profession, there was confidence it would be addressed.

REFERENCES

1. Kiernan S. Code of silence: medical records cloaked in secrecy. *Burlington Free Press.* December 9, 2001. P. 1A.
2. Zolper T. Proposal expands disclosure of doctors' history. Vermonters might gain wider access through Internet. *Burlington Free Press.* February 27, 2002. P. 1A.
3. Zolper T. Bill would open doctors' histories to public. Proposal expends board's disciplinary leeway. *Burlington Free Press.* February 28, 2002. P. 1B.
4. Zolper T. House likes doctors' rules. Bill strengthens medical board. *Burlington Free Press.* April 17, 2002. P. 1A.
5. Zolper T. House agrees to strengthen doctor rules. *Burlington Free Press.* April 17, 2002. P. 1A.
6. Editorial. Doctors of lawmaking. *Burlington Free Press.* April 18, 2002. P. 12A.
7. Mace D. Bill allows for early disciplining of doctors. *Rutland Herald.* May 26, 2002. Available at: http://www.rutlandherald.com. Accessed February 9, 2005.

8. Summary of the 2002 Acts and Resolves. The Vermont Legislature. Act No. 132 (H755). Oversight and Management of the Board of Medical Practice.
9. Associated Press. New law on covering physicians gives public access to information. *Rutland Herald.* July 2, 2002. Available at: http://www. rutlandherald.com. Accessed February 9, 2005.
10. Associated Press. Complaints about doctors are up. *Rutland Herald.* December 31, 2002. Available at: http://www.rutlandherald.com. Accessed February 9, 2005.
11. Kiernan S. Board picks up inquiry pace as complaints against doctors increase. *Burlington Free Press.* December 30, 2002. P. 1A.

PART III

Strategies

CHAPTER 34

Let the Data Speak for Itself

We held a press conference to release our first health status report of Vermonters. Although I frequently spoke to reporters from print, television, and radio, our holding a press conference was not a routine occurrence. But neither was the report, and we knew that we should try to share it widely. The *Health Status of Vermonters* defined the health status of Vermont communities, showed priorities for action to prevent illness, and set measurable goals based on national benchmarks for progress.[1] It was a call to action for Vermont communities. Earlier, in *Healthy Vermonters 2000,*[2] we had published measurable goals and objectives for the year 2000 based on the national *Healthy People 2000.* This document defined priority areas, goals, and measurable objectives for the entire state. But the *Health Status of Vermonters* report took it a step further. And it was not easy getting there.

For years, public health nurses had told me about the differences in health in their areas of the state. In Vermont, we had no autonomous county or local health departments, but handled public health for the state with 12 district offices that housed key local public health programs and provided the ability to respond quickly in case of a public health emergency. The directors of all the districts and I met on a regular basis. These meetings gave me a sense of the extent of various problems throughout the entire state, such as smoking in pregnant women. The nurses and directors would also relate the unique problems they were facing. They knew, and I knew from listening to them for so long, that Vermont had tremendous differences in public health from north to south and east to west. Newport was not like Rutland, and Brattleboro was not like Bennington. Although we "knew" this from our stories and discussions, we had never documented it; so we decided to try. After all, when people hear about national public health problems, or problems at the state level, the problems are still very distant, easy to postpone or ignore. But if we were able to show how health issues were similar or different in our communities, perhaps we could spark interest and curiosity about why this was so, but more importantly, bring health outcomes, both good and bad, much closer to home. If you learned that too many babies in your community were dying or being born at too low a birth weight, and there were scientifically based ways to improve this, wouldn't you want something to be done, and maybe even help? If health problems and priorities for action were documented it might be a way to start community discussions, even controversy, and focus attention on health. If we wanted to know where we were going, we had to first know where we were. There was already a growing interest in community health: maternal and child health coalitions had formed in most areas of the state, and many hospitals had begun to show interest in not only providing health care but improving the health of the communities they served as well.

To create such a report, we had to gather staff from different places in the health department where different pieces of the data resided. We used statisticians, epidemiologists, nurses, and public education experts to define the health of the population, look at the data, size up the differences, and present all this information in a way that would not only get people's attention, but get them to work on the issues. My letter to introduce the report stated that the document went well beyond the purview of medical care by suggesting what could be done by individual citizens, communities, health care providers, and government agencies to focus on prevention and improve our collective health.[1]

We looked at measures of health status: death rates, illness rates, and infectious diseases. We looked at rates of habits and behaviors such as smoking, diet, and physical activity. We examined the distribution of primary care providers, and we looked at demographics such as age, income and education. We looked at more than 20 health status indicators and made comparisons to our 2000 goals, not to state averages. For example, there was little variation in the death rate from diabetes throughout the state when compared to the state average, but when compared to the year 2000 goal, all but one county was worse or significantly worse. Because most of the diabetes was the type associated with being overweight, there was something that could be done about it, both in terms of prevention and treatment. This fact would have remained hidden if we had only noted that rates of death from diabetes were similar all over Vermont.

The areas we chose for the report were the priority areas of *Healthy Vermonters 2000:* heart disease, cancer, environmental health, infectious diseases, injuries, nutrition, physical activity, and access to preventive care, such as the rates for screening for breast cancer and immunizations for children and adults. We looked at differences in heart disease death rates, smoking rates, low birth weights, suicide, diabetes, and breast cancer. AIDS was reported in every Vermont county, but rates of campylobacter infection varied from north to south. Automobile accidents occurred more frequently in some counties than others. Although we could have predicted that there would be differences, we could not have predicted the results.

The next day, after our press conference, the front-page headline of the state's largest newspaper read "Health Study Reveals Contrasts, Illness Rates Vary Widely from County to County." The paper ran a huge story, complete with maps of key health indicators such as heart disease, lung cancer, smoking, obesity, pneumonia, influenza, diabetes, automobile accidents, AIDS, and the percentage of low birth weight babies.[3] The paper also ran an editorial titled "Lives in the Balance" and recommended the report be used by individual citizens, legislators, and health care providers, and be widely distributed to hospitals, doctors' offices, and schools. They noted that our report showed the connection between poverty and poor health. They used the word "unflinchingly" to describe how the information was presented. It was also recommended that it be "mailed to homes, libraries and towns because it reveals how Vermonters can extend their lives by changing their behavior."[4]

We had now changed the perception that the health of Vermont was similar across the state. It was something we knew, but now the data showed it in a powerful way. I was invited to speak to local community groups about health priorities for their areas and practical steps they could take. Public health nurses used the information to help reduce smoking in pregnant women in a county with the highest percentage of low birth weight babies. We couldn't explain why all the differences occurred, but we could give advice on how to improve rates of immunization in older Vermonters and reduce deaths from cervical cancer and AIDS.

Why did this report get so much attention and how did it help public health? National and state health problems are too distant—they are someone else's problem. When the health of your own county or community is so clearly described, it is hard to ignore because it is close to home—right in your backyard. If health is much worse than expected in a certain region, it gets attention and often creates interest in public health issues. Our emphasis was on prevention. We defined a public health issue as any health condition that was common, serious, and potentially preventable. In every county there was at least one health condition that was more prevalent than the our stated goal. With organized community effort, something could be done. This was the clearest way that we knew to generate interest and momentum for public health. The health of our state was different in different communities, and each community had priorities, some similar, and some very different, but all had areas needing improvement. The data confirmed what we knew, and the report presented it in a credible and powerful way. People didn't just have to take our word for it; they could see it for themselves.

Let your data speak for itself. It is a powerful way to focus public attention on health. Data is absolutely essential to define the health of the population. Use universal measures and those unique to your state or local community. We used measurable goals and objectives in updated reports and goals for the year 2010.[5,6]

A former boss used to say that using community health profiles was like a community looking at itself in the mirror, a powerful motivator for action.

Problems are hard to ignore if they are right in front of your face, and they are easier to solve if additional information is provided, guiding individuals, hospitals, health providers, schools, and government agencies to action. Defining the health of the public in measurable terms with goals and objectives, in a format that is clear and understandable, is an essential step in improving the public's health. Not only can you see where you are, where you've been, and where you need to go, you can help focus public attention, community interest, and momentum towards health. The public health nurses were right; we just needed to show their truth.

REFERENCES

1. Vermont Department of Health. *The Health Status of Vermonters—Selected Health Status Indicators, 1988–1993.* Burlington, Vt: Vermont Department of Health; 1995.

2. Vermont Department of Health. *Healthy Vermonters 2000*. Burlington, Vt: Vermont Department of Health; 1992.
3. Health study reveals contrasts. Illness rates vary widely from county to county. *Burlington Free Press*. April 7, 1995:1.
4. Lives in the balance [Editorial] *Burlington Free Press*. April 7, 1995; 6A.
5. Vermont Department of Health. *Health Status Report '02*. Burlington, Vt: Vermont Department of Health; 2002. Available at http://www.healthyvermonters. info/admin/pubs/healthstatus02/health2002.pdf. Accessed March 2005.
6. Vermont Department of Health. *Healthy Vermonters 2010*. Burlington, Vt: Vermont Department of Health; 2000.

CHAPTER 35

The Devil Team

I frequently gave introductory remarks at conferences. No one in the audience wanted an hour-long speech to open the meeting, but I saw each of these invitations as an opportunity to highlight a public health issue—heart disease in women, diabetes, or reducing smoking in children. Each conference was an opportunity to speak about a health priority. To be effective, several points had to be made or emphasized in a brief introductory statement no more than 10 minutes long. I always knew what I wanted to talk about, what aspect of health needed a few extra words of emphasis, and I usually took time to write a first draft for the speech, focusing on the data and concepts that I wanted to highlight. I knew the issues and the facts. In our office were two individuals who reviewed my writing, wrote press releases, developed relationships with the media, and brought clear communication into every public health issue.

My speeches came back marked up in red: "What do you mean when you say this?" "This is too boring." "You said 'enormous' *again*." And although the process was sometimes painful (to me), the final written product was much better and clearer, and in the end, I was better able to take advantage of all those brief opportunities to frame and emphasize public health.

One of the governors I worked for talked about his "devil team," a small group of people who critiqued (or shred) any big idea before it went any further. He told us about his staff that did this work for him, staff whose role it was to play the devil's advocate. Sometimes it was regular staff; sometimes the group was assembled ad hoc. They asked a lot of questions: "Won't people ask how much it will cost?" "Are you doing something new because the old way doesn't work?" "Why are you doing this now?"

When I heard him describe this process, I thought the idea made sense. After all, how many times have you read about an idea or program that was started before it was ready, before it was clearly thought through, before all the consequences, short term and long term, intended and unintended, had been considered? We had several individuals in the department who reviewed every written work, speech, major initiative, publication, brochure, and idea before it went any further. Sometimes a few key staff and public information experts would sit around the table in my office and we tried to find the hidden or not-so-hidden flaws in our ideas. At first, it was important to find the right people to invite to the meeting. Sometimes a larger group was useful to talk about a new program or idea. Different people were invited, depending on the issue.

I often used the word "enormous" to describe anything large, oversized, or problematic. They called me on it every time. They shredded my speeches and some of my ideas. They were not afraid to tell their boss an idea needed work or was unclear. They gave me headaches. The goal never was to be "politically correct," water down the idea, or make raspberry into vanilla, but to make sure each concept, whether it was an idea, a speech, or a final written report, achieved its purpose and got the job done. When I spoke at a ceremony for the AIDS quilt in Vermont, besides the facts and statistics, I needed the right words, the right tone, and the right way to say what I wanted to say. But my ideas went far beyond introductory remarks and speeches; they extended to new programs, initiatives, and putting the vision for public health into practice.

Some people who run organizations have a practice of hiring "yes" people—who love their ideas, no matter how terrible they are, in the misguided attempt to follow the "company line." This can be a big mistake, because it is exactly these individuals who you cannot ever invite to your meeting to discuss a new, bold idea, or really even trust. Your most trusted staff must be able to tell you when you are wrong or need to give an idea a little more work or to just recycle it.

There were probably less than a dozen people in the health department whom I invited to help develop a new idea. Sometimes they were my immediate staff, public relations staff, or experts in their content area. They all shared the same qualities of honesty. They showed their expertise by pointing out the flaws in any proposal. Sometimes they were my worst nightmare in the office. I was always in a hurry, and they slowed me down, made me think some more, made me rewrite something, and say it or explain it better. They helped me, by asking questions for clarification. They made me sharpen my focus and made the final product better. They asked me to explain my new program idea, as if I were talking to the public. They were invaluable. Not only did I avoid trouble that would have been my own doing from lack of clarity, but my work was far better as a result.

If you want to take on big, complicated public health issues and set ambitious but achievable goals and accomplish them, the last thing you need is people who always tell you that your work is great. Seek out those people who are not afraid to critique your work and invite them in to discuss your ideas. They will help you focus your ideas into plans, your plans into actions, and your words into opportunities for public health.

36

The 10-Minute Rule

Margaret A. Moran, MEd

Congratulations! You have just accepted a position as a county health director. You come to this position with a wealth of public health expertise. You may even be an individual with considerable expertise and credentials in public administration. If that is the case, you have a leg up on a number of your colleagues who have climbed the public health career ladder and have finally landed their first senior leadership position. You feel confident in your abilities. Your biggest challenge probably won't be administering the core public health functions and essential services carried out by your county health department. After all you have worked hard throughout your career to build your competency in public health science as well as honing your analytic, policy development, and health planning skills. Your biggest challenge no doubt will be in developing a strong and mutually rewarding relationship with your boss—or in this case your boss*es*, the county board of commissioners.

Much has been written in recent years about "managing your boss" or "managing up." The *Harvard Business Review* devoted an entire issue to "Managing Yourself" with a chapter devoted to "Managing Your Boss."[1] In this article John Gabarro and John Kotter reflect back on their original work on this subject, first published 25 years ago. Generally, articles about managing up depict a relationship between one boss and his or her subordinate as told from the vantage point of the subordinate. The articles are full of tips on how to successfully cultivate and maintain a good working relationship with one's boss in order to obtain the best results for you, your boss, and your organization. Proponents of managing the boss–subordinate relationship argue that managing up is not the same as "kissing up;" rather, it is about strategically striving for mutual understanding and cooperation between two individuals—two individuals who often have divergent perspectives.

Teri Fisher, President and CEO of a management and consulting firm in California, defines managing up as "strategically working with the style and goals of another, blending them with your styles and goals to achieve results and accomplish your career objectives."[2] Despite the plethora of articles on managing one's boss, I have encountered very few articles that discuss the interpersonal dynamics when the boss is a board, let alone a board that is made up entirely of elected officials. I do believe that you can still learn from the tips and strategies derived from these articles, as long as you keep in mind that the execution might be very different.

There are three general rules that are consistent themes in much of the literature on managing your boss.

1. Know your boss.
2. Know yourself.
3. Know your organization.

The focus of this chapter is on the first rule—*know* your boss, understanding who they are and what they want.

When you report to a board of commissioners or a county council, not only is it to your advantage to understand each board member as an individual, it is particularly important to understand the board as a whole. A board of county commissioners can be made up of three, five, seven, or more individuals elected to a defined term of office, generally two to four years. Board members often represent a specific geographic district but are elected at large. As the governing body of the county, the board of commissioners performs legislative, budgetary, and policy-making functions and advocates for citizens at all levels of government. Equally important, the board of county commissioners is charged with establishing the vision for county government as well as defining the level and type of services provided by county government.

Each individual commissioner campaigned on specific issues—land use planning, increasing government accountability, parks and recreation, or a law-and-justice platform. Some may even have championed public health! During their election campaign, he or she probably distinguished themselves from their opponents by emphasizing their professional accomplishments, their civic contributions, and the changes they would like to bring about if elected. They might have also differentiated themselves by upstaging their opponents, making commitments to specific constituencies about increasing services or lowering fees, and if involved in a contentious race, might have played hardball with their competition. Confrontation and controversy might have played well for them on the campaign trail, but once they assume their new seat at the commissioner's table they find themselves in an entirely different environment, an environment that requires a different set of skills, knowledge, and understanding. They are suddenly not the only one on the team. Furthermore, given the electorate's propensity to seek representation from different spectrums of the community, their fellow commissioners are probably from very different backgrounds and experiences. Divergent backgrounds plus different values plus varying agendas can all add up to competing priorities and the potential for ongoing conflict.

Some elected officials have little understanding and little training in the day-to-day processes they must work through to get things done—open meeting laws, public hearings, agenda setting, and dealing with reporters. Yet the minute they are sworn in, they are expected to quickly become knowledgeable about a wide range of issues, interact with a broad spectrum of people, learn about the new role that they have assumed and figure out how to move their individual agendas forward.

Unlike some private company board of directors, elected boards do not have one single unifying goal such as turning a profit. Elected boards are made up of individuals with individual agendas who have to answer to the people who elected them while at the same time conduct the government's business. While it is to your advantage as a county health director to appreciate, know, and understand the unique perspectives and agendas of each board member, your job requires that you take direction from the board as a whole. The balancing act for you is to be attentive to the individual needs of each board member, but to dance to the tune of the full board.

How does one go about dancing to the tune of the full board? One example is what I call "the 10-minute rule." As a county health director I reported to a 3-member board of commissioners. One newly elected board member, a very gregarious commissioner, had been a former county employee in the planning department. His campaign promise was to shape up county government and make it more accountable to the citizens of the county. Prior to being elected to the board of county commissioners he had had significant differences of opinion with the county administrator, the director of the planning department, as well as one sitting board member, which ultimately lead to his decision to run for office. As a former employee of the county, this commissioner had enjoyed an excellent working relationship with several of my deputy administrators (which proved to be a mixed blessing).

When I arrived on the scene as the new health administrator I soon discovered that this commissioner was very much involved in the day-to-day operations of the health department and had forged a close working relationship with the interim health administrator—my deputy administrator for community health. It wasn't long before I observed that the commissioner was routinely found hanging out in my deputy administrator's offices chatting about events and activities that I initially felt were of little import. It soon became apparent that he was making specific requests and demands of my staff that I believed went well beyond simple requests for information. My three deputy administrators, not wanting to alienate a board member—particularly one who was so supportive of our department—were loathe to decline; however they did acknowledge to me that these requests often meant that their own work was often compromised as a result.

I knew that I had to step in and do something. If I were to be responsible for the day-to-day operations of the county health department, then I needed to address the problem by establishing some rules (and tactics if necessary). I needed the board to understand that the only way I could be responsible and held accountable for my department and my staff was for me to provide the direction and support to department staff through the organization's chain of command. I further needed to help the board understand that I took my direction from the board as a whole and that if I were to receive direction from an individual board member I would need to bring the matter before the full board for their consent before taking action. I also needed to place some restrictions on this gregarious commissioner's access to department staff in a way that was respectful of his high need for information, his preestablished collegial relationship with several of my deputies, and his strong interest in learning about public health. While attempting to address his needs I also needed to be sensitive to my staff's desire to be helpful, protective of their respective workloads, and in line with my desire to be held accountable for the administration of my department.

I decided to have a frank conversation with the full board to discuss ways that I felt would meet their needs for information (know thy boss/board), contribute to my overall effectiveness (know thyself), and that would move the county towards achievement of its strategic plan and more specifically our public health goals (know thy organization).

My conversation with the full board was by all rights successful. I acknowledged their need for information and indicated that I understood that in many cases the appropriate provider of that information were staff most knowledgeable in the particular subject matter. I also expressed my understanding that in some cases the timeliness of receipt of said information was best met by going directly to the source. I also explained that for me to be most effective in my role as their health administrator I had a high need to know what was going on in my department, not that I necessarily needed to be involved in all of the details but that I wanted to be informed. I further explained that the department's agenda, derived from the county's strategic plan, was incredibly ambitious and that were we to be successful in achieving our goals, I would need the focus and attention of my key staff and any significant departures from that work plan needed to include me and be vetted through the full board. By this time had a better understanding of the new commissioner. I knew he had the best interests of my department and the organization at heart. I also knew that he did not have the best working relationship with one of his fellow commissioners and that I needed to remain vigilant and not get caught up in a situation that put me at odds with either commissioner which I had observed happening to several of my fellow department heads. I also knew that a light and humorous touch would probably go a lot further than a heavy-handed mandate to cease and desist, remembering that you catch more flies with honey than you do with vinegar.

To that end I proposed (and the board accepted) the "10-minute rule," which simply established the differences between asking for information and directing the work of staff. The rule stipulated that any request that resulted in staff expending *less than 10 minutes* to comply with constituted a request for information. Any request that resulted in staff expending *more than 10 minutes* to respond constituted directing the work of said staff.

I would like to say that each board member operated in full compliance of the 10-minute rule, but to do so would be reconstructing my history. After implementing the 10-minute rule, I continued to find my talkative commissioner lurking in the halls of the health department and attempting to direct staff activities. However he no longer strolled through the front doors, right past my office door, but instead began entering from the back doors of the building and would appear quite sheepish when I encountered him in staff offices and hallways, which simply suggested to me that he was more than aware that I knew and he knew that he was in violation of the 10-minute rule.

Over time his behavior did change. I'd like to think it was because his trust and confidence in my abilities grew and my deputy administrators became more adept at redirecting his overtures or that he simply needed to direct his attentions elsewhere in county government. Then again it could have been a result of my having locked the back doors thereby resulting in him having to walk past my open office door and risk getting caught in the act. I may never know. The moral of my story? Know your boss, know yourself, know your organization, and always have a back up plan.

REFERENCES

1. Garbarro J and J Kotter. Managing your boss. *Harvard Business Review* [Special issue]. January 2005.
2. Fisher, TR. Reach your career goals by managing your boss. Career Journal.com: The Wall Street Journal Executive Career Site. Available at http://www.career-journal.com/myc/climbing/20020424-fisher.html. Accessed July 2005.

CHAPTER 37

When People Are Angry with You or Your Department, Invite Them In

In the 1990s, access to early prenatal care was well below our goals, and late entry into prenatal care had increased. This alarming trend was also seen nationally, and recommendations were aimed toward getting pregnant women into early prenatal care. We needed to identify and address the medical, behavioral, and social forces that put babies at risk for being born at low birth weight, something that carried an increased risk for a premature death in the first year of life. To improve birth outcomes, we needed to identify medical conditions, such as diabetes or high blood pressure, in future mothers, limit risks such as smoking or alcohol abuse, as well as address social factors such as whether there was transportation to get to doctor visits. Although the situation in Vermont fit with the national picture, at the time, ours was further compounded by a shortage of physicians practicing obstetrics in rural areas of the state. And although this crisis in access to health care predated the debate about ensuring universal access to health care through improved health insurance, it raised many of the same issues and barriers that women and young families faced. There were barriers to getting early care, such as lack of insurance, long confusing administrative forms, not enough doctors, and not enough simple and clear educational material to help women with their own health care. We had many problems to solve and no shortage of ideas about what should be done and how we should go about it.

Some advocacy groups and individuals felt strongly that we should construct an entire state-funded system of prenatal care, set up clinics around the state, and use state funds to ensure staffing and appointments for women who needed them. My view, and that of the administration, was that we should try to repair those particular parts of our current system that were broken and build on our current core structure of hospitals, doctors, and nurses. We also believed we should work to remove administrative barriers as well as increase educational efforts, and provide financial means, through health care coverage, to deliver these services. This would cost money, but achieve the same goals—without creating a second health care system just for prenatal care.

No one disagreed that we needed to do something to address this problem as soon as possible, but the advocacy for different approaches was intense, vocal, and public.[1] After a particular period of public debate and increasing unrest, I invited the advocates that were arguing for a new system for prenatal care into my office and listened to their point of view. This was not easy to do.

Powerful, vocal advocates, citizens, policy makers, and others were critical of the department and the overall approach to this public health crisis. It was not easy to face these people in a conference room, sitting across the table from people who had been criticizing the department's efforts publicly, but it was necessary.

Although we did not agree as to how the problem should best be remedied, we were able to constructively discuss the issues and problems. It became clear that despite our disagreement on the solutions, we were all intensely focused on fixing the problems and shared a strong commitment to improving access to prenatal care for the health of mothers and children.[2,3] The road to cooperation was initially bumpy. The legislature had appropriated funds for community grants but would release them only when an acceptable plan was developed by the health department. They released part of the funds,[4] and several months later, grant proposals were requested and grants awarded to communities all over the state for both immediate and long-term efforts to improve access to comprehensive maternity care.[4,5] A hospital-based prenatal care clinic opened in the central part of the state, an area plagued by a shortage of obstetricians.[3] In the same year, the Vermont Department of Banking and Insurance required companies providing health insurance to include coverage for maternity care.[5]

This issue became the focus of a concerted multiyear effort that ultimately included expanding insurance for pregnant women, babies, and young children; financial incentives for health care professionals; grants to communities to enhance local approaches; shortening and simplifying long enrollment forms; and a media campaign.[3] The campaign was designed to educate Vermont women about the importance of early comprehensive prenatal care. It would link them through a phone number in the ads to a public health nurse who would help them receive the care they needed by finding a doctor, enrolling them in insurance and nutrition programs, and being a trusted ally for their health.[3,5] Radio and television advertising, posters, and ads on milk cartons and pharmacy shelves resulted in a flurry of calls to the toll-free number.[5,6] Public health nurses also worked diligently to help women find transportation to care.[3]

Cumulatively, this public health approach, targeting specific barriers that kept women from getting early prenatal care, led to an increase in access to prenatal care and improvements in birth outcomes, particularly among high-risk populations.[5] By 1998, 87% of Vermont women received prenatal care beginning in the first three months of pregnancy.[7] To ultimately improve health outcomes, the health department had to be more flexible in its approach and work to build bridges in areas of disagreement by reaching out to advocates, legislators, hospitals, physicians, and nurses.

It is essential to communicate with partners in public health efforts, the legislature, other government departments, and especially with those who disagree with you. The scope of public health is so broad that there will always be issues that need attention, and there will always be more than one way to solve a problem, deal with an issue, or achieve a public health goal. Advocates, health professionals, policy makers, and individual citizens all have opinions as to what you should do and how you should do it. If you either fail to take action or you chart a different course, there will be individuals and groups that may be upset and angry, and sometimes they will take this argument to the news media or a public forum such as the legislature. When this happens, invite them in.

At the moment when you most want to ignore your ringing phone (because it will be another reporter), hide under your desk, or go on vacation, talk directly to those who disagree with you or who are angry with your department. There is nothing more difficult than asking individuals or groups that are unhappy with you or your leadership to come in for a chat. But you must do it. Sit with them, and listen to what they have to say. Schedule plenty of time for the meeting. You not only will better understand their point of view, but you will also learn why the issue at hand is important to them. Resist the urge to argue for your own approach. After the meeting is over, give yourself a night's sleep to decide whether or not to rethink your strategy and approach to the problem, or whether you should modify your course, even in the slightest way. Being flexible is not the same as compromising your goals.

Sometimes you may decide that your approach is still sound and keep going. More often than not, you may figure out that you really didn't think of absolutely everything, and make minor or major changes to your plans. Some people think this is caving in to public pressure and that you should never try to make all the people happy all of the time. Indeed it is difficult and time con-suming to reach out to interested groups and individual citizens on every single issue, yet despite your best intentions and efforts, you can never think of every-thing if you do so alone.

Long-term relationships are not formed overnight. Initial disagreements may not determine the strength of future relationships you will have with groups and organizations that you work with to successfully address large and complex public health issues. Effective public health efforts initially start from having an open mind and being willing to listen when people disagree with you and your approach. (If you find that you are having such meetings very often, however, you are probably missing something fundamental.) In the case of improving access to prenatal care and birth outcomes, the first step to the development of sound programs and substantial progress was to put issues on the table and try to discuss them. When people are angry with your depart-ment, invite them in. It may be the first small step toward progress.

REFERENCES

1. Dillon J. Health Department Excludes Council From Planning of Prenatal Care. *Rutland Herald.* June 18, 1989; 5A.
2. Hall J. Prenatal Care Proposal is in the Works. *Rutland Herald.* September 2, 1989; 11.
3. Allen S. State plans campaign to help pregnant women. *Brattleboro Reformer.* September 15, 1989; 1.
4. Hall J. Money gets released for prenatal care. *Rutland Herald.* September 26, 1989; 12.
5. Carney JK, Berry P, Thompson E, Brozicevic MM. Improving access to prenatal care in Vermont. *Am J Public Health* 1996; 86(6):880–881.
6. The Associated Press. Prenatal advertising campaign helps Vermont young moth-ers. *Burlington Free Press.* April 21, 1990; 4B.
7. Vermont Department of Health. *Healthy Vermonters 2010.* Burlington, Vt: Vermont Department of Health; 2000.

38

Preventing Childhood Lead Poisoning—Using a Public Health Approach

We met in the basement of the Health Department around a table in the conference room to discuss a report. The Centers for Disease Control and Prevention (CDC) had released its landmark report *Preventing Childhood Lead Poisoning*[1] that spelled out what we knew, what progress had been made, and what public health steps we must now take. Lead poisoning could occur at levels previously thought to be safe. Rates increased most rapidly before children were a year old, and peaked before they were 2 years. The new definition of lead poisoning, based on the scientific studies presented, was now set at 10 micrograms per deciliter, rather than 25 micrograms per deciliter. Our health worry for young children was the effect of lead on the still developing brain and nervous systems: it resulted in increased risks of learning and behavioral problems.[1,2] At such low levels, there were no symptoms; education and screening were now needed strategies.[1,2] One CDC recommendation was to phase in universal screening using a blood lead measurement. In addition, more emphasis would be needed in the areas of primary prevention by reducing exposure to sources of lead that contributed to lead poisoning, a much more difficult task.

For perspective, the CDC talked about the tremendous improvements in lead poisoning that had occurred in the previous 20 years; however, lead-based paint remained a potential source of lead exposure for children, and although the Consumer Product Safety Commission had banned the addition of lead to new residential paint in 1978, houses built prior to then, particularly those built prior to 1960 were likely to contain lead-based paint.[1] Children were the highest priority, especially those aged 6 years and under, and at the national level, the CDC, The Department of Housing and Urban Development (HUD), and the Environmental Protection Agency (EPA) had all released plans to further reduce and eliminate lead hazards.

The CDC report was long, detailed, and represented a substantial change from past documents. We reviewed the report and discussed potential ramifications for Vermont. It was clear that primary prevention, public education, and screening would become our emphasis. We would need a wide array of people to help us. Environmental health issues were complex to explain, and there was significant skepticism, particularly on the part of legislators around similar issues, such as the federal requirements for managing asbestos in schools.[3]

We invited representatives of various parts of public health in Vermont to the basement conference room to discuss approaches and policy. These representatives included the local public health division that covered the entire state, the environmental health program, the epidemiologists and laboratory scientists, as well as pediatricians, concerned consumers, environmental groups, and others.

We were concerned that physicians might not initially be supportive because of the potential workload increase that screening children for lead poisoning might cause. My staff and I attended one meeting of the Vermont chapter of the American Academy of Pediatrics, where we were met not with hostility, but with a great deal of skepticism and questions about the science, the CDC report, and why this could be problem in Vermont. Because there had been little lead poisoning seen at a level of 25 μg/dl, and because there was a perception that this was a "big city" problem, what we learned from the pediatricians' comments and questions guided us in what we needed to do.

There were isolated stories of individual lead-poisoned children. One physician in New Hampshire refused to let a Vermont child be discharged from the hospital after treating the child for severe poisoning. Isolated reports increased as public awareness rose with the information provided at the federal and state levels. But we really didn't know the true prevalence of lead poisoning in Vermont children at the new level. Although we knew that this was likely a problem for us, as our housing stock was old, we needed to find out exactly how big, to help us better target our efforts. A group from the health department–public health nurses, chemists, epidemiologists, statisticians, and I–designed and implemented a lead prevalence study.[4] The percentage of all Vermont children with lead levels of 10 μg/dl or more was 9%; it was almost 15% in the children enrolled in the state's Medicaid program, a proxy for families with limited income. Almost 2% of Vermont children had a level greater than 20μg/dl. The percentage of children with elevated lead levels in the state's most populous county was less than the percentages seen in the rural parts of the state.[4]

What we found was contrary to commonly held perceptions about the extent and potential risks for lead poisoning in Vermont children. This information served as the foundation for our efforts to inform the public in a specific way and to help educate physicians and other health professionals as we worked to focus attention on this issue. Communicating around this issue was not simple; we needed to educate professionals and the public, but not cause alarm. We had to figure out how to begin to phase in and promote screening, but we were already seeing controversy around how best to accomplish this, through a voluntary approach or through mandating screening, something that had been done nearby in Massachusetts.

We held a conference in the statehouse, and there was a huge turnout. Controversy raged over the approaches recommended by prominent national and local environmental groups. The governor prioritized addressing this problem and called for legislative action.[5]

It was clear that preventing lead poisoning was potentially very complicated and would take some time. It was also clear that our usual partners, the hospitals, doctors, and nurses, were needed to help us. But we also needed to develop new and strong relationships with many other groups and organizations—and fast. In Vermont, the greatest source of lead poisoning was our old housing stock. The myth that this was an urban problem had been shattered by our prevalence study, as had the notion that this was not a problem for our rural areas. It became quickly apparent that we needed to take this problem to the legislature, as we needed new authority for public health in this area.

One of the immediate problems was the testing itself. Physicians, now that we had some scientific evidence, became some of our strongest champions. But our efforts to expand health insurance for kids, and incorporate needed primary care and preventive services into the work of pediatricians, family physicians, and nurse practitioners around the state proved impractical. We had eliminated well-child clinics provided by the health department because health insurance for children was expanded. But our ideal strategy to incorporate lead screening into physician offices was still too cumbersome. The capillary testing method could produce false positive results, because the skin could easily be contaminated with small amounts of dust and careful and time-consuming skin cleaning was required to eliminate this factor. This was not very practical to do in a brief visit to a busy physician's office. Physicians had to sometimes send young children to the hospital lab, which even if it was in the same building, may or may not have a skilled person available to test a very young child. It was easy to imagine a parent with young children visiting a doctor's office being asked to go somewhere else for the blood test—they just might not go. We were concerned that this might not be an optimal arrangement to have kids screened.

The director of the division of community public health, the division that provided local public health throughout the state, convinced me that this really was a job for public health, at least right now. We received a federal grant, and public health nurses began offering free lead-screening clinics for children. These clinics were publicized, held all over the state, and parents and children were met with the trusted face of a Vermont public health nurse. This was a major step in getting children screened.

The Health Department published lead-screening guidelines with recommendations for universal screening of all 1-year olds and older children based on risk factors in the environment.[6] These recommendations were updated in subsequent years.[2] It was estimated that about half of all children tested were being tested at the Health Department's free screening clinics. Interventions varied, based on the test results: if a child's blood level range was 10–14 µg/dl, parents received written information about reducing potential exposure to lead; at a slightly higher level of 15–19 µg/dl, parents received educational materials and were offered a home visit by health department workers or trained volunteers to help parents with practical advice about ways to reduce lead exposure in the home, reinforce the importance of good nutrition, and reiterate the need for follow-up testing. At levels over 20 µg/dl, parents were offered education and a complete environmental assessment of their home that included paint, dust, soil, and water sampling.[6] Much of the health department emphasis was on educating the public through its Web site, through fact sheets, and through a campaign designed to reach a diverse audience that included health professionals, well-educated parents, and parents with limited ability to read. Materials were developed with the philosophy that materials that were easy to read and understand would help raise public awareness, prompt requests for more detailed information, and help to get children screened as recommended.[7] A toll-free hotline was established to make it easier for the public to ask the health department any questions related to lead and lead poisoning.

We worked with the legislature, with strong support from the administration, in the passage of Act 94, the "Act Relating to Childhood Lead Poisoning Screening and Lead Hazard Abatement."[8] Our work on this bill provided much opportunity for education and discussion of childhood lead poisoning and its ramifications as the bill traveled through the health and welfare, finance, natural resource and ways and means committees on its way to passage and the governor's signature. The bill gave new authority to the health department as well as laid the policy framework that would guide the direction of public health and other agencies, groups, and organizations involved. Testimony was heard from public health experts, the state department of housing, pediatricians and the medical society, the housing and conservation board, the historic preservation representative, the housing finance agency, national and local environmental groups, the Vermont health care authority (who were determining possible plans to assure health care access), the state department that licensed child care centers, along with parents, landlords, homebuilders, subcontractors, visiting nurses, and others.

One area we were particularly concerned about was the possibility that as public awareness was raised about the importance of this as a health issue, well-meaning homeowners or contractors might inadvertently poison children through improper handling of lead-based paint. The Federal Residential Lead-Based Paint Hazard Reduction Act in 1992 allowed states to develop training, certification, and licensing programs for contractors working with lead-based paint.[8] The CDC report emphasized the need for experts to properly manage these potential health hazards.[1]

There were potential tensions ahead particularly between ways to manage health risks from lead and still address needs for affordable housing. Many of the national and Vermont findings and statistics were written into the text of Act 94. One strategy used by some legislators in developing legislation is to outline legislative findings, the background that provided statistics, data, and background on an issue, so that the reader can follow the logic of why a bill does what it does. It is helpful to other legislators when the bill comes up on the floor for a vote; the background of the problem is right there. From a public health perspective, the background information demonstrates that the committee not only understands, but supports the issue, and sends a message of its importance. Legislators and governors are elected every two years in Vermont, but many complex issues take much longer to solve; such background can be helpful for future years. The findings of the bill laid out the health issue: lead poisoning was widespread in American children; it listed and described the health impact of low levels of lead poisoning; and approximately 124,000 Vermont homes likely contained significant amounts of lead-based paint, with an estimate that between 84% and 88% of housing in two large areas of the state were built prior to 1978.[8] At this point, more than 300 cases of lead poisoning had already been reported to the health department, with some severely poisoned children seen in rural parts of the state.[8] There were also two unique aspects of managing this health problem in Vermont— the number of structures listed or eligible for classification as historic places, and the need for affordable housing. From the start, the potential tensions between health and affordable housing were recognized and anticipated: the bill stated that Vermont should develop "reasonable procedures for preventing lead poisoning and should determine the implications of lead-hazard reduction for the health of children, the affordability, safety and quality of housing, and owners' and lenders' liability."[8]

After much testimony from others in public health and health care and myself, an entire section of the bill was devoted to public education, and the legislative process was helpful in spelling out through the law what specific steps were needed to accomplish this goal. Media efforts and clearly written materials would be developed and distributed to health care sites, government programs, child care and preschools, realtors, subcontractors, and apartment owners.

The bill also directed that beginning a year later, all health care providers who provided primary medical care would be required to ensure parents of young children receive counseling regarding the "availability and advisability" of lead screening, according to the state's guidelines.[8] This was an area of disagreement between environmental groups and health professionals and public health. National and local environmental groups wanted lead screening to be mandatory, that doctors and other health providers would be required to make sure it happened. This was done in some other states, and they felt it was the strongest message about screening. Our view was that it was potentially a false sense of security, when you say you've required it— well, there you've done it. But to really achieve universal screening, it was important for public health to work closely with health professionals, to develop the educational materials needed, provide public education, and conduct lab testing and free clinics if needed. To get children screened, you needed to raise awareness that such screening was important, provide access to health care, and remove barriers to children receiving these services. So, our thinking went, if you had to figure out all the steps to get kids screened, and health professionals were committed to work with you, why would you need a mandate? We didn't feel that we did, and I spent much time talking with representatives, in the hallways and cafeteria, to promote a collaborative, rather than a regulatory, approach with our health care partners, who were already working closely with us. In the final version of the bill, we succeeded in getting the language that we preferred, but not without a threat for a mandate if two years had passed without substantial progress. The bill laid out provisions for steps to follow in the event a child was severely poisoned, and there was also a provision for the study of housing and liability issues, complex questions raised by housing agencies, landlords, and attorneys, and insurance companies.[8]

The Lead Paint Hazard Commission was also created to study and report on issues related to preventing lead poisoning and safe, affordable housing, including liability issues for both owners and lenders.[8] The commission included representatives from health and housing, historic preservation, housing finance agency representatives, the state housing authority, and the housing and conservation board. There were members appointed by the governor, including health professionals, a parent of a lead-poisoned child, an environmental or consumer organization, a contractor, an owner of target housing, and a lender. The committee met, extended its time because of the complexity of the issue and made recommendations for the next phase of our efforts.

Such factors as costs, impact on affordable housing, and related issues could not yet be precisely determined, and this thoughtful approach would help us develop "reasonable procedures" as the law directed us, not to remove all lead and not to make children homeless, in the process of reducing exposure to lead. The two priorities, health and housing, were related, and the commission gave us some additional time to develop a Vermont solution to a complex issue.   ·

The Lead Paint Hazard Commission held many meetings and struggled with the complex and delicate balance between liability and consumer rights, available housing and risks of lead poisoning, and the perspectives of parents, landlords, insurance companies, housing agencies, and environmental groups. It was a fascinating process, and as a member and vice-chair, I was educated on issues well beyond my usual purview. Testimony was taken and the complex interplay of health, housing, liability, insurance, legal, and other issues made the creations of practical and timely approaches challenging. A report was given to the legislature, and another bill was crafted. Act 165 was passed by the legislature and signed into law by the governor in 1996.[9] It was the end of two year's work by the commission and the testimony and debate of health advocates, environmental groups, insurance companies and regulators, realtors, bankers, environmental consulting companies, tenants, landlords, parents, and others.

The idea of the commission and ultimate bill was based on the premise that the goal was to develop a low cost, "do-it-yourself" prevention-oriented approach to allow property owners to reduce health risks related to lead paint.[9] Of the severely lead-poisoned children in Vermont, most lived in housing units with potential lead-based paint hazards, nearly 90% in rental housing. Vermont had received a HUD grant for $3 million to rehabilitate close to 500 housing units to pass dust clearance tests.[9] It confirmed what we already believed: lead-based paint, related to the age of our housing was a determinant of lead poisoning in severely poisoned Vermont children.

The law included the commission's recommended "Essential Maintenance Practices." These practises were designed to: protect children from lead poisoning. They also protected property owners by giving increased liability protections to property owners in compliance by allowing easier access to insurance, and by allowing owners to comply through preventive maintenance, saving money by forgoing more costly abatement. The law targeted older rental housing and child care facilities, specifically those built before 1978, and allowed exemptions for transient residences, motels, and others.[9]

Essential maintenance practices included such things as checking the conditions of painted surfaces, looking for and identifying areas where paint is in poor condition, periodically performing special cleaning, putting in window-well liners to prevent lead dust from being spread during the opening and closing of windows, and being careful during renovations.[10] It required owners of rental properties and child care facilities built before 1978 to inspect the condition of paint and perform essential maintenance, sign an affidavit that it had been done, provide tenants with an educational brochure about lead poisoning, post notices that ask people to report damaged paint, and make sure anyone performing the essential maintenance practices has completed a training program. Although the health department had extensive enforcement authority related to all potential public health risks and hazards, it was emphasized that the approach would work to educate and ensure that people complied with the law voluntarily.[10]

The Vermont Health and Housing departments had worked together to prevent childhood lead poisoning, and the Vermont Housing and Conservation Board had financial assistance programs. From 1996–2000, more than 8000 people had completed training in performing the Essential Maintenance Practices.[11] The health department continued its focus on public and health provider education, free screening, and implementing the aspects of the law that related to public health. Lead screening increased from 27% of 1-year-old children tested in 1994 to nearly 70% in the year 2000, and at the same time the number of lead-poisoned children decreased from about 11.7% in 1995 to 6.3% in 2000.[11,12]

Although it was difficult to evaluate the specific contributions, collectively it was clear that such a comprehensive and multidisciplinary, or public health approach, using public and provider education, efforts to prevent lead hazards in older housing, screening in public health clinics and health care offices, and a true and sustained partnership with both the health care and housing community, was essential to these results. The bottom line was that more kids were getting screened and fewer poisoned. Was the job over? Of course not, as older housing continues to age, efforts must continue, and lead screening must remain an essential part of preventive health care for all children. In addition, screening rates in Vermont were much higher in 1-year-old children than in 2-year-olds,[13] and given the age at which blood lead levels peak,[1] additional emphasis on screening at both ages is needed. But the overall approach, involving a broad group of people and focusing on practical approaches to addressing a complex, serious, but potentially preventable public health problem, was a success for Vermont children.

The Institute of Medicine cites the essential need to develop partnerships to address public health issues in the 21st century[14] and defines an ecological approach to health as being "Multiple strategies are developed to impact determinants of health relevant to the desired health outcomes."[15] We called this, in practice, a public health approach; it was an approach that relied not only on the many day-to-day relationships needed to impact public health problems and their roots, but on developing new partnerships when needed, as well. The CDC changed the landscape about lead poisoning, and required a prompt, but comprehensive, response to successfully deal with this issue. Physicians responded in force when shown the severity of the problem in Vermont. Sustained partnerships between health and housing, as well as health providers, parents, advocacy groups, child care providers, lawmakers, and many others, contributed to raising public awareness, designing and implementing programs, and sustaining our efforts. The legislature embraced the severity of the issue and responded with new laws, some controversial, as both health and housing advocates tried to get at the most serious source of potential lead exposure in Vermont.

Each public health issue is different, as is each public health response, complicated because of size, complexity, and the many contributing factors that need to be remedied in order to see positive results. But what all public health issues have in common, and require, is a thoughtful approach to determine all the necessary partners and getting them around the table, (in our case a basement conference table), to discuss what we needed to find out, where we needed to go, and how we might get there–all together.

REFERENCES

1. Centers for Disease Control and Prevention. Preventing lead poisoning in young children. Atlanta, Ga: US Department of Health and Human Services; 1991. Available at http://www.cdc.gov/nceh/lead/lead.htm. Accessed March 21, 2005.
2. Vermont Department of Health. Lead [Resource Guide for Parents]. Burlington, Vt: Vermont Department of Health. Available at http://www.healthyvermonters. info/hp/lead/leadparents.shtml. Accessed March 17, 2005.
3. Holtzman B. Debate swirls around asbestos issue. *Rutland Herald.* May 6, 1990; 1E.
4. Paulozzi LJ, Shapp J, Drawbaugh RE, Carney JK. Prevalence of lead poisoning among two-year-old children in Vermont. *Pediatrics* 1995;96: 78–81.
5. Allen S. Experts warn of lead danger. Governor calls for legislative action. *Burlington Free Press.* December 18, 1992; 1B.
6. Vermont Department of Health. Lead Poisoning Prevention in Vermont [Vermont Department of Health Disease Control Bulletin]. Burlington, Vt: Vermont Department of Health; January 1999. Available at http://www.healthyvermonters.info/dcb/011999.shtml. Accessed February 27, 2005.
7. Dorey LF, Erickson N, Garbarino, Carney JK. Could lead be poisoning your child? Abstract presented at American Public Health Association meeting. Washington, D.C; October 1994.
8. Acts of the 1993–94 Vermont legislature. Act No. 94. An Act Relating to Childhood Lead Poisoning Screening and Lead Hazard Abatement. Montpelier, Vt; 1994. Available at http://www.leg.state.vt.us. Accessed March 17, 2005.
9. Acts of the 1995–1996 Vermont Legislature. Act No. 165. An Act to Prevent Childhood Lead Poisoning in Older Rental Housing and Child Care Facilities. Montepelier, Vt; 1996. Available at http://www.leg.state.vt.us. Accessed March 17, 2005.
10. Vermont Department of Health and the Vermont Department of Housing and Community Affairs. Preventing childhood lead poisoning in rental properties and child care facilities. [Fact sheet]. Burlington, Vt; 2004. Available at http://www.healthyvermonters.info/hp/lead/act165fact.pdf. Accessed March 21, 2005.
11. Vermont Department of Health. Lead poisoning in Vermont [Disease Control Bulletin]. Burlington, Vt: Vermont Department of Health; May 2001. Available at http://www.healthyvermonters.info/dcb/052001.shtml. Accessed March 21, 2005.

12. Vermont Department of Health. *Health Status Report '02.* Burlington, Vt: Vermont Department of Health; 2002:17. Available at http://www.healthyvermonters.info/admin/pubs/healthstatus02/health2002.pdf. Accessed March 21, 2005.
13. Vermont Department of Health. Childhood lead poisoning prevention program [Disease Control Bulletin]. Burlington, Vt: Vermont Department of Health; May 2004. Available at http://www.healthyvermonters.info/dcb/052004.shtml. Accessed July 19, 2005.
14. Institute of Medicine. *The Future of Public's Health in the 21st Century.* Washington, DC: National Academies Press; 2003:4.
15. Institute of Medicine. *Who Will Keep the Public Healthy?* Washington, DC: The National Academies Press; 2003:7.

Sometimes the Toughest Battles Are on the Inside: Assessing and Managing Environmental Risks

The problem might never have been discovered if soil contamination was not found when a new school was being built on a site that the Windsor School District bought in 1976. The site had been previously owned by the State of Vermont and had housed a prison and wood-treatment operation. Part of the purchased land had also been turned into athletic fields.[1] Just a year later, the Vermont Agency of Natural Resources, Vermont's environmental agency, found dioxin on the site, including the football field. As of 1999, about $4 million dollars had been spent in cleaning the site. Costs included engineering costs, testing for contaminants, and removal of contaminated solids. The school district had spent nearly $1 million.[2]

The state of Vermont operated a state prison in the town of Windsor, Vermont, until 1971.[3] The land was owned by the state of Vermont at that time. Between 1954 and 1958 the Vermont Department of Corrections (DOC) had a wood-treatment facility it operated on the property. The wood treatment performed by the state prisoners during that time included the use of kerosene and pentachlorophenol, and it was believed that contaminants from this facility made their way into the soil and groundwater.[1] Part of the state-owned land, including the part where the wood treatment was performed, was sold to the Windsor School District in 1976.[3]

In 1995, the school district began to initiate action, requesting the Vermont Department of Corrections to share in testing and any needed remediation costs. The school district also requested the Vermont environmental agency to intervene. The Agency of Natural Resources, through letters from the commissioner of the Vermont Department of Environmental Conservation to the commissioner of the Vermont Department of Corrections, told the Department of Corrections to investigate the site to determine how much contamination was present, determine the risk to the public, and investigate needed actions to remedy the contamination problem. Excavation of the most severely contaminated soils was also required, and the DOC hired private companies to do this.[3]

The legislature had given the authority for the management and enforcement of hazardous waste laws to the Secretary of the Agency of Natural Resources, under which fell the Department of Environmental Conservation, the department overseeing this work.[3,4] Testing from monitoring wells showed the presence of pentachlorophenol (PCP), kerosene, and dioxin, and a letter written by the Waste Management Division of the Vermont Agency of Natural Resources in May 1997 described this as "significant long-term human health risk at the site due to the release of contaminants from the past wood-treatment operation," and that "Long-term contamination of groundwater is expected to persist at levels above drinking water standards for possibly thousands of years."[3] Further, according to court documents arguing appeal for responsibility to the Vermont Supreme Court, in July 1997, the Agency of Natural Resources concluded that "Contamination present at this site presents a threat to public health and the environment and that it is necessary to take immediate remedial action to minimize the risk."[3] Such actions included both excavating highly contaminated soils and covering other contaminated areas.[3]

PCP or pentachlorophenol[5] is a manufactured chemical and biocide or pesticide. It was widely used as a biocide in the 1970s, but is no longer found in wood-preserving solutions or insecticides and herbicides available for home use. It is used as a wood preservative for railroad ties, fence posts, and power line poles. One health concern for human exposures to technical grade PCP is because it may contain such toxic impurities as polychlorinated dibenzo-p-dioxins (CDDs) and dibenzofurans.[5] According to the Agency for Toxic Substances and Disease Registry (ATSDR), there is "weak evidence that PCP causes cancer in humans."[5] The International Agency for Research on Cancer (IARC) has classified PCP as possibly carcinogenic to humans, and the Environmental Protection Agency (EPA) has classified it as a probably human carcinogen, but it is felt that some of these adverse effects may be due to the impurities present in the PCP.[5]

One group of the possible contaminants of PCP are chlorinated dibenzo-p-dioxins (CDD), which are a family of 75 compounds called polychlorinated dioxins.[6] The CDD with four chlorine atoms at positions 2,3,7,8, on the dioxin molecule is called 2,3,7,8-TCDD (tetrachlorodibenzo-p-dioxin). This is one of the most toxic of the CDDs, and CCDs that have similar toxic characteristics to 2,3,7,8-TCDD are called *dioxin-like* compounds. Scientists and toxicologists using results from animal studies relate the toxicity of dioxin-like compounds as a fraction of 2,3,7,8-TCDD, called a Toxic Equivalent Factor (TEF). The pentachlorophenol (PCP) used to preserve wood contains some of the more highly chlorinated CDDs.[6] Studies of workers exposed to very high levels of 2,3,7,8-TCDD suggest an increased risk of cancer.[6] The Environmental Protection Agency (EPA) has classified 2,3,7,8,-TCDD as a possible human carcinogen alone and a probable human carcinogen in combination with other compounds. In addition, noncancer effects, such as reproductive damage and birth defects in animals, are associated with exposure to 2,3,7,8-TCDD.[6]

In Vermont, responsibiliy for the environmental risk management is located in the Agency of Natural Resources (ANR), specifically in the Department of Environmental Conservation. The environmental risk assessment office is located in the Department of Health, part of another agency, the Agency of Human Services. Although statutory authority and ultimate responsibility for risk management rested with the state environmental agency and the health department role was advisory, it was essential for the health department toxicologist and risk assessor to have a close working relationship with the environmental agency such that there would be cooperation in the most complex and difficult situations. Understandably, these situations were difficult, complicated, and sometimes costly.

The health department became involved in the public health risk assessment of this situation after contamination was found as the new school was being built. The presence of PCP from the wood treatment in the 1950s made the risk assessor and toxicologist want to also look for dioxins, possible contaminants of pentachlorophenol used as an herbicide or insecticide in this process. Both compounds were of great public health concern, with potential for harm in the short term and long term, particularly cancer risks. In contrast to a pure regulatory approach, the public health approach meant understanding what real and practical exposures were happening. Some experts equate risk assessment to "assessment" and risk management to "policy development" and "assurance" in a public health framework.[7] Contaminants present in fields where children played or in water that people drank were of great concern. The history of people's use of the area was also important: was this a community where people moved in and out frequently, or did people often live there for generations, factors that might be important to determine the real extent of exposure and subsequent health risks.

This particular situation was further complicated by the fact that not one, but three state departments were involved. Our department's health findings would impact what the department of corrections (another department in the same larger agency as the health department) would have to do, likely under recommendation or order from the environmental agency, who had the authority and responsibility to enforce the hazardous waste laws passed by the legislature. The health department staff visited the site and worked with officials in other departments and consultants that they hired.

Tensions simmered then brewed after contamination was initially found and discussion began around the level of cleanup. The health department used standard conservative practices or assumptions that protected the most vulnerable populations, such as children. Taking into account various potential sources of exposure and the appropriate duration of exposures, the health department customarily used a level not to exceed an excess lifetime cancer risk of one in a million. This would be protective of health and seemed appropriate based on what they learned from meetings, conversations, and visits. In contrast, individuals from the corrections department wanted cleanup to a less protective level, which would require less remediation and considerably less costs. There were disagreements in meetings between the different departments. While staff made appearances at public meetings, I was busy ensuring that the administration understood the impact of exposure to such contaminants in this setting, despite the fact that two different departments in the same agency had differing opinions, and that three different state entities were all involved. Ultimately, cleanup efforts proceeded in a way protective of health, and the environmental agency took responsibility to ensure subsequent remediation was properly done.[8] However, because of the complexity, and ongoing discovery of further contamination,[9-14] discussions and legal actions continued for a number of years over costs and who would be responsible.[1,2,3]

Environmental risk assessments are complicated and often difficult to manage and communicate with the public. The Agency for Toxic Substances and Disease Registry (ATSDR) gives an overview in their citizen's guide to explain the differences in the approaches to reclaiming contaminated sites. The guide also explains the agency's role in public health.[15]

ATSDR makes the distinction between risk assessment and a public health assessment, noting that "risk assessments are often conducted without considering actual or possible exposure" and such assessments don't measure "the actual health effects that hazardous substances at a site have on people."[15] In contrast, ATSDR notes that a public health assessment "also factors in information from citizens about actual exposures" and "functions like a clinical evaluation of a community."[15] In such an approach, it is important that local conditions for each situation be considered, using science and what exposures people might actually have, rather than a cookbook assessment of theoretical risks. Such public health assessments require judgment, and are challenging, because they must protect public health in real world conditions. Similarly, other authors make a distinction between environmental risk assessment and surveillance-based public health, highlighting the contrast between the toxicological properties of a single substance and adherence to a regulatory standard versus a public health or population-based approach that involves assessment, policy development, and assurance.[7]

Sometimes, in public health, the toughest battles are on the inside. This situation was complicated by the fact that three different departments of state government were involved and contamination occurred decades previously. In Vermont, risk assessment recommendations and risk management decisions were performed by two different state agencies, who worked well together for the benefit of the public, despite the fact that occasionally a very complicated situation arose. In addition, separating risk assessment and risk management provided a check and balance to the pressures, particularly economic, that face all state agencies. It is at least theoretically possible that having health risks assessed and managed by a single agency or department, in a time of limited resources (which is just about always) would make it more difficult to protect health because the same department that would assess risks would be financially responsible for the management of the ones that they found. In this situation, the people of Windsor, particularly children at the schools, benefited from the collaboration between the environmental and health agencies involved and the public health approach used by health department staff in trying to understand this complex problem. Health department staff involved in the assessment, quantification, and communication of health risks were conscientious and made extensive efforts to understand the real uses and risks, not just theoretical risks of contamination with compounds that can pose serious risks to health, as when dealing with substances that have the potential to cause cancer.

Why did we all work so hard to make sure potential health risks were addressed? Because we were dealing with carcinogens and because staff saw with their own eyes mothers with children in strollers, older children playing in water at the site, kids on the playing field, and people of all ages using the surrounding space, and knew any exposures that were present would likely be there along with the children growing up, maybe for generations. Latency for health problems such as cancer is long, measured in years or decades, and the decisions that we make and sometimes fight for, will impact people and their health for years ahead, long after administrations change and staff move on. So, in many ways, making such decisions and implementing them to protect health is even more important. Although at times, tensions were high, the situation difficult, and the work required extensive, we were working to protect public health in the best possible way.

REFERENCES

1. State held responsible for Windsor contamination. Abigail Nitka. *Rutland Herald* February 27, 2002. Available at http://www.rutlandherald.com. Accessed April 8, 2005.
2. Windsor wants to consolidate school cleanup disputes. Tracy Schmaler. *Rutland Herald* November 26, 1999. Available at http://www.ruthlandherald.com. Accessed April 8, 2005.
3. State v. CNA Insurance Companies (No. 99-276); 172 Vt.318; 779 A.2d 662, Filed July 20, 2001. Available at http://www.dol.state.vt.us. Accessed April 10, 2005.
4. Vermont Statutes Annotated:10 VSA 8003(a),(12), 6604, 6604a, 6610a(a), 6615.
5. Health consultation. Agency for Toxic Substances and Disease Registry (ATSDR). Pole, Incorporated Wood Treating Facility, Oldtown, Bonner County, Idaho. Available at http://www.atsdr.cdc.gov/HAC/PHA/poleshc1/piw 1.html Accessed April 10, 2005.
6. ATSDR Public Health Statement for Chlorinated Dibenzo-p-dixoins (CDDs) Available at http://www.astdr.cdc.gov/toxprofiles/phs104.html Accessed April 10, 2005.
7. Novick, LF and GP Mays. Public Health Administration: Principles for Population-based Management. Aspen Publishers, Inc. Gaithersburg, Maryland. 2001. Chapter 26 Environmental Health Administration pp 604-622.
8. The Associated Press. Agency to clean up contamination. *Burlington Free Press.* July 17, 1997; 6B.
9. The Associated Press. Pesticide residues found in school field. *Burlington Free Press.* August 13, 1995, 4B.
10. The Associated Press. Traces of dioxin found at site of Windsor school. *Burlington Free Press.* November 18, 1995. 4B.
11. The Associated Press. Soil cleanup plagues Windsor school. *Burlington Free Press.* February 2, 1997; 8B.
12. Southern Vermont Bureau. More Chemicals Found at School. *Rutland Herald.* September 11, 1997; 18.
13. The Associated Press. Contamination discovered on Windsor football field. *Burlington Free Press.* May 10, 1998; 3B.
14. The Associated Press. Windsor finds more contaminated soil. *Burlington Free Press.* September 3, 1998; 5B,
15. A Citizen's Guide to Risk Assessments and Public Health Assessments. Agency for Toxic Substances and Disease Registry. Available at http://atsdr1.atsdr.cdc.gov/publications/Citizen's Guideto Risk Assessments.html. Accessed April 10, 2005.

40

House Calls in Public Health

When we think of "house calls" in health, we think of a style of medicine that has nearly vanished, one that conjures up the image of a physician traveling to a patient's home, sometimes in a rural setting. However, this concept of house calls in public health continues to be an essential one for public health practice. To gather an accurate perspective on many public health issues, it is essential. You have to go where the action is, during a problem or crisis, but also as part of your routine. How you communicate, on a personal level, during visits with different groups, individuals, organizations, or health facilities, and the information you learn from such visits, can help in understanding issues, identifying community needs, and solving public health problems in the real world.

We had authority over the licensing of hospitals (actually through the board of health), as well as varying responsibilities related to health planning and the Certificate of Need Process. One of the smaller hospitals in the state, Rockingham Memorial Hospital, in Bellows Falls, Vermont, was having financial difficulties. Although licensed for 47 beds, its patient census had dwindled to two or three per day.[1] Although emergency services would remain open 24 hours a day,[2] and there would be outpatient services for local residents, the hospital would eventually close. Even a hospital whose census had been declining for some time had history, roots, and strong supporters. A state representative, who was born in that hospital called to ask if I could do anything. I didn't know if I could do anything, but I told him that I would come down. I made a trip there, to visit and walk around the hospital (which by then was very near closure), to see the facility, and talk with local physicians and nurses there, and with administrators from the hospital. I also visited a nearby hospital as well, to see if there were opportunities for the two hospitals to work together; perhaps basic community health services could continue, but be provided in a different way. Although I knew the statistics from the reports, after my tour and meetings, I had a much clearer picture of the situation.

The hospital later closed. Its struggles were the same that faced many small rural hospitals—a declining number of patients. In this case, declining numbers were partially due to the fact that there was a large medical center and six small hospitals in the region.[1,3,4] Although my visit didn't change anything, as the hospital had been declining in census for years, it was still important to go, to visit, to spend time understanding the situation, not only on paper, but in person. It was important to the people served by the hospital and their representative who had called me; the hospital had been an important part of the local community for many years. It was important for me to visit to best understand the situation,

I had an understanding that couldn't be gained from statistics or health planning reports.

At another time, when I was attending a hospital meeting, an administrator from Vermont's smallest hospital introduced himself and asked if I would consider being the speaker for the hospital's annual meeting. I told him that I would have to check my schedule. He called soon after, as I had not said no (he told me), and I agreed to speak. At the time I wasn't a much practiced speaker with public audiences, but tried to accept invitations whenever there was interest about health. The hospital, which had a short book about it called *The House That Became a Hospital*,[5] was called Grace Cottage Hospital, in Townsend, Vermont. It was small, and from sitting on the committee that reviewed hospital budgets across the state, I knew that this hospital had an incredibly small budget compared to the rest of Vermont's hospitals. Substantial funds for this hospital came from an incredibly energetic auxiliary and through immense community support. A joint house and senate resolution[6] honored the hospital for 50 years of medical service, and their founding physician, Dr. Carlos Otis, figured out how to get the financial backing to better serve the surrounding communities with comprehensive health services. The name "Grace" was the wife of the primary benefactor, and Grace Cottage Hospital had opened in 1949.[6] The hospital was literally a house turned into a hospital. According to the hospital history,[7] 900 guests attended the hospital opening and the delivery of a baby by Dr. Otis marked the beginning of the hospital's long and important service to the surrounding communities. Adjacent houses were donated and added for nursing and residential care homes, and the facility was modernized with a new wing, following concerns about the lack of emergency exits from the second floor, where the babies were delivered, and the need to modernize its facilities. I had the occasion to visit many times over the years, and as a speaker when invited.

On the night of the event, I was staying in Grafton, Vermont, and we were having a weekend retreat, called the Grafton Conference on Health Care. I excused myself from the evening activities and after supper set out on the road from Grafton to Townsend. It was dark, and there was no one else on this road. After a while I wasn't sure if I was lost, so I stopped for directions at a house, and then kept going. The event was crowded, and I spoke for a little while about cancer prevention and smoking. Sitting in the front of the audience was Dr. Carlos Otis, the founder of the hospital. I was showered with baked goods and good wishes when I left. The community support was evident not only in the fundraising thermometer outside, but in the size and attitude of the crowd. I remembered the evening and my visit for a long time afterward.

I had several occasions to deal with this hospital over the years, related to emergency medical services, questions about location of services, and the building itself. Because of the time it took me to drive from Burlington, I decided to spend more of the day on one visit seeing the updated facility. I toured the hospital and nursing home facility and saw the memorial garden outside the hospital. Despite its size, in comparison to other hospitals, there was clear evidence of the personal style of care and success in meeting many needs of patients in their community.

I traveled to other parts of the state as well, to hospitals in Newport, St. Johnsbury, Central Vermont, Middlebury, and Rutland, whether to talk with a medical staff, county medical society, community groups organized to improve health in the hospital area, or in response to a growing heroin crisis at community forums.

From my office in Burlington, in close proximity to Vermont's academic medical center, such trips seemed time consuming and potentially a distraction from all the day-to-day pressures of the job, particularly on those days where I felt like an air traffic controller, had deadlines ahead, or correspondence piling up. It would be all too easy to talk on the phone (which was done all the time anyway), use written or electronic communication, or rely on the reports of staff in local offices. All these means of communication were invaluable to manage the day-to-day issues that occurred in public health over an entire state. There is, however, no substitute for an occasional visit.

During an urgent situation personal visits were a must. Unless there was some compelling reason not to, if a crisis occurred it was always best to show up in person. I helped public health nurses give measles shots, went to the town having the Legionnaires disease outbreak to go on the local radio program about the issue, and another time went to hear angry citizens at hearings about environmental contaminants in drinking water. These community visits, what I called public health house calls, were just as important when there was not a crisis. Although not an every-week occurrence, I would schedule these trips, get in the car and go, because I remembered these visits and knew the perspective they brought to my work would remain for weeks, months and years after.

REFERENCES

1. Mace P. Hospital will cut services. *Rutland Herald.* June 23, 1990; 1. Page 1.
2. Mace P. Emergency room will remain open at hospital. *Rutland Herald.* June 29, 1990.
3. Allen S. Hospitals' Troubles are Danger Sign for Others. *Rutland Herald.* September 4, 1990; 6.
4. Mace P. Hospitals sign new contract. Springfield Takes over Rackingham. *Rutland Herald.* September 29, 1990; 5.
5. Sonnenfeld M, Leigh D. *The House That Became a Hospital.* 1990.
6. State of Vermont. No. R-174. Joint Resolution Congratulating the Grace Cottage Hospital on 50 Years of Medical Service (J.R.H.134). Available at http://www.leg.state.vt.us. Accessed March 2, 2005.
7. Grace Cottage Hospital and Otis Health Care Center Web site. Available at: http://www.gracecottage.org. Accessed March 2, 2005.

CHAPTER 41

Remember the "Public" in Public Health—Distributing KI

One afternoon in the months following September 11, 2001, I picked up my ringing phone and was connected to a citizen in southern Vermont, who lived not far from Vermont Yankee, Vermont's nuclear power plant. She asked, "Why don't you give out potassium iodide to the public?" I told her that we focused on prompt evacuation in the event of an emergency. I said we had been participating in preparing for emergencies for many years and that our plan called for giving potassium iodide (KI) to emergency workers who would be entering a plume of radioactivity. I told her that I was confident of our emergency response capability as we had required mock drills each year. She then asked me, "what if a terrorist bombed the power plant or a plane flew into the plant? What would happen?" she continued to make her case for potassium iodide distribution to the public. As I listened, I instinctively reached down to the beeper on my waist that kept me connected to our statewide emergency response, 365 days a year.

After we hung up, I thought about it some more. As health commissioner, I was part of the required team that responded to any unusual events or activity related to the nuclear power plant and participated in required federal preparedness exercises. I had the responsibility to advise the governor about evacuation in the event of a release, potential release, or other major problem at the plant. We practiced, we drilled, and we were experienced. If anything, we recommended evacuation early, very early. But it was after September 11, 2001, that everything suddenly changed. She was right. A plane hitting the plant or an unexpected event that was so sudden might mean that even in the best conditions, our experienced team couldn't get the public evacuated fast enough.

During this time, as part of every state's review of emergency procedures, many states with nuclear power plants revisited emergency preparedness, including the use of potassium iodide. After some further discussion, the decision was made to begin developing a way to safely distribute KI to the general public. It was not a substitute for emergency directives, such as evacuation or sheltering, but something in addition–something we could do to be best prepared. We reviewed the work of the three federal agencies involved with this issue: the Food and Drug Administration (FDA), Federal Emergency Management Agency (FEMA), and the Nuclear Regulatory Commission (NRC),[1,2,3] and discussed how we might do this. We also tried to estimate the number of people who would fall into the 10-mile radius of the plant, whether at home, at work, in school, or participating other activities.

The governor wrote to the head of the NRC in November, indicating our interest in the KI issue. News articles also talked about the FDA and its revision of guidelines for potassium iodide.[4,5] The FDA had highlighted the risk of thyroid cancer, higher in young children, after exposure to radioactive iodine (I-131) largely from data from Chernobyl and the subsequent experience in Poland where KI was used with large numbers of people.[1] The timing was also important; the FDA emphasized that for best protection the KI should be taken before or during exposure to radioiodine, but even taking it three to four hours later could offer some protection.[1]

The timing was also critical for practical aspects of emergency planning. Evacuating people during a real emergency takes time, and in the event of a release of radioactive iodine, people, especially children might get KI too late to be effective. We needed to develop a strategy that distributed KI ahead of time—"predistribution," if we were going to be effective.[6] We considered people having KI at home, in their car, or at work in advance of any problem, in addition to having it available at the reception center for people evacuating in an emergency. To do this would require much public education, because it would be disastrous for people to delay when an evacuation was ongoing, looking for a KI tablet. It would also be necessary to clearly communicate this measure during an emergency response.

In January 2002, all governors were notified of the availability of potassium iodide on a first come, first serve basis, with the ability to request two tablets per person in the 10-mile emergency planning zone around a nuclear power plant. At the end of January, I formally requested more than 92,000 doses, and we estimated that about 20,000 residents would be eligible for predistribution.[6]

Our goal was to develop a practical plan, one that was tightly linked to our existing emergency response plan in Vermont. The plan required predistribution, much public information about any potential risks and benefits, and involvement of public health nurses, because their ongoing work at the local public health district office would make them integral to working with the community. We wanted public input for the plan to make sure we would implement a plan that would really work.[6] A draft plan was posted on the health department Web site and well publicized through local paper.[5] Materials were developed for the public that emphasized the FDA's information regarding safety and effectiveness, the specific role of KI, and its role in emergency preparedness. Specifically emphasized was that the use of KI was not a substitute for emergency directives such as evacuation. Charts with proper dosing and special instructions for very young children and pregnant women were developed. Materials were developed for health professionals based on comments received during the public comment period.[6,7]

The program for the distribution of KI began in April 2002.[8] One dose per person in the 10-mile emergency planning zone could be obtained with applications available through the health department, pharmacies, employers, and others as well as on the health department Web site. Public education was emphasized through statewide and local news coverage in TV, and radio, newspapers. Posters were placed where people go—town offices, grocery stores, laundromats, and libraries. Also, extensive efforts were made to reach members of the community through employers, government agencies, pharmacies, schools, hospitals, physicians, and churches.[6] After the first five months, more than 1000 individuals had received KI, and an estimated 3000 to 4000 doses had been distributed to schools.[6] Subsequent health department efforts included direct mailing to households in affected towns, with tablets being available at the local health department office or at local pharmacies. Clear, concise information about KI continues to be available on the health department Web site.[9]

Remember the *public* in public health. It is essential to listen to their calls, read their letters, and involve them in your plans, to make sure what you are trying to do will really work. In public health, we tend to think and talk about populations, but populations are just groups of people, real people. The weeks and months after September 11, 2001, were frightening and required a renewed effort to revisit emergency preparedness in many areas of public health, in every community, in every state. Citizens expect you to do everything in your power to help, and that is your responsibility. There is always something more you can do.

REFERENCES

1. CDER. *Potassium Iodide as a Thyroid Blocking Agent in Radiation Emergencies.* Washington, DC: Department of Health and Human Services, Food and Drug Administration, Center for Drug Evaluation and Research (CDER); November 2001.
2. Federal Emergency Management Agency. *Federal Policy on Use of Potassium Iodide (KI). Federal Register.* 2002;67:1355–1357.
3. US Nuclear Regulatory Commission. *Consideration of Potassium Iodide in Emergency Plans. Nuclear Regulatory Commission. Final Rule. Federal Register.* 2001;66:5427–5440.
4. Wald M, Revkin AL. Radiation exposure. FDA revises treatment guidelines, emphasizing benefits of potassium iodide. *Burlington Free Press.* December 17, 2001; 1C.
5. Clark M. New guidelines bring anti-nuke pill closer to Vermonters. FDA updates KI dosages. *Brattleboro Reformer.* December 13, 2001; 1.
6. Carney JK, deFlorio F, Erickson N, McCandless R. Enhancing nuclear emergency preparedness: Vermont's distribution program for potassium iodide. *J Public Health Manage Pract.* 2003;9:361–367.
7. Armstrong P. State seeks comment on nuclear pill distribution. *Brattleboro Reformer.* February 5, 2002; 1.
8. Henry T. State readies to dole out anti-nuke polls. *Brattleboro Reformer.* April 2, 2002; 1.
9. Vermont Department of Health. Vermont's distribution program for potassium iodide tablets. Available at: http://www.healthyvermonters.info/hp/yankee/ki.shtml. Accessed June 10, 2005.

42

Mercury—You Can Still Protect the Public When There Are Things You Can't Control

A state representative had written me a letter about mercury and requested the health department to issue a fish advisory like the state of Maine had done. We reviewed results from available fish tests, and the possible move by the federal Environmental Protection Agency (EPA) to change to a standard potentially much more protective of health. Tests had been done on fish the previous summer, and more than 500 fish were scheduled to be taken and analyzed from 35 lakes.[1] A fish advisory was issued in 1995, and refined and expanded as more information from Vermont fish caught in Vermont waters was obtained.

In 1999, the health department advised pregnant women to limit the amount of tuna that they eat.[2] A publication was targeted to pregnant women because they were most susceptible and also because public health nurses, who saw pregnant women in the Women Infant and Children's Clinic (WIC), noted occasional high consumption of commercially available fish, particularly tuna. The state toxicologist[3] noted that people were reporting high daily intakes of canned tuna, and decided it would be best to give pregnant women additional information. This information was based on the exposure limits established by the U.S. EPA, which were stricter and more protective of health than those of the Food and Drug Administration (FDA).[2,3] The guideline was in the form of a small colorful brochure called "Mercury in Fish, What You Should Know If You Are Pregnant, Planning to Be Pregnant, or Nursing a Baby."[4] The brochure explained how mercury builds up in older and bigger fish, as well as explaining the potentially harmful effects on babies and young children. We didn't tell people to stop eating fish, but just to be cautious of the fish that were eaten and to consider all sources of fish when making dietary choices. The brochure recommended pregnant or nursing women not eat swordfish or shark and offered limits for tuna consumption on a weekly basis. In addition to this specific focus, the health department's fish advisory covered various fish, different water bodies, and defined the size of portion of a fish at a meal. The addition of tuna and other commercial fish, to the advisor, using the EPA level of protection, added an additional level of protection and public information regarding mercury.[4]

Mercury occurs in the environment in several forms: metallic or elemental mercury, inorganic mercury, and organic mercury.[5] Elemental or metallic mercury is the liquid metal used in some types of thermometers and electrical switches, as well as thermostats, fluorescent light bulbs, and some blood pressure monitors.[5,6] When mercury combines with carbon, the compounds formed are called organomercurials or "organic" mercury. The most common of the organic mercury compounds found in the environment is methyl mercury. From a public health perspective, methyl mercury can build up in some commonly eaten fish, both freshwater and saltwater, to levels much greater than in the water.[5] Thimerosol, used as a preservative, is metabolized to another organic mercury compound, called ethyl mercury.[5] There are many federal agencies involved in making recommendations about levels of mercury exposure, and most states issue guidelines, recommendations, or advisories, as well as issuing state laws regarding mercury. Recommendations are also made by the federal Environmental Protection Agency, Food and Drug Administration, Occupational Safety and Health Administration (OSHA), the Agency for Toxic Substances and Disease Registry (ATSDR), and the National Institute for Occupational Safety and Health (NIOSH).[6] The EPA, FDA, and OSHA having regulatory roles.

Most of the information used to make federal recommendations or standards is based on research about health effects of methyl mercury.[5] However, agencies such as the Centers for Disease Control and Prevention (CDC) remind the public that safety margins are included in the creation of such guidelines or recommendations, and should be understood in the context of duration and level of exposures, rather than a line above which harmful effects occur immediately.[5]

In humans, the nervous system is sensitive to mercury, and the most potentially harmful effects occur from methyl mercury and mercury metal vapors because exposure to these forms of mercury can reach the brain. Kidneys and developing babies are also particularly vulnerable to effects of mercury. Children may be at increased risk, for example, when consuming fish containing high levels of mercury because they may eat more per body weight and have a nervous system that is still growing and developing.[5,6]

In the environment, methyl mercury is mostly produced by bacteria and fungi in the environment. Up until the 1970s substances containing organic mercury compounds were used as a fungicide to protect grains, but were banned when the adverse health effects of methyl mercury were uncovered.[6] Mercury can enter the environment from the normal breakdown of minerals in rocks and soil as well as mining and the burning of fossil fuels; ATSDR estimates that total annual mercury releases from human activities ranges from one third to two thirds the total mercury released.[6] Such activities as fossil fuel combustion, mining, and solid waste incineration contribute to elemental mercury released into the air.[6] Most mercury in our environment is metallic and inorganic mercury. Microorganisms can convert inorganic mercury to methyl mercury, which can accumulate in the food chain, first in smaller, then larger fish.[6] Potential exposure to humans comes from diets high in fish from contaminated waters, particularly in larger and older fish. Methyl mercury is the form most easily absorbed through the gastrointestinal tract, and after consumption of fish (or other foods) contaminated with mercury, methyl mercury can enter the bloodstream, and can move, in pregnant women, from mother to fetus, potentially impacting the nervous system, which is sensitive to the harmful effects of mercury.[6] Lessons about harmful effects of mercury were learned from large-scale poisoning in pregnant and nursing mothers exposed to very high levels of methyl mercury in contaminated grains used to make bread in Iraq and in seafood in Japan.[6]

At the health department, we reviewed mercury levels in fish every year and looked at the database as fish were added. Health department experts met with the Department of Environmental Conservation staff in the state environmental agency to review the database and identify gaps. Fish were collected each year, if possible addressing gaps in water bodies or types of fish. The filet tissue of the fish were analyzed, by making a "fish puree," and the information was added to the information collected to date. The overall strategy was to be as specific as possible, and accurately define risks for consumption of fish from Vermont bodies of water. A simple and blanket fish advisory would not have been credible, and it would have been unacceptable to all those who, well, enjoyed fishing and eating fish. Fish advisories targeted women of childbearing age, where a fetus might be more sensitive to harmful effects of too much mercury consumption, children aged six and under, and adults who weren't in another category.[7,8]

Communicating potential health risks from mercury in fish was a delicate balance—educating the public about mercury, but not eliminating the consumption of fish, an excellent source of protein, by issuing a blanket or overzealous warning. The best and most specific information about Vermont fish in Vermont's bodies of water provided the most accurate information in a way that protected health but didn't eliminate a food from the diet. However communicating this information was not always easy. Examples of strategies used were fish and wildlife manuals distributed with sale of fishing licenses, publicity through the media, and postings at water bodies. Making the fish advisories specific, but not so complicated that they were ignored, was a challenge, and clear communication of this information was essential.

Environmental advocacy groups noted that commercially available fish such as tuna were not included in fish advisories for Vermont waters, and public health nurses told us stories of pregnant women daily eating large amounts of tuna, and feeding large amounts to young children, so we added tuna to the advisory as well.[4] Vermont had an increasing number of refugee populations, some of whom ate large quantities of fish as part of their usual diet. After working with local community leaders, health department staff felt it was imperative to make fish advisories available in many different languages. The fish alert posters, large and user friendly, were made available in Russian, French, Spanish, Serbo-Croatian, and Vietnamese, as well as English.[7]

Vermont's efforts to reduce the impact of mercury went beyond public health. In addition to the health department, much policy advocacy came from a mercury advocacy group, the Mercury Policy Project, and other environmental groups, and extensive discussion and debate about Vermont laws regulating mercury occurred during this same time period. In addition, Vermont's environmental agency conducted a thermometer swap, and the administration's support of these activities contributed to the growing public awareness and legislative efforts to decrease the harmful effects of mercury in Vermont wherever possible.[9,10] In 2001, pharmacies in Vermont participated in a statewide mercury thermometer exchange sponsored by the Vermont Agency of Natural Resources, the state's environmental agency. Vermonters were able to bring mercury-containing thermometers to pharmacies and swap them for a free digital thermometer. The campaign was called "Catch the Fever" and was extremely popular, and was part of the overall Vermont efforts and initiatives of the state's Mercury Education and Reduction Campaign. The Department of Environmental Conservation, part of the environmental agency, also initiated a school science and lab clean-out project, which had, as of 2001, removed more than 400 pounds of mercury from Vermont schools. Mercury spills had occurred, some serious, in schools and the effort was designed to prevent similar future occurrences. The same agency also collected mercury used in farm equipment.[9,10] With funds from the legislature, the Vermont Agency of Natural Resources bought 13,000 new digital thermometers, and worked to educate the public about sources of mercury in household products.[9,10] Nearly 1400 older glass mercury thermometers had been swapped in a short time period for newer digital versions, and many Vermont pharmacies, on their own, stopped selling ones containing mercury.[10]

The Vermont legislature passed a mercury labeling law in 1998 that required warning about mercury on fluorescent lamps and packaging. This law was controversial at first, but following intensive litigation, (with amicus briefs filed by nine other states), and when the U.S. Supreme Court would not hear the case, the trade group representing most lamp manufacturers planned to extend labeling across the United States.[11] Similar legislation was discussed or passed in some other states, and at the time 10 states warned pregnant women and young children to limit intake of canned tuna.[11] The Environmental Protection Agency estimated in 2004, that one of every three lakes in the United States and almost a quarter of the rivers had enough contamination to warrant limitations on fish consumption, with 44 states having fish consumption advisories in place.[12]

Nationally, childhood vaccines were also under review and thimerosol, a preservative used in some vaccines since the 1930s, has been greatly reduced or eliminated in most childhood vaccines as a precautionary measure, following recommendations by the Public Health Service, American Academy of Pediatrics, and vaccine manufacturers in 1999. This was done following passage of a law called the Food and Drug Administration (FDA) Modernization Act in 1997, which instructed the FDA to review risks of all mercury-containing food and drugs (CDC). During the review, the FDA concluded that mercury intake from vaccines containing thimerosol in the first six months of life might exceed the Environmental Protection Agency (EPA), but not other federal agencies, and as a result major organizations and vaccine manufacturers agreed to reduce or remove it as a precaution.[5]

Vermont continues its efforts to influence and reduce exposure to mercury through legislation and continued public education, both from an environmental and public health perspective, and a law was passed in 2005 to take additional steps to reduce in-state sources of mercury.[13]

There is always something that you can do to better protect public health. In the case of mercury, raising public awareness and updating fish advisories each year, including tuna, was one way to protect the public when we had no real direct control over all the sources of mercury that ended up in the fish in Vermont waters. Public health efforts were not in isolation, but were a part of many efforts by other state agencies, advocacy groups, and the legislature. Fish advisories had to be repeated, written in many different languages, and posted where people fish.[14] Public health nurses could use this information as they talked with pregnant women about their nutritional needs. Information for the advisories was based on the most specific science that we had, making sure we had a growing bank of data of mercury levels in Vermont fish in Vermont water bodies. We were able to speak specifically about possible risks, rather than issue a blanket warning. Such warnings are some of the most challenging, trying to strike a balance between crisp credible warnings to protect the public, but not drive them away from fish, a great source of protein.

REFERENCES

1. Bazilchuk N. State may issue fish warning. *Burlington Free Press*. April 5, 1995: 1A.
2. Bazilchuk N. Mercury warning expand to ocean fish. *Burlington Free Press*. April 3, 1999: 1A.
3. Dillon J. State advises pregnant women to limit tuna. *Rutland Herald*. October 2, 1999. Available at http://www.rutlandherald.com. Accessed May 7, 2005.
4. Vermont Department of Health. Mercury in fish. What you should know if you are pregnant, planning to be pregnant, or nursing a baby. Burlington, Vt: Vermont Department of Health; 1999, 2004.
5. Centers for Disease Control and Prevention. Mercury and Thimerosal. Q's and A's. Available at http://www.cdc.gov/nip/vacsafe/conserns/ thimerosal/faqs-mercury.html. Accessed May 21, 2005.
6. Agency for Toxic Substances and Disease Registry (ATSDR). Public Health Statement for Mercury. March 1999. CAS# 7439-97-6. Available at: http://www.atsdr.cdc.gov/toxprofiles/phs46.html. Accessed May 21, 2005.
7. Vermont Department of Health. Health alert on eating certain types of fish. Available at http://www.healthyvermonters.info/hp/fish/fish. shtml. Accessed May 21, 2005.
8. Hazard on the menu (Editorial). *Burlington Free Press*. July 31, 2000; 4A.
9. Sneyd R. State offers trade on worrisome mercury thermometers. *Rutland Herald*. January 24, 2001. Available at http://www.rutlandherald.com. Accessed May 7, 2005.
10. A healthy fever (Editorial). *Burlington Free Press*. February 9, 2001; 4A.
11. Mills S. Vermont mercury labeling law to be applied nationwide. *Rutland Herald*. January 18, 2003. Available at http://www.rutlandherald.com. Accessed May 4, 2005.
12. Heilprin J. Most states have polluted fish in waters, EPA reports. *Rutland Herald*. August 25, 2004. Available at http://www.rutlandherald.com. Accessed May 4, 2005.
13. State of Vermont. The Vermont Legislative Bill Tracking System. S.84 Comprehensive management of exposure to mercury. 2005–2006 Legislative Session. Montpelier, Vt: State of Vermont; 2005. Available at http://www. leg.state.vt.us. Accessed May 21, 2005.
14. Crawford M. Fish mercury warning to be posted. *Burlington Free Press*. May 8, 2003; 1B.

43

Data Has No Constituency, or Does It?

Data has virtually no constituency. In the legislative process, there is no advocacy group lining up to testify in support of more statisticians, computers, or epidemiologists. In the competition for scare resources, health care for underserved people; food and housing programs; and services for alcohol, drugs, HIV, and mental health will all win the competition for funds. Advocates for needed funding for services and programs come to hearings to speak about personal challenges for themselves, friends, and relatives. They are effective in making sure that dollars go immediately to services that help people.

These programs are needed, valuable, and an essential part of public health, but so is the ability to carry out the overall mission of public health: monitoring the health of the population, providing sound public health policy and planning, as well as providing the overall assessment function recommended by the Institute of Medicine.[1] "Infrastructure" is a word that carries no weight, may connote an increase in government size and people, and doesn't immediately translate to those services that can help people, or the public, in the immediate future. Data and the resources needed to assess and monitor the health of the population, set priorities, and evaluate programs are essential to carry out in an efficient and effective manner, part of the mission of public health and of our core responsibilities.

So how do we help people who are making decisions about policy and funding see the value of data and the benefits to public health? We have to prove it. We have to link it to real programs or real services or, most importantly, real issues that are important to people. We have to make data personal. Not personal in the sense of making confidential information public, but in the sense that data is cemented and inextricably linked to things that impact the health of the public. We must tie it to the issues. Talk about it in the same breath as you talk about cancer or diabetes or smoking or obesity. Talk about limitations and strengths. Talk about what you will do with the data once you get it.

In public health practice, we often have to find creative ways to see if we are successful. We use simple evaluations, such as before-and-after progress reports, such as comparing numbers or rates of young children screened for lead poisoning, disease reports of hepatitis or salmonella, or percentages of children using marijuana. We never have time or resources to conduct another study; we must figure out how to gather what data we can, make sure it is clearly communicated and presented, make sure it is technically accurate and sound, and make sure it is timely.

Vermont was found to have a high breast cancer death rate. It was reported by the Centers for Disease Control and Prevention[2] and prompted focus and attention on the issues of why this was happening and what could be done about it. During this same time, a cancer coalition had formed and was helped by a federal grant. The coalition, staffed by the department of health, brought together the expertise of academics, state agencies, health agencies and providers, nonprofit agencies, and many others. One of the recommendations of the coalition's plan[3] was to develop a statewide population-based cancer incidence registry for Vermont to learn more about cancer incidence (not just deaths), understand risk factors, and determine the effectiveness of cancer programs. Cancer was also a priority area for *Healthy Vermonters 2000,* our roadmap for improved public health for the year 2000.[4]

A cancer registry bill was introduced into the Vermont legislature. It took only a couple of weeks after it was introduced for it to pass the Vermont House of Representatives, go quickly through the senate, and be signed into law by the governor. It directed the health commissioner to establish a cancer registry in the department of health, defined what was included, and directed that a training program be developed for participating health care facilities, and a quality control program be established for the data collected. It prescribed reporting requirements and timelines, protected the confidentiality of the information, and included a provision to collect information from facilities and states outside Vermont where Vermont residents received care. It directed cooperation with the National Institutes of Health and the Centers for Disease Control and Prevention in the sharing and use of cancer incidence data. In the findings, the legislature, wrote that cancer was the second leading cause of death in Vermont and that Vermont ranked in the top 10 states for breast, prostate, and other cancer death rates. The general assembly also wrote that statewide cancer incidence data was needed to better understand cancer in Vermont.[5]

The bill was short and clear, based on current data and statistics from health department staff and others, and the process seemed so simple, but it was the result of long and serious work by the cancer coalition, the department of health, cancer advocates, and many others. The cancer coalition's work provided a broad group that supported this registry as a priority for cancer prevention and control efforts, a consensus that such data was essential for Vermont to effectively prevent, detect early, and treat cancer. A federal grant had provided the resources to initiate the planning work, develop and staff the coalition, and develop a simple and clear plan that laid the groundwork for this registry. Legislators in Vermont were involved and highly supportive, as was the administration.

During this same time period, there was a growing network of breast cancer survivors who worked and organized at the state level and in Congress. They organized locally and across the nation, advocating for research, and gathering support to track cancer through the development and funding of registries.[6–9] Vermont Congressman Bernard Sanders and Senator Patrick Leahy worked to sponsor the Cancer Registries Act. The legislation was introduced after several key breast cancer advocates who organized a letter campaign and one woman, a cancer survivor, brought 13,000 letters from Vermonters to state congressmen.[6] The letters requested that money be given to states to establish better tracking systems for cancer. The cancer registry bill passed Congress with the help of Vermont breast cancer survivors.[10]

Our congressman and senator responded by sponsoring the act and also working to secure funding for Vermont and other states. Vermont was one of 37 states to receive cancer registry funding and they announced Vermont's award in a statehouse ceremony with us and the CDC.[11,12] The news coverage gave us another opportunity to speak about cancer, the high death rates, and how the registry would help. Because we were small, compared to other states, it would take time to gather enough data to make accurate conclusions, but the importance of this work was now widely understood, from Vermont to Washington and back. Three strong women, working with hundreds more, armed with sacks of mail, helped launch one of the key data initiatives in public health designed to help Vermonters and most importantly, reduce cancer deaths.

In Vermont, work on the registry began. It would take time to provide accurate data, but the need was clearly understood. Advocacy for the fight against breast cancer by many Vermont women garnered widespread support, as did the ongoing work of a dedicated coalition with a focused list of priorities, support from the legislature, governor, and Congress. Federal funds had helped initiate the background work and launch the program, and it had enabled all of us to bypass the difficult task of gathering funds of this magnitude from state resources. Hospitals around the state, knowing that a registry would take additional resources and staff, still supported the bill and the registry. The health department was ready and committed to doing the work.

During this time, data had a constituency because it was tied to a public health issue that was not well enough understood and was killing Vermont women. Advocates argued for better treatment and cures as well,[13] and although there was the potential for conflict regarding the emphasis on early detection, or breast cancer screening, by the health department as the primary strategy, there was always consensus on the fact that cancer was the second leading cause of death in Vermont and breast cancer was killing too many Vermont women.

The efforts needed to develop and implement a large registry, including training, data quality, and the need to capture every newly diagnosed cancer case for state residents, was a long-term commitment to detailed work. Along the way, we looked at registries from other states to determine how we should present the data and make sure it was translated into clear and useful information, so it could be used as intended, to better understand trends, target areas for additional work, monitor the effectiveness of our programs, and ultimately impact cancer, our public health goal. We decided to format the data into the type of information and document that was easily understood by the public. Background tables and detailed information would be available, but we wanted to use the data to convey useful information to the public, physicians, nurses, and policy makers about public health in the same manner that our data had been used to educate the public about public health in areas such as prenatal care, access to health care, smoking, and the many other areas included in our goals for improving public health listed in *Healthy Vermonters 2000* and *Healthy Vermonters 2010* and our reports on the health status of Vermont communities. Accurate data was a given, and this was the responsibility of the program collecting the registry data, with advice from researchers and other coalition members. The challenge was in how to present the data to let it speak for itself: how could the data direct our focus, and the focus of all those working with us, to take the next steps, and make further progress on the issue.

We decided on a short document, 20 pages long, with a Vermont-green cover, that summarized the first three years of the Vermont Cancer Registry.[14] We included information about cancer, the most common types for women and men, and how our rates compared to available national data. Causes of cancer, the role of prevention and early detection, and basic information about treatment, surveillance, cancer clusters, and the concept of latency were all included. Cancer incidence and deaths were presented and compared, and references and information sources were included. In addition, detailed information, statistics, and maps were provided for common causes of cancer and deaths from cancer for both men and women, focusing on breast, colorectal, lung, and prostate cancer. Information about effective screening was presented, along with risk factors, such as smoking for lung cancer and information about controversy in screening recommendations, such as those for prostate cancer.

Cancer rates had been calculated for 23 different cancer sites, and for the first time, we had information about the incidence, the number or rate of newly diagnosed cases of cancer, as well as deaths from cancer. The rate of colorectal cancer incidence was found to be statistically worse than the U.S. rate.[14] Vermont had a higher incidence of cervical cancer than the United States, a statistic pointing to the need for widespread use of Pap tests. Incidence rates for lung and larynx cancer were also statistically worse that the rates for the United States. Lung cancer was the leading cause of cancer deaths for both men and women; this gave additional urgency to our ongoing efforts to reduce smoking.[14]

Vermont's breast cancer incidence rate was not higher than the rate in the rest of the United States, and the breast cancer death rate was declining. This information reinforced our current emphasis to make screening tests, mammograms, and clinical breast exams widely available to women at recommended ages and intervals, as well as access to state-of-the-art cancer treatment. The worry that our high death rates from breast cancer were due to more cancer occurring were put to rest by the information from the registry.[14] The first use of this important data was a report that helped us focus our efforts and continue our fight to improve public health in the area of cancer.

It was front-page news. The top headline read "Vermont Cancer Rates at US Average—Study Puts State 23rd in Breast Cancer Deaths."[15] The detailed article went on to summarize findings from key cancer types and showed maps of lung cancer incidence for men and women for Vermont counties, and provided statistics on incidence and deaths from lung, prostate, colorectal, and breast cancer. Newspapers around the state[16] ran articles as well, highlighting the statistic that breast cancer rates were no higher than the average United States rate and that overall cancer rates were no higher than in rest of the United States.

A later report emphasized that Vermont's colorectal incidence rate was higher than the U.S. rate, and that only about a third were diagnosed at an early stage.[17] This information highlighted the need for more screening to detect colorectal cancer earlier, at a time when only about half of adults were screened and cancers were only diagnosed in earlier stages a third of the time. Our cervical cancer incidence was higher than the United States rate, further emphasizing the need for Pap tests, especially for women after age 50. In contrast to colorectal cancer, over 60% of breast cancers were diagnosed at a localized stage,[17] supporting the ongoing need for early detection to try and identify breast cancer at a time when treatment would be more successful. Lung cancer continued to be the leading cause of cancer deaths for both women and men, and was now the leading cause of new cancers, rather than breast cancer, in Vermont women.[17]

If widely disseminated, made public, and circulated to health groups and organizations, hospitals doctors and nurses, Vermont communities, and policy makers, such information had the potential to focus attention on better understanding, preventing, detecting early, or successfully treating cancer in Vermont. The story of cancer in Vermont is clearly not over, but the use of data, specifically the cancer registry, was critical to increasing more intense, accurate, and focused public health efforts.

Data has no constituency, or does it? For big efforts, a cancer registry or other large data initiative, successful efforts take planning, coalition building, and patience. Funding from a federal grant was essential for this project. The need for data was clearly tied to the issue—breast cancer, and the advocates in Vermont, who were often survivors themselves, gave the data a face, a name, an identity. The data became personal; these were women in Vermont, fighting a disease we knew little about in our own state.

But, although this example resulted in a registry that has great potential to help understand and impact cancer in Vermont, the process was the exception, rather than the rule. Other registry initiatives, such as a trauma registry, were attempted and failed. At the time, I wasn't sure whether the timing for registries had passed, (as they were resource and labor intensive), or that the issue didn't have the depth of grassroots support that had been so compelling for breast cancer and the creation of the cancer registry.

It was always difficult to garner resources for data; seeking federal grants for essential surveys was a good strategy as was linking the data to the issue at hand. If you want to prevent childhood lead poisoning, you need to track children screened. If you want to understand new infectious diseases, you have to figure out how to find and count them if they are there. During debates on health care reform, data was seen as valuable in efforts to control costs, and we found that if we talked about prevention and public health using literature linking it to reduced health care costs, there was always more interest. We worked especially hard during a severe fiscal recession in Vermont to make sure our public health foundation of data and statistics wasn't demolished by the economic pressures and realities of the competition during the budgeting process. We knew that if it went, we would never, ever, get it back. Funds are hard to come by because of the competition with other types of services, other government departments, and the need to continually show the relationship of data to health benefits for the public.

However, one thing we finally realized after a long time, is that data does have a constituency that is essential to changing the culture around health issues, by bringing public focus, setting priorities, and helping data drive policy, all difficult tasks. The constituency for public health data was the press. And if we were able to gather and clearly communicate the data we had, from one source or multiples sources, we were then able to use it to educate the public about important health issues. Without an additional dollar, that realization helped us use our limited and precious resources in the best possible way to educate the public and improve public health.

REFERENCES

1. Institute of Medicine. *The Future of Public Health.* Washington, DC: National Academy Press; 1988.
2. CDC. Progress in Chronic Disease Prevention. Chronic Disease Reports: Deaths from Breast Cancer among Women, United States, 1986. *MMWR.* 1989;38:565–569.
3. Vermont Coalition for Cancer Prevention and Control, Vermont Plan for Cancer Prevention and Control 1990–1995. Burlington, Vt: Vermont Department of Health. 1989.
4. Vermont Department of Health. *Healthy Vermonters 2000.* Burlington, Vt: Vermont Department of Health; December 1992.
5. State of Vermont. Acts of the 1993–1994 Vermont Legislature. No.90. An Act Relating to a Cancer Registry (H.177). Available at http://www. leg.state.vt. us/DOCS/1994/ACTS/ACT090.HTM. Accessed May 2, 2005.
6. Ferguson E. Vermonters rally for cancer research. *Burlington Free Press.* October 10, 1991; 7A.
7. Soga A. Leahy, Sanders propose measures to fight breast cancer. *Burlington Free Press.* December 13, 1991; 3A.
8. Sanders calls for research on cancer. Bill would pay for statewide registries. *Burlington Free Press.* January 7, 1992; B1.
9. Tracking cancer to its sources (Editorial). *Burlington Free Press.* January 13, 1992; 6A.
10. Ferguson E. Congress approves cancer registries. VT women played role in passage. *Burlington Free Press.* October 9, 1992; 6A.
11. Copans L. State awarded $1.3 million to start a cancer registry. *Rutland Herald.* October 1, 1994; 1.
12. Wallace A. $1.3 million grant to boost cancer registry. *Burlington Free Press.* October 1, 1994; 1B.
13. Blackburn M. Group of VT women take case to capital. Group: Breast cancer a health emergency. *Burlington Free Press.* May 3, 1993; B1.
14. Vermont Department of Health. Cancer in Vermont. A report of 1994–1996 cancer incidence data from the Vermont Cancer Registry. Burlington, Vt: Vermont Department of Health; January 2000. Available at http://www. healthyvermonters.info/hs/epi/cdepi/cancerregistry/CancerInVT.pdf. Accessed March 3, 2005.
15. Bazilchuk N. Vermont cancer rates at U.S. average. *Burlington Free Press.* February 1, 2000; 1A.
16. Associated Press. Vermont's breast cancer rates no high than U.S. average. *Rutland Herald.* October 20, 1999. Available at www.rutlandherald.com. Accessed May 4, 2005.
17. Vermont Department of Health. Cancer in Vermont. A Report of 1995–1999 incidence data from the Vermont Cancer Registry. Burlington, Vt: Vermont Department of Health; March 2003. Available at http://www. healthyvermonters.info/hs/pubs/2003/2003cancerInVT.pdf. Accessed March 31, 2005.

44

Be There

In the 1990s, tobacco control in Vermont focused on changing the culture around the use of cigarettes and other tobacco products. It was an active time for antitobacco coalitions and the legislature related to tobacco prevention and control. It was at the time before all the tobacco-related industry documents became public and prior to the funds made available through the Master Settlement Agreement following the national work of state's attorney's general and antitobacco advocates. There was little money available, and what there was, was used to develop efforts among school-aged children to educate their peers.

In addition, there was a coalition, which changed its name repeatedly through the years, that included the major health-related nonprofit organizations, concerned citizens, legislators, health professionals, and others. It was a very fluid organization, and it was a time of tremendous legislative activity in public health, and in many areas of tobacco prevention and control. There was an ongoing momentum of back-and-forth communication between health officials, coalition members, and legislators of both (and sometimes three) political parties on health issues, both during and outside the legislative session. Many legislators had introduced and signed on as sponsors to a variety of tobacco prevention and control bills during this time, and there was both great interest and energy. Because current funds were meager, and state funds were hard to come by, it seemed like the policy opportunities provided the best strategy to tighten up laws where needed, and to work to change the culture around tobacco use, to one that better promoted health. Further, the public nature of these legislative activities, and their debates, provided much needed media attention and opportunities to promote public health and provide information about smoking in children and adults, the health effects of tobacco use, and the health benefits of quitting.

One representative became very interested in tobacco advertising, and asked for journal articles and more information about this area. It was a time when cartoon characters, with exaggerated features, were being used in tobacco advertising and researchers were comparing children's' recognition of them to well-known cartoon characters, such as Mickey Mouse, in children as young as 3 years old.[1] Although such literature did not prove that these cartoon characters with exaggerated features caused children to start to smoke, it brought such advertising to consciousness among people concerned with health and preventing smoking in children—that children at an early age could recognize characters promoting tobacco products that were legal to sell to adults. This created much discussion and became an area of interest for public health-minded legislators.

However, the issue of tobacco advertising was a complex one, one that had a long history, and that was regulated by federal law. Although there were no television ads marketing cigarettes, there was much concern about ads on billboards during sporting events and the use of these cartoon characters to promote tobacco products. The representative understood from her research that legally, it was very difficult, if not impossible to write and pass a law at the state level that could affect these factors. There was only a very narrow window to write a law that limited cartoon advertising in commercial advertising, and from a public perspective, communicating this perceived limitation of speech would be nearly impossible.

However, despite all this, a bill was introduced with 19 sponsors in the House of Representatives that attempted to do just that.[2] A companion bill in the Senate, with four senate sponsors, likewise tried to limit the use of cartoon characters in advertising. At the time, we didn't think that anyone believed such a bill would pass, but many involved legislators decided that the severity of the health issue warranted attempting it. At the outset, there was no doubt that such legislation would be controversial, but the seriousness with which the bill was taken by the industry propelled the debate.

The bill was titled H.295, an Act Relating to the Use of Cartoon Characters in Advertising to Minors. The bill's purpose was to prevent the use of cartoon characters to advertise addictive substances prohibited to minors. It listed the vulnerabilities of minors and how they were susceptible to forms of advertising and promotion. The bill prohibited the use of a cartoon character in an advertisement or display of a product if the product was an addictive substance and the product could not be lawfully purchased by a person under the age of 18. The language stated that the definition of "cartoon character" would be narrowly interpreted, and there were exceptions noted on labels and in photographs. The attorney general or state's attorney would have enforcement authority.[2]

The bill was introduced and sent to the house health and welfare committee, and the committee decided to take up the bill for testimony and discussion. Tobacco advocates testified about the issues of children smoking and available literature on tobacco advertising and children. At one point the committee invited a tobacco industry representative to testify. Tobacco lobbyists, individuals representing tobacco companies, were present in the statehouse, and often did their work in the hallways and the cafeteria, and testified on some occasions, but not often. They were sometimes observers in the committee rooms, and sometimes active participants during these discussions. For this particular bill, there was an individual arriving from outside of Vermont to provide testimony against the bill. I received a call and was asked to come down to the statehouse in Montpelier and sit in the committee room during this testimony, not to speak, but just to be present, and provide moral support. I did just that, and took a seat on one side of the room, in the small number of folding chairs lined up along the walls of the small committee room.

The committee room was on the third floor of the statehouse, at the end of the hallway, and had tables put in a square shape, with the representatives sitting around the table. The committee chair sat directly across the room, as the door opened into the committee room, and the individual testifying sat directly opposite, just as you opened the door. On the glass panel in the door was the committee name, Health and Welfare, along with a printed scheduled of testimony for the current week. The room had several large windows on two sides of the room, and on the left as you entered was a board with bill numbers tacked up on a bulletin board as bills were introduced and sent to the committee. The room was large enough to hold the committee, and a single narrow row of guests sitting in folding chairs against the walls behind the representatives, but not much else.

I sat in my folding chair, near a window at the side of the room, behind the committee members at the table and watched as the committee sat and began questioning the witness. People sitting along the sides were not part of the discussion, unless asked by the committee chair or other representatives. Most of the discussion occurred between the committee and the person sitting in the chair to testify. Everyone else sat and listened, and often took notes.

The individual testifying was a woman, probably in her thirties, dressed well, with matching accessories in black, far more formally dressed that the usual person providing testimony to Vermont legislative committees—she was actually just a little too well dressed, something that was very noticeable. She provided her testimony against the bill, and talked about how the advertising done by the tobacco companies was not aimed at children, only at people old enough to smoke. She mentioned that she had children, and indeed gave the appearance of a person of the right age to be a parent.

One of the representatives, and a bill sponsor, during the woman's testimony, passed me a note. I opened it and it said, "What should I ask her?" I sat and thought for a minute of a few areas—and passed back the paper after I had written, "Ask her if smoking causes lung cancer." The testimony went on about the bill and advertising and questions were beginning to be asked by committee members. At one point, the representative who had passed the note asked the witness if smoking caused lung cancer. The witness paused and moved around in her chair a bit and began to talk about her personal opinion at which point she was asked for the opinion of the client she represented. She answered something to the effect that there wasn't enough scientific information to tell.

Well, committee members were now awake and the collective questioning of the witness grew more intense, even angry. One representative leaned forward in her chair to ask further questions. This was the health and welfare committee, the committee that was very knowledgeable about scientific evidence about the health effects of tobacco use and was very supportive of public health. The witness's testimony unraveled at that moment, a single question, removing even a shred of credibility from a person trying to bring her own role as a parent to the aid of her client who opposed the bill. In fact, her testimony probably contributed to the bill being voted out of committee, and going to the floor of the house of representatives, something felt most unlikely at the start. There was no doubt that the bill was controversial, prompting newspaper editorials against it, directed at the broader protection of free speech, and commentaries written back in return, talking about smoking and health. The bill was debated, modified, and amended, though with the basic original provisions passed the house of representatives by a vote of 75 Yes votes to 67 No votes.[3,4] It was then sent to the Senate, where it was sent to the judiciary committee (called also by its nickname "The Cemetery") where it failed to receive any further action and died in committee.

Was this bill enforceable? Would it greatly benefit public health? No one would ever know. It was controversial to start, and remained so in its brief, but intense debate. It was introduced and debated in the context of a series of bills over a short number of years that would indeed strengthen the policy foundation for Vermont's efforts to reduce tobacco use, and represented the broad support, momentum, and extent to which many representatives and senators were willing to explore all available means to protect children's health. The bill, even at its introduction, attempting to go through a narrow window in its efforts, was not felt to be credible by many, but the debate and discussion provided ample opportunity for tobacco and public health advocates to repeat again and again information about the impact of tobacco use on public health and the dangers of smoking. The reason the bill went as far as it did, though, was because of the committee's intense response to a witness who tried to oppose the bill in a committee well versed in the science about smoking and health by taking a position counter to current science.

Sometimes a single question, and more importantly, a single answer, can determine a committee's response and whether or not an issue is gently discussed or propelled out of a committee room. In this case, the committee's knowledge and concern for public health was underestimated. Although the bill did not pass, the discussion continued to keep smoking and public health on the minds of the public and the legislature, critical to the ultimate goal of reducing tobacco use in Vermont.

REFERENCES

1. Fischer PM, Schwartz MP, Richards JW, Goldstein AO, Rojas TH. Brand logo recognition by children aged 3 to 6 years. Mickey Mouse and Old Joe the Camel. *JAMA*. 1991;266:3145–3148.
2. State of Vermont. H.295. An Act Relating to the Use of Cartoon Characters in Advertising to Minors. Bill as Introduced. Available at: http://www.leg.state.vt.us/DOCS/1994/BILLS/INTRO/H-295.HTM. Accessed March 11, 2005.
3. State of Vermont. An Act Relating to the Use of Cartoon Characters in Advertising to Minors. Available at: http://www.leg.state.vt.us/DOCS/1991/BILLS/House/H-295.HTM. Accessed March 11, 2005.
4. State of Vermont. The Vermont Legislative Bill Tracking System. Roll call vote Detail. 1993–1994 Legislative Session. H.0295. Montpelier, Vt: March 16, 1994. Available at http://www.leg.state.vt.us. Accessed March 11, 2005.

Controversy Is an Opportunity to Focus Your Message

There was a report on television about controversy in screening for breast cancer, questioning whether or not there was a benefit for women 40 to 50 years old. We were busy promoting advice to increase the number of Vermont women who received mammograms and clinical breast exams in an effort to raise awareness that early detection of breast cancer could save lives. We promoted this message in a variety of ways over an extended period. During this time, controversy arose, based on studies reported in the scientific literature about whether or not breast cancer screening, specifically using mammography, was effective in women aged 40 to 50 years. This controversy became public and received national attention. We had been emphasizing that the risks of breast cancer were highest for women as they got older and emphasized the importance of mammography and clinical breast exams for women 50 years and older. We were careful to monitor the recommendations of national organizations for the 40- to 50-year-olds as they changed. When the controversy about women aged 40–50 years erupted, I was concerned because if the information was confusing, women might stop getting mammograms. So, when asked by the press about the 40- to 50-year-olds, I decided that we would use a different strategy. I talked about the benefit of new studies and advancements in the science of our understanding about the most effective screening or early detection methods to detect breast cancer early, but also said we must not forget that the risks for breast cancer increased with age and that the recommendations for women 50 years and older hadn't changed. I took the opportunity of the controversy to remind Vermont women of our strong and unwavering recommendation for women 50 years and older to get an annual mammogram and clinical breast exam, and that early detection could save their lives. This controversy gave us an opportunity to again reiterate our message about these screening recommendations.

The health department launched a condom advertising campaign, targeted at 20- to 29-year-olds, and the largest television station in Vermont wouldn't run it. Health department staff had reviewed data from public surveys and found that in young people engaging in behaviors that would put them at risk for chlamydia, HIV/AIDS, or unintended pregnancy, more than a third did not think they had a risk of getting HIV.[1]

Epidemiology and HIV/AIDS program staff, working with federal funds, developed a media campaign to raise awareness and educate this target group about how to prevent sexually transmitted diseases and HIV. Focus groups were held over a year's time with young adults who would be the recipients of such a campaign to get feedback on what types of messages would work and how to best deliver them. The advice given was to not use scare tactics or preachy health messages.[2] The intended message for young adults engaging in high risk behaviors was direct but humorous, and included television, radio and newspaper ads, intended to break the ice in talking about condom use. There were three television stations, and the largest one would not run the campaign, despite the fact that the ads would be on at 10 P.M. I met with the executive vice president of the station, but to no avail. When we launched the prevention campaign, one of the articles focused on the refusal of the TV station to run the ads, and gave a good description and rationale for the campaign.[2] In the next week, the state's largest paper wrote an editorial applauding the campaign and the need for it.[3] The department's first AIDS campaign, "Don't forget your rubbers" many years prior was understandably controversial at the time, but despite the fact that such a high proportion of young adults in Vermont were unaware of the risks of contracting HIV or chlamydia, it was still controversial, and the state's largest television station was still not comfortable with a direct but needed public health message. However, their refusal provided another opportunity to articulate the number of people with AIDS in Vermont, the need for prevention, and how to prevent it.

Controversy is an opportunity to focus your message. Health is of great interest to the public, with rapid advances creating tremendous opportunities for public health. The danger of all this information, however, is with so many individual studies coming out, and some of them conflicting, in the absence of ongoing and strong public health messages by credible spokespeople, the public will find the health messages confusing or contradictory.

In the case of screening for breast cancer, we were concerned that given conflicting evidence, or when there is perceived uncertainty, disagreements, or frank arguments among educated scientists, that women might simply wait for them to figure it out, a potentially dangerous delay. In the face of a new study every day, conflicts between articles and scientists will arise, expectedly, as new science develops. Consensus statements and the groups that make them use criteria and weigh the different study designs, the evidence, and makes decisions to recommend or not, or say when there is not enough evidence. The media reports, focusing on individual studies, don't make this distinction, and may result in confusion and perceived mixed messages. Advances in science and health are a great thing, but there needs to be strong and consistent public health messages about what we do know and advice for what you should do today, even as the science advances and the controversy continues.

In the case of preventing HIV, despite the fact that such prevention messages and use of the word "condom" had been common for years, there was still controversy, even when the message would be aired late in the evening. However, in both these examples, the controversies provided opportunities for public health education: to reiterate statistics, talk about the health issue, and the importance of prevention.

Sometimes, controversy in public health is viewed as a distraction, something that gets in the way, or is to be avoided at all costs. However, there are times, and opportunities, to use a controversial moment, scientific article or issue, to frame a public health issue and repeat sound advice. Public health should look for and take advantage of these opportunities to make strong statements on health and reinforce messages that will benefit the public.

REFERENCES

1. Vermont Department of Health. *Healthy Vermonters 2000, Progress Report.* Burlington, Vt: Vermont Department of Health; 1996:10–11.
2. Geggis A. Health department launches condom campaign. *Burlington Free Press.* June 21, 1997; 1B.
3. Starting the conversation [Editorial]. *Burlington Free Press.* June 28, 1997; 10A.

CHAPTER 46

Find New Ways to Involve the Public

When the legislature is considering a possible new law, committees hold hearings in their usual or sometimes larger committee rooms, take testimony, and sometimes also hold public hearings, especially on controversial topics, or on pending bills that would represent a large change in direction or policy for the state, such as in areas of health care or education. Sometimes, depending on the issue, hearings are sparsely attended, and other times, they are crowded, loud, and controversial. There may be media attention to the issues and television and newspaper reports of individual comments or overall tone of such meetings. State agencies also try to involve the public in different ways to get feedback or gain support for proposed initiatives. There are many different ways to gather public input, and we were participants or organizers for many sessions designed to involve the public in our plans.

The emergency medical services (EMS) division of the health department thought that Vermont's statewide EMS system needed an update. They had hired a consultant from Maine, who gave a harsh critique of Vermont's EMS system[1] and an editorial described it as being in "critical condition."[2] There were many issues at the time, such as dependence on broad use of volunteers across the state, the difficulty local squads had in financing their services and keeping up with regulatory requirements, changing standards of best EMS practice, and the lack of a comprehensive plan.[1,2] 3500 flyers were sent out inviting EMS providers, legislators, town officials, and citizens to help plan the future of Vermont's EMS system. Five public hearings were scheduled in a 3–4-week period, in different locations throughout Vermont.[3] They were scheduled in the evenings, usually at a local school, and we traveled to a variety of different sites in Vermont to get ideas and input on the future plan. News articles irritated the EMS program staff by highlighting controversial comments, rather than the big picture,[3,4] but overall the hearing process helped us, especially when there was a concrete idea or suggestion presented to the group to react to. This was a specialized audience, one that had a vested interest in what we were doing, and comments were focused on the topics at hand. Money was a frequent request,[4] to which we always asked what would be done with additional funds, to gauge the level of planning and priority setting that had been already done for the local region.

Why not just do a statewide plan from the health department office in Burlington? Critical considerations for any statewide plan were local control by EMS squads and unique aspects of each Vermont community served by EMS providers and the challenges they faced. Not only would such a centralized plan not work, it would not have addressed the broad range of needs, some common, some locally unique, that created the network of emergency services for our entire state. Updating the needs for EMS services for Vermont was not an easy process, but one that helped find commonalities and differences. This was my first experience in trying to improve a statewide aspect of public health, and it left me with a lasting impression about the strengths and weaknesses of the methods that we used to involve the public. Over several years, we used a number of different approaches to gather public input in a variety of areas of public health.

I sat in a hearing in one of the large statehouse meeting rooms as a member of the Commission on Tobacco, Alcohol, and Substance Abuse Addiction, around the large wooden tables, in a format similar to legislative hearings. Several members of the administration were part of the commission that was established for the purpose of "studying and making recommendation for the development of coordinated effective and adequately funded system for preventing tobacco, alcohol, and substance abuse addiction and treating such addictions when they occur, in a humane, carrying and effective manner."[5] Vermont had a growing substance abuse problem, particularly in the area of opiate addiction, and during this time, there was much public activity and debate on the resources needed, coordination within government and with the private sector, and the tensions between investing more heavily in prevention when there were so many needs for substance abuse treatment. It was not uncommon for the legislature, before it adjourned in May or early June, to convene special commissions or task forces to look at complex, costly, or controversial issues, and report back to the legislature the following January, prior to any major decisions about funding or policy change. Such commissions had staffing from the legislature and ceased to exist when their work was done.

What I remember most clearly about the testimony for this commission was what I saw as I sat at the table listening to the testimony. Witnesses gave compelling stories about how they were addicted to alcohol or drugs, and described in vivid detail the struggles that entailed, and how they were able to resume a productive life in recovery after having received treatment, all naming the same treatment facility. In this case, citizens providing testimony to the commission reiterated the need for more treatment and recovery services, but were also advocating for a particular treatment facility to be funded. The targeted lobbying for a particular facility was intended to give the appearance of consumers providing general input about treatment to the committee. The commission heard from a wide range of interested parties and government agencies and consumers who had received treatment, and looked at the wide range of issues before crafting its report to inform the legislature.[6]

During the same time period, we were asked by the governor to assemble a task force on heroin, called the Heroin Action Committee, to convene stakeholders and gain consensus on priorities, and hold public meetings throughout the state. During this time there was tremendous focus on a growing heroin problem and its impact on Vermont, but there were policy differences between the administration and legislators involved in the issue.[7] Nearly 40 people met at the department of health including state and local police, judges, treatment providers, physicians, schools, health care, teen centers, corrections, and many other organizations. In contrast to the style of hearings held by the legislative commission, this work focused on trying to gain consensus on priorities, and developing specific actions that could represent priorities for funding throughout the coming year, whether by grants or through the administration and legislative budget process.

The group met and agreed that a comprehensive approach was needed that included prevention, treatment, and law enforcement, and that the focus must include alcohol, marijuana, and other drugs as well as heroin. The committee came up with specific priorities in the areas of prevention, treatment, and enforcement that would be used at a series of public hearings around the state. Such ideas as putting a substance abuse counselor in every Vermont school, residential treatment programs for youth, and drug courts were part of the list of specific priorities for public reaction.[8,9]

In the fall, six public forums were held, along with a youth leadership group, to discuss potential strategies.[8,9] At the meetings, participants were given an overview of the problem in Vermont and asked: What impact was heroin, alcohol, marijuana and other drugs having in the region? What were the top priorities in the areas of prevention, treatment, and enforcement? What suggestions or next steps were needed to move forward with the top priorities? Smaller groups in the three areas were then used to gather detailed feedback. The impact of heroin, growing in severity with regular reports in the news media about crimes, overdoses, and its impact on young adults and families, was seen all over Vermont.

The hearings were well attended, with about 400 community members attending, and provided much detailed feedback. They showed that the two overarching themes—that a comprehensive approach was needed and that we must address more than heroin—were well supported across the state.[8,9] In addition, there were regional and local differences in concerns and in proposed priorities; young people at a forum for high school students reinforced the view that alcohol and marijuana were most commonly used, and solutions to heroin must address these other drugs as well. In Vermont's largest county, work was ongoing toward the opening of a methadone treatment facility, whereas in another county, a petition with 1200 signatures opposing methadone was rolled out along the carpeted meeting room and more than 150 postcards presented against a methadone clinic.[9] Other meetings in the northern part of the state highlighted the challenges of the economy and rural areas. Southern Vermont residents were concerned about close proximity to other states and interstate highway access to and from more urban areas.[9]

When all was done and the report was presented, we had a much clearer picture of similarities and differences throughout the state, and priorities for prevention, treatment, and enforcement. This was a difficult time with the growing heroin crisis, and there was much debate and discussion among the public, government departments, and the legislature as to the best means to stem the tide, but it was essential for the public to have opportunities for involvement, as ideas were discussed and developed.

During one summer, Vermont's public health nurses took to the streets and roads of Vermont to interview more than 3000 Vermonters. They were gathering essential information for a state health plan called for by the Vermont legislature.[10] In crafting this plan, it was essential to involve the public. This was something that created some careful thought and discussion within the department. Public input and discussion could take many forms: large public gatherings in towns, public hearings at the statehouse, and requests for comments about proposals, and all had strengths and weakness. Sometimes lobbying for specific interests or groups came in the guise of public testimony. Public hearings held in the evenings attracted people who were able to go out in the evenings, and might not include the parents of small children, senior citizens not wanting to drive at night, or people working second shift. The question that I asked myself and my staff was "How could we get information from citizens in Vermont that actually would reflect what the public might think?" We needed a new approach.

Who better to get information about health from the public than Vermont's public health nurses? In Vermont, public health is organized as the state department of health with 12 local offices located throughout the state, with no autonomous county or local health departments. Public health nurses were located in the state central office and in all the 12 districts. They were involved in everything from maternal and child health, home visits, the investigation of disease outbreaks, and potential environmental risks to health. They were capable, flexible, energetic, and trusted in their communities. When we had a controversy around a needle exchange program in one part of the state, the local office director became the health liaison for a contentious issue in the community. When pregnant women in Vermont weren't receiving prenatal care at all or very late, a media campaign was launched that showed a public health nurse giving a strong health message and offered a toll-free number. Public health nurses were indispensable, and I considered them the backbone of our public health system.

During that summer, public health nurses went out to every Vermont town, asking two questions: What is needed to improve the health of Vermonters? And what keeps us from improving health in Vermont, whether for an individual or family, community, or the entire state?[10] We needed a better understanding of not only what was missing and needed, but what were the barriers that needed to be removed or addressed in order to get there. The nurses began their interviews with a broader view of health than previously used; they showed a pie chart that described five broad areas that impacted health: the environment, human biology, habits and behaviors, social and economic factors, and health care.[10] This was not a statistical exercise; the information was qualitative, structured, yet open-ended and gathered by face-to-face interviews.

The credibility of the public health nurses ensured both an adequate and honest response, and we gave them broad latitude about the important places to visit in their communities, since they worked there and knew them best. They spoke with doctors, hospital administrators, dentists, school officials, parents, town clerks, business owners, and day care providers. They talked to organizations and groups involved and interested in health. They spoke with shoppers, people on the street, other government agencies, senior citizens, and legislators. They went to schools, general stores, farmer's markets, golf courses, hair salons, laundromats, beaches, police stations, post offices, restaurants, and senior centers. They went to state fairs and swimming pools. They interviewed government workers, leaders of advocacy groups, town officials, educators, and legislators. They did this all without fanfare or much publicity. Quietly and steadily they went to towns all over Vermont that summer to talk to the people there.[10] And the information we received, gave me confidence that, while not knowing what every single person thought, we had a good idea of what health issues were on people's minds.

When decisions were being made about the use of Vermont's Master Settlement Agreement funds, a tobacco task force, created by the legislature with the governor's support, held six hearings around the state, as well as a youth forum, to discuss what should be done with the tobacco settlement money Vermont was to receive.[11] The evening forums were advertised as to what to do with $30 million dollars per year. The meetings started with a brief introduction from one of the task force members and then broke up into smaller groups for more detailed discussions. Media reports frequently highlighted the meetings and gave opportunities to reinforce the importance of tobacco prevention and cessation prior to the fate of the funds being decided in the upcoming legislative session.

During this time, we had taken the approach of sending out health department staff to Vermont communities to gain information on aspects of tobacco prevention and control where we might need more emphasis and to see if the elements of the Center for Disease Control and Prevention (CDC) Best Practices for Comprehensive Tobacco Control Programs[12] resonated with the public. Staff from all 12 health department district offices around the state talked to nearly 3000 Vermonters throughout the state, between the 4th of July and Labor Day.[13]. Most Vermonters were concerned about the use of tobacco in their own community. Smoking rates among both young people and adults were consistently overestimated, especially by smokers and young people,[13,14] which fit with our notion that we had to correct the misperception that many people smoked—a notion that had been accentuated over time by tobacco advertising. Of the CDC's elements of a comprehensive plan, there was much support for smoking cessation efforts for pregnant women, youth-designed programs or events, school programs, smoking cessation programs, and enforcement of state tobacco laws to keep young people from smoking.[13] Antismoking advertising campaigns had less public support. When we were working to establish a comprehensive tobacco prevention and cessation program for Vermont, we were prepared to explain why antismoking advertising campaigns were important in our efforts, forewarned of questions that would likely also be on legislator's minds.

Find new ways to involve the public. As we carry out our mission to protect and improve public health, we have to find new and better ways to involve the public in our plans. There are many ways to do this, and it is important to fit the approach with the task at hand. Sending our draft plans for comment and publicizing the reasons why we needed the public's help, public meetings, interviews by public health nurses and health department staff, may all be appropriate for different issues at different times. After September 11, 2001, we used our Web site as an additional means to gather public input on a plan to distribute potassium iodide (KI) to people living and working in the area of Vermont's nuclear power plant. There are many ways to gather information to make your work better and more effective. Each of these has trade-offs, and you have to decide, before you start, what your goals are. Are they to educate the public about an issue, test your ideas and strategies, see if your data reflects people's perception, and gather support for an initiative or idea that may be initially controversial or need additional resources in a competitive environment? Do you want noisy public events or quiet information gathering, an approach conducted more behind the scenes?

There is no one-size-fits-all style or approach to involving the public in your plans. And there are also risks: if you successfully fuel public support for an issue, and it doesn't get funded or no actions are taken, your credibility is at stake. You must know what you want to achieve before you begin, and you must finish what you start. For something as comprehensive as a state health plan, a level of detail was needed that was gathered by our public health nurses. For heroin, it was important to educate the public about effective prevention and treatment options as well as gathering their focused priorities in small group portions of public meetings. For tobacco, where much funding was at stake, it was essential for us to know what we would do with funds and why, not just that more funds were needed, and gauge the level of public knowledge and support for science-based strategies. Involving the public is fundamental to achieving your goals, but how you choose to go about the task depends on the issue and what you need to achieve. The openness with what you are doing and how you are thinking about an issue is critical to credibility and trust for your role in public health.

REFERENCES

1. Gottschalk M. Vermont Emergency Care needs help, study says. *Burlington Free Press.* September 15, 1988; 1A.
2. Critical Condition [Editorial]. *Burlington Free Press.* September 20, 1988; 10A.
3. Gottschalk M. EMS hearings intended for comment, not debate. *Burlington Free Press.* November 15 1988; 1B.
4. Gottschalk M. Rescue personnel raps state. *Burlington Free Press.* December 14, 1988; 1B.
5. State of Vermont, Legislature. Act 63. An act making appropriations for support of state government, included language for "studying and making recommendations for the development of coordinated, effective, and adequately funded system for the prevention and treatment of alcohol and substance abuse additions when they occur in a humane, caring and effective manner." Montpelier, Vt: State of Vermont; 2001.
6. *Report of the Commission on Tobacco, Alcohol, and Substance Abuse Addiction. The Impact of Substance Abuse on the State Budget.* Montpelier, Vt: Legislative Counsel; December 2001. Available at http://www.leg.state.vt.us/reports/reports2.htm. Accessed April 2005.
7. Sneyd R. Heroin treatment in dispute. *Burlington Free Press.* February 15, 2001; 1B.
8. Carney JK, Perras TE, Bellino JC, Piasecki MA, Dorey LF. Vermont's heroin action committee: public involvement in setting priorities for action. Abstract presented at 130th Annual Meeting of APHA. Philadelphia, Pa: November 12, 2002.

9. Vermont Department of Health. Governor's Heroin Action Committee Report. December 2001. Available at: http://www.state.vt.us/health/_admin/pubs/2001/hac2001.htm. Accessed April 7, 2005.

10. Vermont Department of Health. *Vermont Health Plan. A Call to Action.* Burlington, Vt: Vermont Department of Health; 1999. Available at http://www.state.vt.us/health/healthplan99.htm. Accessed April 2005.

11. Tobacco Task Force. Blueprint for a Tobacco-Free Vermont: Final Report. Montpelier, Vt: Vermont Tobacco Task Force, 1999. Available at http://www.leg.state.vt.us/tobacco/finalreport.pdf. Accessed March 28, 2005.

12. CDC. *Best Practices for Comprehensive Tobacco Control Programs.* Atlanta, Ga: CDC; August 1999.

13. Remsen N. Poll: Fewer smoke than people think. *Burlington Free Press.* September 30, 1999; 1A.

14. Vermont Department of Health. Vermont Best Practices to cut smoking rates in half by 2010. Burlington, Vt: Vermont Department of Health, 2000. Available at http://www.healthyvermonters.info/hi/tobacco/pubs/tobacco2000.htm. Accessed April 2005.

CHAPTER 47

Don't Just Preach to the Choir

Nearly every profession and discipline has its own language. Patients hear complicated medical phrases during visits to a hospital or doctor's office. Microbiologists speak easily about microorganisms that are hard to pronounce. We all know of attorneys who speak "legalese" and professors who speak in complicated linguistic terms when simple words will do. We have our own language in public health, with terms such as "assessment," "policy making," and "assurance," terms we all understand, although they may carry many different meanings to those not in our field. To an epidemiologist, nearly every risk is, well, relative. We talk about "essential public health services" and "core functions," which don't refer to eating, sleeping, or breathing, but instead include preventing epidemics, promoting healthy behaviors, responding to disasters, monitoring the health of the population, and so on. There are many different reasons that complicated terminology exists in different disciplines and professions, but in public health the use of such language can prevent us from developing the kinds of broad relationships that are needed to protect and improve public health and develop valuable and long-term constituencies and colleagues in public health.

We tend, as a habit, to preach to the choir, and speak to those other professionals or groups who understand our language and whose work, at least in part, intersects with some of our own. It's easy to understand why; it's easy, it's comfortable, and it becomes a habit. We talk in our strongest terms, in our loudest singing voices to those who will nod their heads and agree. It's a hard habit to break, but to improve public health, we have to think of new audiences to convince, new people to explain health to, new constituencies to develop, to work with us in many areas of public health, some of them global, some more specific to the issues. There are examples and strategies to help think about who we work with and how we communicate with them.

To reduce childhood lead poisoning, we had to work closely with, and convince, Vermont physicians that this was a real and serious problem. We actually had to prove it to them by conducting a prevalence study and talking about the results. We had to show them the data and prove our case with science. And even more importantly, to get at the root of the problem, we had to invite new people to the table, people who were not our usual colleagues, and we had to get to know and work side by side with the housing community, because the most important risk factor for severe lead poisoning in children was the age of our housing stock and the possibility that lead paint had been used. It took some time. We spent time together in meetings, task forces, in the legislature, and later worked together when each of us was applying for grant funds. We shared the same interest in protecting the health of young children without making them homeless, and our priority became theirs and vice versa.

In our fight against tobacco, we worked with physicians, nurses, and hospitals, and statewide educational programs developed by the University of Vermont's College Of Medicine to help people quit smoking. We worked with the American Cancer Society to develop and promote a toll-free number. But we also thought of another group of health professionals who saw patients more often than physicians—dentists, and worked with them to develop another new approach to reinforce our critical health message. We had an excellent working relationship with the state dental society and an ongoing relationship with dentists to improve access to dental health throughout Vermont, especially for children. Dentists and dental hygienists had a critical role to play in tobacco prevention and cessation because they saw patients on a regular basis and were skilled in educating patients about their health. The dental society convened an advisory committee and developed a program to provide training to dental practices in tobacco prevention and cessation. They did this in the dentist's own office and the program was funded by funds from the tobacco Master Settlement Agreement.[1]

The dentists first developed a curriculum that included lectures, slides, and written materials that focused on the training needs of these professionals. Specially trained dental health professionals recruited dental practices and began to train staff in dental offices throughout the state. Continuing education credits were offered as an incentive to increase participation. About half of all dental practices in Vermont were trained in just over a 2-year period.[1] Dental offices were now part of our war against tobacco, and when individuals saw TV ads about the quit-smoking toll-free number, they might later hear something similar during a dental visit. These efforts were not only inexpensive and practical, they broadened the use of consistent messages about smoking through many different channels. We had new partners in the difficult task to cut smoking in half by the year 2010.

Promoting increased consumption of fruits and vegetables was also a priority for public health. We worked with federal agencies and schools to promote consumption of five fruits and vegetables per day. It was a priority area of *Healthy Vermonters 2000*[2] and *Healthy Vermonters 2010,* our blueprint for improved public health.[3] Reported fruit and vegetable consumption was initially less than two servings per day, and educational efforts tried to raise awareness of the importance of fruit and vegetables in a healthy diet. With limited funding, schools were linked to grocery stores by creating partnerships between local stores of three major grocery chains and local elementary schools. Each store contributed three servings of fruit and vegetables per child each school day for a month. The teacher used the produce of the day in all subjects in the classroom, and children were taught about and exposed to new fruits and vegetables in the classroom environment. Parents, schools, and local grocery stores benefited from this new partnership. We took the message to schools and grocery stores to find new ways to promote health.[4]

In another example, each year health promotion staff would organize a workplace wellness conference, inviting in national speakers and businesses in an effort to create new avenues for health promotion. An introduction at these conferences provided an opportunity for me to speak with representatives from many different types of businesses from different parts of the state. We brought our Healthy Vermonters theme to the workplace, and focused on protecting health and preventing injuries, low-cost strategies to improve worker's health, and many other topics. The workplace was an ideal location to provide health messages,[5] with such settings having been used to promote the benefits of early detection for breast cancer. The availability of health promotion information whether related to quitting smoking, being physically active, eating a better diet, and understanding the importance of cancer screening, could only help promote health through places where people spent so much of their time. We also focused on protecting health, such as preventing repetitive motion or other injuries. Educational strategies in the workplace gave a new place to promote health, as well as the opportunity to create new partnerships.

We worked with church groups, cancer survivors, environmental advocacy groups, businesses, grocery store chains, health professionals in many disciplines, allied health professionals, school principals, school nurses, veterinarians, game wardens, maple syrup producers, dental hygienists, every government agency imaginable, people with HIV, police, children, and individual citizens. Strategies to develop multidisciplinary approaches to public health issues, such as cancer, tobacco, and preventing lead poisoning, required many different and sometimes new partnerships to impact the issue.

The Institute of Medicine cites the need to develop new partnerships as an area for action and change for public health in this century.[6] Our own strategies involved thinking about who should be involved that we hadn't yet thought of and why would they be interested? Grocery stores served local communities, and what benefited health in elementary schools was also good for their stores. Workplaces want healthier workers, and practical, low-cost strategies to keep the workforce healthy and to promote both business and health. In addition to these "win-win" situations, over time, more and more organizations became partners in public health. I thought about them as our "colleagues in public health," essential to successfully addressing a health issue and being another voice for public health in our state. We tried to translate public health technical language into words that would reach farther than those in our department, farther than our traditional colleagues. We realized that it is important to not just preach to the choir, but to go outside the usual partnerships and consider new colleagues in public health.

REFERENCES

1. Carney JK, Garbarino KM, Ivey RT. Oral health means no tobacco: Vermont dental health professionals join the statewide effort. Abstract presented at the 130th Annual Meeting of the American Public Health Association, November 13, 2002. Philadelphia, Pa.
2. Vermont Department of Health. *Healthy Vermonters 2000.* Burlington, Vt: Vermont Department of Health; 1992.
3. Vermont Department of Health. *Healthy Vermonters 2010.* Burlington, Vt: Vermont Department of Health; 2000.

4. Ewing JF, Wick JR, Carney JK, Flynn BS, Harvey-Berino J. 5-A-Day: A unique partnership between education, business, and health. Abstract presented at the American Public Health Association annual meeting, Washington, DC, October 1994.
5. Blackburn M. Official: employers have best shot to deliver health message. *Burlington Free Press.* October 13, 1993; 1B.
6. Institute of Medicine. *The Future of Public Health in the 21st Century.* Washington, DC: The National Academies Press; 2003.

48

Walking the Extra Mile for Children's Health—Door-to-Door Lead Screening

Reducing childhood lead poisoning in Vermont was a tremendous challenge. It was an ambitious but achievable goal of *Healthy Vermonters 2000* to reduce the percentage of children who had elevated lead levels.[1] Not only did we have to overcome the misperception that this was an urban issue, that we were immune from these problems, we had to convince physicians, parents, and legislators. We worked hard with health and housing groups, parent advocates, and many others to change course, set policy, pass needed laws, get kids screened, and prevent lead poisoning in children all over the state. Some efforts, including widespread public education, those involving policy, and free screening clinics, were extended statewide. Some efforts were local.

Many state health departments had been trapped in the conflicts between providing direct care, usually to those without health insurance, and carrying out what others call the "essential public health services" of public health,[2] everything from preventing epidemics and responding to disasters to providing direct services as needed, and linking people to health services.

In Vermont, we had made conscious policy choices to expand access to health care, first for pregnant women and young children, and later to include nearly all children and many adults. As a consequence, we decreased funding and capacity to have "well child clinics," clinic visits that were similar to those provided in physician's offices. We worked hard to create partnerships with private physician offices, as the policy of covering more and more children increased financial access. Public health carried out its core duties of assuring quality and accessibility of health care through a collaboration and partnership with health providers throughout the state.

One of the duties of the health department was still to "provide direct services as needed," and when we were trying to prevent lead poisoning in Vermont children, we took a look at all the steps needed to include lead screening in the basic preventive health care intended for all young children. After the Centers for Disease Control and Prevention (CDC) called attention to the new and lowered definition for lead poisoning,[3] it became clear that if harmful effects on children's learning and behavior could be seen at lower levels, the emphasis had to shift to prevention, not an easy task. Educational efforts aimed at physicians and parents, new laboratory methods, free screening, laws to protect people during renovations by the use of standards and certification for workers, were just some of the needed steps.

In Vermont, most of the potential for lead poisoning was from the age of our housing stock—we had much housing built prior to 1978. Pre-1978 rental housing subsequently became a focus for legislative action and educational efforts. We also decided that, despite our reluctance to duplicate efforts available in physician offices, the demand for testing was so great, and the testing so time consuming (inadequate cleaning of the skin before a screening test could lead to a falsely positive test) and the public health issue so urgent that we decided to promote free lead-screening clinics run by public health nurses to bridge the gap in health care services until we could incorporate these screening tests into regular preventive care in doctor's offices.

Our partnership with housing agencies and local communities continued to grow and strengthen around preventing lead poisoning, and despite the fact that more children were being screened in free clinics, we decided to go door-to-door to try and screen more children at high risk. We worked with the city of Burlington, Vermont's largest city, to identify and screen children at risk of lead poisoning. Nearly three quarters of the housing stock in what was called the "Old North End" was built prior to 1939 and likely contained lead paint. The mayor estimated that 80% of the more than 5000 homes and apartments contained lead-based paint. Both door-to-door lead screening and lead hazard reduction was part of this effort. A public information strategy gave the neighborhood advance notice of the campaign, and a press conference with the mayor, director of the housing and conservation board, and myself let people know this was happening. Local television stations and newspapers carried the story.[4,5]

Public health nurses and environmental risk assessors from the health department worked as a team going door to door in the 30-block area of the city's oldest section. Free lead testing was offered to any child under age six, done right there in his or her own home. It was also noted whether or not the residence contained chipping or peeling paint. Public health nurses provided information about lead poisoning and what the results meant to residents of the children they screened. Limited funds and loans were available to prevent lead paint from causing health problems in young children.[4]

During the screening campaign, nearly 90 children were tested for lead poisoning, with nearly 80% not having been screened before. Almost half had levels over 10 μg/dl, the definition of lead poisoning. Five children were found, and later confirmed, to have levels higher than 20 μg/dl, the definition of severely lead poisoned.[5,6]

This effort was done during a week in the summer. Public health nurses went door to door in these neighborhoods, providing parents with information about lead poisoning and practical steps they could take to reduce their children's exposure to lead. They came prepared to take a capillary blood screening sample from eligible children, which involved careful cleaning of the child's finger and taking a small amount of blood after a finger stick. They talked to individuals and families home that week. They didn't know how many children there were or if the children had already been screened. But they found many children who never had a lead test and many parents who were not aware of the health issue.

We thought that our public information efforts and efforts to provide free screening clinics had been extensive. Despite this, the vast majority of children the nurses tested had never been screened, results showed that nearly half met the definition of lead poisoning, and some severely poisoned children were found. Working with the City of Burlington, part of the city was identified that would likely have the majority of housing with lead-based paint, and the nurses took it from there. As symptoms would not occur until levels were much higher, these results gave the opportunity to intervene with education, environmental advice, or remedies, and permit follow-up with these families to minimize the effects of lead exposure on the child's health. Elsewhere in Vermont, public health nurses reached out in this way in their local communities, finding many children who had never been screened for lead poisoning.[7] Media coverage helped provide advance warning and public education, and although our effort was not necessarily time efficient, based on what we found, it was needed.

Sometimes you just have to walk the extra mile. Even when you think you are making it easy for people to understand about a public health issue and even make the service free, sometimes that still isn't enough. It's not that simple to improve health, because there are many additional barriers to good health, even after people have health insurance. We learned over the years just how big those barriers can be, and that if you want to improve the health of the entire population, you needed to work very hard to get through all the reasons that people were not receiving services, in this case screening for lead poisoning.

We did not know exactly why these children had not been screened before, we could only guess. Despite efforts to reach the public in easy to understand language, despite free clinics and a toll-free number, information about preventing childhood lead poisoning did not reach every Vermont family. Transportation may have prevented some from going to a clinic. We did not know why, but knew that despite all the efforts made, that sometimes you have to make an extra effort, walk the extra mile. Sometimes, in public health, you just have to go door to door.

REFERENCES

1. Vermont Department of Health. *Healthy Vermonters 2000.* Burlington, Vt: Vermont Department of Health; 1992.
2. Turnock BJ. Public Health: What It Is and How It Works. 2nd ed. Gaithersburg, Md: Aspen Publishers, Inc; 2001:327.
3. CDC. *Preventing Lead Poisoning in Young Children: A Statement by the Centers for Disease Control and Prevention.* Atlanta, Ga: US Department of Health and Human Services; 1991.
4. Bazilchuk N. Lead-prevention program to blanket Old North End. *Burlington Free Press.* August 29, 1995; 1B.
5. Carney JK, Garbarino KM, Keating KO. Reaching children at risk: door-to-door lead screening. Abstract presented at the annual meeting of the American Public Health Association. New York, NY: November, 1996.
6. Bazilchuk N. Children show high lead levels. Problem plagues Old North End. *Burlington Free Press.* October 7, 1995; 1A.
7. O'Connor K. Lead Poison Screenings For Children. *Rutland Herald.* August 19, 1996; 11.

49

Pertussis—If You Look, You Will Find It

A small news article in mid-December carried the headline "Whooping cough kills 15-month-old" and warned residents of three Vermont counties—Essex, Orleans, and Caledonia, to immunize their children against whooping cough. The health department toll-free number was listed and symptoms were described.[1] In early December, two cases of pertussis were confirmed in young children in the northeastern corner of Vermont, called the Northeast Kingdom. The bacterium that causes pertussis, or whooping cough, Bordetella pertussis was also identified in an unimmunized child who had died.[2] Whooping cough was highly contagious, with vaccination of young children offering the best protection, and the health department investigated reports of cases and recommended antibiotic treatment for both adults and children in close contact with infected individuals to reduce the possible spread, severe illness, and even death in very young children.[2] A day later, newspapers around the state carried further details,[3-6] and the state's largest paper carried the headline "Victim of whooping cough belonged to sect: Island Pond church shuns medical treatment".[7] The article stated that the child who died was one of many unvaccinated children belonging to the Church at Island Pond. The physician at the local health center was interviewed and related his discussion of childhood immunizations with members of the church since the death of the child. The state epidemiologist, being careful not to discuss confidential information, talked about "the unvaccinated group", how the health department and the local physicians were working together and had given the antibiotic erythromycin to people to prevent further disease spread. He also told the reporter that since there were three cases of pertussis, (including one in a vaccinated individual) a more general public health warning was indicated. In addition, contact with schools and day-care centers was also recommended.[7] In order to determine the cause of the unexpected death the deputy state medical examiner was also involved, and spoke gently to the reporter about the situation.[7]

Deaths, especially of a child, were uncommon, and prompted intense scrutiny from the news media, and although the state epidemiologist was careful to speak generally, reporters had gathered detailed information about the child involved, and also about the church community. It was often difficult to make a rapid and precise diagnosis of whooping cough, because the early symptoms were like so many other common respiratory illnesses. But pertussis was confirmed, and indeed if many children were not vaccinated, there was a very real and serious risk to other members of the church community, and maybe further. The reporter chronicling the situation noted that this particular church had, at least in the past, not been accepting of medical treatment and dealt with health issues within their own community, historically not even registering births or deaths with the state. The church, according to news reports, also had its own cemetery.[7]

Pertussis, or whooping cough, is a highly contagious disease, caused by the bacterium Bordetella pertussis and is characterized by severe coughing spasms, called paroxysms.[8] The incubation period is about a week to ten days, and symptoms start with those seen with a cold or mild respiratory infection.[8] Very young children, particularly infants are more likely to have a more serious illness, have complications, need to be cared for in a hospital, and are more likely to die.[8]

The community where the child died, and where whooping cough was suspected, had not had a peaceful relationship with the state. The Northeast Kingdom Community Church (also called the Island Pond Church and the Community at Island Pond) was located in the northeast kingdom of Vermont, in a town called Brighton. On June 22, 1984, there was a raid on the Community Church by state officials. Vermont state police, social workers, and others went to 20 homes at daybreak investigating reports of child abuse, gathering up more than 100 children, and taking them by bus to the courthouse in Newport. The District Judge ruled against the state, the children could not be detained, and the state did not appeal.[9] This episode happened long before the pertussis investigation, but because of the intense controversy around this event, relationship between the Community Church and the state was not one of trust. In Vermont, the health department, although it had local offices throughout Vermont, was indeed a state agency, and the handling of the investigation had to be done respecting what had happened there in the past.

Handling this situation would be complicated as past practices involved a preference to handle health problems within the community whenever possible. Efforts to promote immunizations, would likely be counterproductive, and probably create a wall to further cooperation. However, community residents had been working with a local physician and the state epidemiologist told one reporter that "we're encouraged by the rapport we have developed with the population at risk." Warnings had been well publicized in the newspapers in the immediate area as well as in all counties in the northeastern corner of Vermont, as there were now more suspected cases.[3] The warning included the advice to be sure their children had up-to-date vaccinations, detailed symptoms, and the toll-free number of the health department. The state epidemiologist also reminded people that immunizations could be obtained free at the local district offices of the health department located in Newport and St. Johnsbury.[3] One newspaper reported at least 10 suspected cases in the Northeast Kingdom,[3] and later news reports informed the public that the outbreak was still being investigated.[10]

In this unique situation, it was necessary to act with incomplete information, when a child had died, with a diagnosis that was difficult, time moving too fast, and a lingering distrust of the state. The usual approach would not have worked, with public health being more prominent and the state epidemiologist playing an active, visible role. But because there was still a level of distrust of the state, health department staff worked quickly and quietly with a local physician and local public health nurses in nearby areas. Epidemiology staff had to work more in the background, and facilitate the best possible management of the situation through local personnel. The strategies to issue public warnings about the disease being confirmed, remind the general public about the need to make sure children were up to date on immunizations, and provide antibiotics to limit the spread of illness among this closely-knit community, were the best options at the time. From an epidemiology perspective, one looks at numerators and especially denominators, but there was never a denominator, and never a clear picture of the total number of children at risk, as the state epidemiologist described them as the "unvaccinated group."[7] The situation was closely monitored for some time,[10] having already taken its toll.

Although this happened in 1989, it was the beginning of a long-term public health relationship with pertussis, and the challenges faced in preventing harm in young children, something seen across the country. Nationally, until the mid-1900's, pertussis was a major cause of childhood deaths in our country, decreasing with the introduction of pertussis vaccine, and increasing since the 1980's.[8] The history of outbreaks tended to by cyclical, with epidemics every three or four years, and in 1996, there were nearly 8000 cases reported to the CDC, the highest number since 1967.[8] Pertussis can occur in people of any age, vaccinated or not, although vaccinated children often have milder illness, and infants are more likely to need hospitalization and die[8]. One of the difficulties in tracking and reducing the spread of pertussis, is that older teenagers and adults may be misdiagnosed as having another type of coughing illness[8], because the early symptoms are similar.

Pertussis has been seen in older children and adults, in vaccinated individuals. In Vermont, in 1996, an outbreak of pertussis was described and several key factors that helped us manage further outbreaks and contribute to national efforts [11]. In the first six months of 1996, ten confirmed cases of pertussis were seen in Vermont. Later in the same year, three cases were seen in very young infants, less than four months old. An alert was sent to Vermont physicians in primary care and emergency departments to remind them of pertussis, in patients of all ages. During the remainder of that year, a total of 280 pertussis cases were reported, for an incidence rate of 47.6 per 100,000 people, and it was noted that the highest rate occurred in children aged 10 to 14 years old. Nearly a quarter of the cases were in individuals older than 20 years. Symptoms were similar to those previously described and included coughing spasms (paroxysms) most commonly, with coughs lasting an average of more than a month. Nearly 70% of the school-aged children had received four of more doses of Pertussis vaccine.[11]

The intense education strategy was to keep physicians fully informed and included alerts mailed during three separate times, along with mailings to school nurses, school principals, child-care providers, and many others. In schools where children were diagnosed with whooping cough, letters were sent home to parents to let them know about the illness in their child's school, remind them of the symptoms, and encourage them to seek medical care if such symptoms were present. Guidelines for precautionary antibiotics for close contacts were followed, and other small group settings such as clubs and after-school activities, were identified to find contacts of ill children.[11]

During 1997, cases decreased dramatically, but in 1996 the rate of pertussis in Vermont was higher than any other state in that year,[11] despite a record number of reported cases nationally.[8] Although difficult, the use of cultures to confirm clinical cases helped and public health education efforts helped to raise awareness throughout the state. Vaccination rates in Vermont are some of the highest in the nation, but the high numbers of cases in school aged children, when immunity was believed to wane and vaccines not able to be given, contributed to the complexity of dealing with this situation. The ultimate goal of the public health response included maintaining high immunization rates, public and professional education, testing and using appropriate antibiotics was to protect very young infants.

Pertussis didn't go away. In 1998, 72 cases had been confirmed as of December, and eight in Caledonia County, part of the Northeast Kingdom. The local paper wrote an article about the cases seen in the county, how it is potentially fatal in very young children and how it is spread, and what symptoms were important to look for.[12] Our epidemiologist talked about the previous two bad years, and that she felt that we had the second highest incidence of documented pertussis in the country because we did a better job at finding it. School nurses in the area reiterated vaccine recommendations for the diphtheria-pertussis-tetanus shots.[12] News reports[13] including an editorial, reminded the public that "An Old Foe Persists".[14]

In 2001, 113 confirmed cases of pertussis were reported in Vermont, [15] and during the period of 1997-2001, Vermont ranked first or second nationally in pertussis rates or incidence, with cultures accounting for 45% to 58% of the confirmed cases. This happened despite the fact that Vermont had strict definitions and criteria used to define and document cases. Did Vermont have more pertussis than other states, or did we just look harder? When this was studied a bit further, we decided that we had been taking many steps over the years to raise the awareness level about the possibility of pertussis among physicians and nurses in our state.

The death reported in 1989 started the cascade, followed by outbreaks in 1993 and 1996, and a total of 10 articles were published in the health department newsletter used most by clinicians in the state. In addition, statewide alerts were mailed to health professionals and there was much media coverage to raise awareness among the general public. The health department laboratory did not charge for testing, and as in other areas, public health nurses in all parts of the state helped arrange testing by linking health care practices and the health department epidemiology unit and our public health laboratory, making it easier to confirm diagnoses. All confirmed cases received extensive follow up, with letters, and preventive antibiotics when indicated, and our relationships with school nurses promoted excellent communication and reporting of children who might be ill with pertussis.[15]

In addition, the source of the reports of pertussis gave us hints as to how well we were educating the public and health professionals. During the time period of 1997–2001, cases of pertussis reported to the health department were most often reports from testing sent to the state public health laboratory; but patients (or people coming into close contact with someone ill with pertussis) commonly reported their illness, as well as reports coming to us from school nurses and physicians. We decided that it was not very likely that Vermont had more pertussis than other states, but instead that we had just done a more intensive job of raising awareness to health care professionals and the public, so that people would think about it more often when there was a prolonged coughing illness, and more likely get tested and diagnosed. And the more cases suspected resulted in more cases being detected, and on and on, called (in Vermont) the "snowball effect".[15]

In 2002, a statewide alert reminded the public that more than 100 cases of pertussis had been reported to the health department and reminding the public and physicians of the symptoms and what to do.[16] Fact sheets were available, describing the disease in non-technical language and we expected to see reported cases of pertussis in Vermont in the future. Fortunately, the Federal Food and Drug Administration has approved a vaccine to help protect adolescents from pertussis,[17] a single booster shot to adolescents from aged 10 to 18 years old, and it is hoped that at least some of what we saw, diagnosed, and managed, will be preventable sometime in the future. Efforts continue among physicians to remind their peers that pertussis is not just a disease seen in children and the importance of recognizing this in adults is to prevent transmission to vulnerable infants.[18] In 2005, CDC reported that whooping cough is endemic in the United States, with epidemics every 3-4 years, and that nearly 26,000 cases were reported in the United States in 2004, representing the highest number since 1959.[19]

Preventing epidemics and the spread of infectious diseases has been a cornerstone of public health, and one of the areas best understood and supported by the public. In the last 10 to 15 years, however, we have seen renewed challenges in this area of public health, unlikely to stop in the near future. The challenges of new infectious diseases, challenges in animal and human health, vaccine limitations and shortages, virulent forms of common bacteria, multi-drug resistant forms of infections and old infections showing up in new places, whether geographically or in different age groups where they might not be immediately suspected, presents new and urgent challenges and continues to test our ability to pivot and respond quickly to protect the public.

In addition to educating health professionals to be alert, the parallel challenge of educating the public on these issues is even greater and essential to the most effective practice of public health. A surveillance system for infectious diseases is only as good as the communication that goes with it—if the test is not performed, it can't be reported. For some communicable diseases, such as pertussis, you have to look for the disease, be aware of it, and think of it, all during busy days when many other common diseases produce similar symptoms. In public health, one of our roles is to make sure health professionals and the public know to look for a disease and understand the symptoms. From our experiences, we learned that if you look hard, you will find it—by educating health professionals, parents and schools, and the public, when the opportunities arose, through the media.

Sometimes it takes more than the usual efforts, the usual system, and the usual comfort, to find and take steps to prevent infectious diseases, in this case to prevent serious illness or death in our youngest citizens. One of the risks of being aggressive in our efforts to raise awareness, educate physicians and the public about a contagious illness, and seeing the Vermont snowball effect[15] is to have to explain why our state has all this whooping cough. In reality we didn't think that we did, but that we just looked harder to find it, and when the public is used to hearing you talk about an illness, why it is important to understand the symptoms, get medical attention if they have them, vaccinate their children, and call for more information, and they trust your work, they will also understand when you explain why the rates may look higher than some other states. We always believed that it was better to find the disease and try and do something about it, rather than maybe have a false sense of security and that public confidence would be much higher in a department that was on the case, each and every one, despite the fact that resources were limited, in order to best do their job. With whooping cough, we looked hard to find it, found it often, told physicians, nurses, and the public about it, because we felt it was our best way to protect public health.

REFERENCES

1. The Associated Press. Whooping cough kills 15-month-old. The *Burlington Free Press*. December 13, 1989.
2. Vermont Department of Health. Pertussis Outbreak in Vermont. Disease Control Bulletin. December 1989
3. Whooping Cough Warning Out. Caledonian-Record. December 13, 1989; 1.
4. The Associated Press. Whooping Cough Cases Reported. Rutland Herald. December 13, 1989; 13.
5. The Associated Press. Baby's Death in Island Pond Prompts Warnings. Rutland Herald. December 15, 1989; 12.
6. Baby who Died of Whooping Cough Member of Church at Island Pond. Caledonian-Record December 14, 1989; 2.
7. Hemingway S. Victim of whooping cough belonged to sect. Island Pond church shuns medical treatment. *Burlington Free Press*. December 14, 1989; 1.
8. Centers for Disease Control and Prevention. Guideline for the Control of Pertussis Outbreaks. Chapter 1, Background. Centers for Disease Control and Prevention: Atlanta, GA, 2000.
9. Northeast Kingdom, Island Pond, Brighton, VT. Town History (courtesty of the Center for Rural Studies). www.vermonter.com/nek/islandpond3.asp Accessed June 7, 2005.
10. The Associated Press. Whooping Cough Investigated. *Rutland Herald*. February 5, 1990; 8.
11. Centers for Disease Control and Prevention. Pertussis outbreak – Vermont, 1996. Morbidity and Mortality Weekly Report 1997; 46:822-6.
12. Whooping Cough Escalates in Area. The Caledonia-Record. December 10, 1998. Available at http://www.caledoniarecord.com. Accessed February 27, 2005.
13. The Associated Press. Whooping cough rate up. *Burlington Free Press*. December 9, 2000; 3B.
14. An Old Foe Persists. (Editorial). *Burlington Free Press* December 9, 2000; 6A.
15. Schoenfeld, SE, Zanardi, LR, Carney JK. Pertussis Vermont: Seek and you will find it? Abstract presented at 37th National Immunization Conference, Chicago, IL, March 17-20, 2003.

16. Vermont Department of Health. Health Officials issue statewide pertussis alert. News alert. Burlington, Vt: Vermont Department of Health; October 23, 2002. Available at http://www.healthyvermonters.info/admin/releases/102302pertussis.shtml Accessed May 18, 2005.
17. First Combination Vaccine Approved to Help Protect Adolescents Against Whooping Couth. U.S. Food and Drug Administration, FDA Talk Paper, May 3, 2005. www.fda.gov/bbs/topics/ANSWERS/2005/ANS01354.html
18. Dworkin MS. Adults are Whooping, but Are Internists Listening? Ann Intern Med 2005; 142:832-835.
19. CDC. Recommended Antimicrobial Agents for the Treatment and Postexposure Prophylaxis of Pertussis. 2005. MMWR 54(RR-14); 1-16.

A Vision for Health Planning

In Vermont, healthy planning has taken on different forms, shifted to a variety of free-standing agencies and government departments, and struggled to address the increasingly complex and costly health care needs of the population. The Certificate of Need was the basis of health planning for many years and decisions were made, at different times, by the Vermont Department of Health, a Certificate of Need Review Board (with an additional Certificate of Need Appeals Board), the Health Policy Council, a Vermont Health Care Authority, and later folded into the state Department of Banking, Insurance, Securities, and Health Care Administration (BISHCA). Health plans were titled Health Resource Management Plans (HRMP or "Hurrump" for short), the State Health Plan, Health Resource Management Plan, and most recently the Health Resource Allocation Plan.[1] Various forms of public oversight have been utilized, from a broad-based body called the Health Policy Council to a Public Oversight Commission. In the various forms, responsibilities included reviewing Certificate of Need applications. Debates symptomatic of the difficulty in controlling health care costs and improving access to needed health services in a largely rural state frequently entered these discussions in the 1990s during many efforts, both legislative and administrative, to improve access, quality, and control costs of health care.

Throughout this time, we worked to improve our ability to interject public health and the improvement of health into the debate on health care, and particularly costs, with varying degrees of success. Our presence and expertise in health promotion and disease prevention, was evident in the HRMP, but less so in Certificate of Need discussions. During one particular change in the law, the responsibility for producing the state health plan was shifted to the Agency of Human Services, the umbrella agency containing the Department of Health.[2]

We were directed by the legislature to "adopt a state health plan that sets the goals and values of the state."[3,4] The legislature directed the creation of a different kind of health plan, one that took a broader view of health, that included health care, but also the other factors that impacted health. Public input was sought by health department public health nurses who traveled throughout the state asking citizens open-ended questions about what was needed to improve health and what keeps us from improving it. Barriers to the improvement of health were identified and became an important part of the plan.[3,4]

Emphasis was placed on those aspects of health care that improved health, such as primary and preventive care, and the other factors that impacted health in the broadest sense. This shifted the plan from a sole focus on the health care delivery system (though there was much about health care included), and emphasized all areas related to improving health outcomes, defined by the scientific and public health literature, and buttressed by public input.[3]

We emphasized the need for community and social change, and educating the public to be wiser consumers of health care and how they could prevent premature illnesses in themselves and their families. We noted the enormous expenditures by our nation per capita on health care, but that only a tiny percentage was spent on preventing these same conditions. The challenge was to increase the way we prevented diseases and promoted health, while at the same time, assuring access to high-quality health care services.

Before the public health nurses interviewed a single person, we started with a simple chart that looked like a pie with five wedges—one wedge each for all the broad categories that impacted health: human biology and genetics, habits and behaviors, our changing environment, economics and social factors, and health care.[4] There was no way that we knew to precisely estimate the size of the wedges, so we made them all equal size, the intent being to frame the type and role of health care services in improving health outcomes. Personal habits and behaviors included smoking, alcohol use, nutrition, physical activity, seat belt use, hand washing, and others. The environment included workplaces, safe food products, drinking water, housing, indoor air, and emerging infectious diseases. Biology included inherited or genetic risks, aging, and new diseases. Economic and social factors included income and jobs; education, cultural, racial, and ethnic diversity; and community assets. Health care included access to primary and preventive care, health insurance, emergency care, counseling, dental care, health care quality, and control of infectious diseases.[4]

This framework was presented to the public by public health nurses during their interviews across the state, when they interviewed over 3000 citizens. This framework was also presented in special interviews with government officials, legislators, hospital administrators, nonprofit organizations, advocacy groups, and health and education leaders. People were asked questions about what was needed in each of these broad areas, and what was getting in the way of improving health.[3,4] These attempts to gather qualitative information across Vermont supported the extensive range of factors that impacted health, with goals that were consistent with *Healthy People 2010.*[5]

All this information was used, along with measures of the health status of the population, to develop recommended actions in each area. Each of the broad areas contained further categories and actions, data for related health status indicators and trends, simple descriptions of the relationship of the issue to improving health, along with direct quotes from people interviewed.[4]

The broad category of human biology included such needed actions as further reducing the infant mortality, ensuring that all Vermont women obtain early comprehensive prenatal care, ensuring child care was consistent with early education principles, promoting healthy behaviors throughout life, and assuring adequate geriatric care. In the area of the new genetics the action needed was to integrate genetics research into medical and public health practice, and use new discoveries in genetics to strengthen public health messages. In the broad category of habits and behaviors, health actions for children and adolescents focused on helping youth make positive choices in their teen years, emphasizing the problems of smoking, alcohol, and marijuana use. Specific attention was paid to the challenges of 18- to 24-year-olds. Nutrition and phys-ical activity measures at all ages were emphasized. In the area of the environ-ment, recommended actions included expanding disease surveillance, judicious use of antibiotics, tracking diseases in Vermont's animal population, and the relation of animal and human health. Vermonters interviewed understood the link between education and income to health and the health of their families. Recommended actions included encouraging communities to use data to set goals to improve their community's health, and increasing civic participation and social connections.[4]

The section on health care included the role of primary care, preventive care, dental health, access and quality of care, control of infectious diseases, and links to public health, all aspects of health and medical care that had potential to improve health outcomes. Emphasis on preventive health care was emphasized, including those clinical services with documented efficacy to pre-vent or detect diseases early in their more treatable forms, such as immuniza-tions for children and adults, as well as improving insurance coverage in these areas. Emphasis on primary care in a rural state was essential, and one of the challenges facing Vermont was to address those areas of the state that remained fragile with respect to a supply of primary care professionals. Improving oral health involved not only dental care, but understanding the cost saving poten-tial of community fluoridation. Assuring an adequate supply of dentists and dental hygienists was cited as an action, as was increasing the role of these health professionals in preventing tobacco use. Links between public health and health care, which had resulted in high childhood immunization rates and high rates of early prenatal care, demonstrated the effectiveness of these strate-gies, but the growing impact of chronic illnesses and their risk factors in an aging society made these linkages even more urgent.[4]

The cumulative list of actions needed in all these areas was long, but they highlighted the importance of the links between habits and behaviors, social and economic factors, the environment, human biology and genetics on health, in addition to those elements of health care that have the greatest impact on improving the health of the population. During this time, there was also tremendous momentum in human services, with the larger umbrella agency working to mobilize Vermont communities and each year define the social health status of Vermont communities in a way that focused on measur-able outcomes and focused community energy to both health and well-being of communities in Vermont.

Why all the changes in health planning? Part of the difficulty stems from the federal history of health planning, and the costs and complexities of the health care system. In parallel, though, there was much support given to improving health outcomes, both from a public health perspective and one that empha-sized and quantified the social factors strongly linked to health. However, health planning stills means different things to different people and is weighted heavily towards health care planning.

So how does all this relate to health planning and improving the health of the population? The health plan we developed put forth a vision, but it still needed a much stronger connection to the existing health care delivery system, where most data (particularly regarding costs) and planning activity had occurred. Although ties between primary and preventive care and public health were strong, defining and articulating the links between those factors that determine how healthy we can be as individuals, families, and communities, needed to be stronger. And, in an environment focused on outcomes and costs, there needed to be even stronger quantitative links and more public education relating the science that links broad determinants of health to health outcomes, particularly in the areas of social, educational, economic, racial, ethnic, and cultural factors. Such data would make it easier to bridge the health care, public health, and human service gaps. More recent efforts try to better link health planning and resource allocation, has incorporated the assessment of community needs.

We need to figure out how to better integrate the entire discussion of health care with a focus on health. A vision for health includes a vision for health care, but must also do more, much more, to improve the health of our population. Most health spending is directed to medical care and related research, with estimates exceeding 90%,[6] despite the fact that behavior and environmental factors contribute to nearly three quarters of the preventable deaths in our country.[7] Although health care is a critical determinant of health, with lack of health insurance creating a huge barrier to health care (along with potential gaps in mental health, substance abuse, dental health, and preventive care), social, educational, economic, environmental, and behavioral factors are also major contributors to the public's health, particularly with regard to preventable diseases and conditions.[8]

One of the six recommended areas of action and change for public health in this century is to adopt a public health approach that "considers the multiple determinants of health," recognizing the importance of this and other recommended changes as broad trends occur, such as continued the growth and aging of our population, along with increasing racial and ethnic diversity.[8]

Did our approach succeed? Have we shifted health care planning to health planning that systematically incorporates the broad determinants of health? Not yet, but the process used to define it, including the public's knowledge of these factors and their responses, and the fact that a plan was put on the table, put us one step closer.

REFERENCES

1. State of Vermont. Acts of the Vermont Legislature. 2003–2004. Act No. 53 (H128) An Act Relating to Hospital and Health Care System Accountability, Capital Spending, and Annual Budgets. Montpelier, Vt: State of Vermont; 2004. Available at http://www.leg.state.vt.us. Accessed May 2005.
2. State of Vermont. Acts of the Vermont Legislature. 1995–1996. Act No. 180 (S.345) An Act to Coordinate the Oversight and Regulation of Health Care and Health Care Systems. Montpelier, Vt: Available at http://www.leg.state.vt.us. Accessed May 2005.

3. Carney JK, Moffatt SG, Berry P, and Wilcke BR. A new vision for health planning: Abstract presented at 128th Annual meeting of APHA. November 14, 2000. Boston, Ma.
4. Vermont Department of Health. *Vermont Health Plan, A Call to Action.* Burlington, Vt: Vermont Department of Health; 1999. Available at http://www.state.vt.us/health/healthplan99.htm Accessed May 2005.
5. U.S. Department of Health and Human Services. *Healthy People 2010.* Available at: http://www.healthypeople.gov. Accessed September, 30, 2005.
6. McGuiness GM, Williams-Russo P, Knickman JR.The case for more active policy attention to health promotion. *Health Affairs.* 2002;21:78–93.
7. McGuiness GM, Foege WH. Actual causes of death in the United States. *JAMA.* 1993;270:2207–2212.
8. Institute of Medicine. *The Future of the Public's Health in the 21st Century.* Washington, DC: The National Academies Press; 2003:1–45.

PART IV

Challenges

51

Outcomes Are the Bottom Line for Public Health

In many of our public documents and reports, I wrote a personal letter at the beginning to introduce the document. As we introduced our priorities for the year 2010, I wrote in my letter "Dear Vermonter, with the start of a new decade, I am pleased to present *Healthy Vermonters 2010,* our blueprint for continuing to improve the health of Vermonters. We are making progress! Working together we have met or made substantial progress toward more than two thirds of the goals established in *Healthy Vermonters 2000,* the predecessor to this document. For example, since 1990, breast cancer deaths are down, fewer teens are smoking, and childhood lead poisoning has decreased."[1]

This document, called *Healthy Vermonters 2010,* published by the Vermont Department of Health, laid out goals and measurable objectives for the year 2010.[1] The premise was based on the national *Healthy People 2010,*[2] which contained 467 measurable objectives in 28 focus areas and 2 overarching goals to increase the quality and years of healthy life and to eliminate health disparities for all Americans.

It was no coincidence that goals were met or progress made in two thirds of the measurable objectives written in *Healthy Vermonters 2000.* The original process, begun in the early 1990s was a first for public health in Vermont. Not only did the health department invite individuals from outside the health department to participate, but the department worked in partnership with these participants to develop goals and measurable objectives for public health in Vermont.

At the time, the process to review available data and set priorities was designed to not only facilitate communication among different programs and areas of public health within the department, but to begin a longer-term process to connect the health department's work to that of many other groups, agencies, and individuals focusing on improving public health, as well. When I started work in public health in Vermont, I had originally asked myself how I would know if we had succeeded, and ultimately I decided that measurable improvements in health outcomes defined success in public health and my ability to lead the department. *Healthy Vermonters 2010,* although initiated by the health department, was the product of many different groups' and individual's efforts. It was done by working within a broad framework of public health and using national *Healthy People 2010* and Vermont data.

The basic agreement underlying the entire process was that one group, individual, or organization could not hope to impact problems as large and complex as preventing cancer and heart disease, reducing tobacco and alcohol use, or infant mortality. It was recognized that such complex problems, often with broad roots, would not be improved without sustained efforts from a wide range of Vermonters, involving many groups and organizations and extending much farther than the department of health.

In addition, addressing these complex issues would require specific emphasis on needs and barriers for people with limited incomes and education. Methods to successfully impact public health and achieve specific measurable objectives, such as increasing the percentage of primary care providers who counsel about smoking, diet, and cancer screening, would require systematic partnerships with all aspects of health care. One example was that reducing lead poisoning in Vermont children would require working with housing agencies.

These priorities and objectives would need to, over time, be incorporated into policy and planning at many levels. We had to develop and maintain partnerships, ensuring that the priorities of our partner groups included public health. Was it possible to get housing agencies, working to provide more affordable housing, to now think about childhood lead poisoning as a priority? Could we strengthen our relationships with schools such that their health education efforts included science-based curricula designed to prevent HIV, smoking, alcohol and drug use? Could we measure and shift the focus in primary care settings to also include attention to clinical prevention, known to prevent or detect early such conditions as breast and colon cancer? Could we engage legislative representatives and senators, from all political spectra, in an ongoing manner to help us in our efforts to protect and improve public health, an area highlighted in *The Future of Public Health*?[3]

The short answer was yes. The measurable objectives told us where we were and where we needed to go. Our goals told us what we wanted to achieve. The skills we developed by taking the most current scientific and public health knowledge and applying it in the real world through our work with many other groups and organizations would determine our success. Further, by making the goals and objectives our public roadmap or blueprint, we were defining accountability for public health and for ourselves. Our success would be ultimately measured by the results, and our ability to achieve those results depended on our ability to bring others along in the effort.

Although we followed the framework of the Institute of Medicine (IOM) report *The Future of Public Health*[3] that defined the responsibilities of the government public health agency, in assessment, policy development, and assurance, (though I never used those terms outside the building), I realized that achieving this was no small task. The first step was to define a way to set priorities and measure our success. In this framework the accountability for public health in Vermont would be through the results. This approach was a long-term strategy that carried some risk, as we didn't have the resources or the responsibility for the priorities of all these other organizations, but was a way to focus attention on results.

The next step was to put our strategy into practice. The goals that we set for the future were indeed ambitious, but they were achievable if we collectively focused our efforts both within the health department and outside the health department to reach our goals. Addressing these issues, and determining their solutions often involved many groups and organizations requiring a truly multidisciplinary approach, also called an "ecological approach," but what I simply called a "public health approach." Using this approach, we relied on the many day-to-day relationships that we had already developed (or needed to develop) to define, based on the best available science and best practice, our roles and responsibilities in addressing a specific and measurable public health goal.

During the subsequent years, we produced progress reports, highlighting areas where we were making progress and where we were falling short. We outlined simple and focused strategies, based on science and best practice, and incorporated these into easy-to-read documents. Using our data from different sources in different ways, we looked for ways to best define and understand each health issue. We knew which areas we were flying blind in and needed more information, but we never succumbed to the notion that we could not make any progress without another study or more money for an information system. Decisions always had to be made with data that had limitations, and we understood the trade-offs against time and additional resources and the urgency of the problem.

When we released *Healthy Vermonters 2010*, we noted that we had made progress toward or reached more than two thirds of the original objectives.[1] Lawmakers, health care professionals, hospitals, schools, law enforcement, housing agencies, advocacy groups, non-profit organizations, and Vermont's news media all played a role. This meant fewer deaths from breast cancer, less teenagers smoking, declines in childhood lead poisoning, and more flu shots in older Vermonters. More women were getting mammograms and pap tests, alcohol-related motor vehicle deaths were down, child abuse was decreasing, access to early prenatal care had improved, and infant mortality had declined. Childhood immunization rates were among the best in the country. Laws were expanded in the areas of immunizations and clean indoor air. Heart disease and stroke deaths were down and the number of schools teaching HIV prevention had increased. These examples showed us and others that it was indeed possible to make real and measurable progress in many areas of public health.

Results matter and improvements in health outcomes enhance credibility for public health and create momentum. But credibility doesn't only come from success. One editorial writer called our efforts an "unflinching assessment of public health, in plain numbers, as well as aggressive goals for doing better."[4] There was not all good news, and it was just as important to give the bad news in the same breath. Forty percent of adults age 50 years or greater had never had a screening test for colorectal cancer, our second leading cancer killer; nearly a third of youth had used alcohol before 13 years of age; and half of our college students were binge drinking. Only a quarter of adults got regular exercise. Adult smoking, smoking during pregnancy, youth marijuana use, and obesity showed little or no progress and were emphasized as priorities for the next decade.[1] The list of partnering organizations was large and growing, and news coverage reported areas of progress and areas needing more work, emphasizing prevention over treatment. Our largest local paper wrote an editorial called "Blueprint for Better Health"[5] that talked about the priorities for the next decade, and emphasized the need to reduce adult smoking, adolescent drinking, and drug use.

The national process to define *Healthy People 2010* goals and objectives was lengthy and balanced the ideal and the achievable.[2] The use of national data, such as the Behavior Risk Factor Survey (BRFS), provided a way to look across states and counties. But observers noted that our record showed improvements in the delivery of services such as adult immunization or mammograms had been easier to attain than changes in behaviors. Further, where such behavior changes have shown improvements, such as in seat belt use, it has been the result of a multidisciplinary approach.[6,7] Given what we know about the "real killers" of the public–tobacco, poor diet, physical inactivity, and alcohol misuse[8,9,10]–and our variation in health outcomes across the country, it has been argued that these are missed opportunities for health improvement or "public health opportunities in waiting."[7] In Vermont, we tried to highlight the differences in our counties,[11] to better facilitate work at the community level. When a health status report noted that northern Vermont counties had obesity rates significantly worse than the year 2010 goal, one newspaper repeated public health concerns, advising county residents to "get moving".[12]

So what do you do when there is no data? Some authors make the case that before the BRFS we had no way to make national comparisons in many areas.[7] But while efforts are being made to improve data quality, and most certainly to make what data we have into meaningful and usable information, we have to use what is available and sometimes devise our own approaches. We adopted the two overarching goals of *Healthy People 2010* in our *Healthy Vermonters 2010* documents: to increase the quality and years of healthy life and to eliminate health disparities.[2] But our second overarching goal was more difficult to assess: our 1990 census estimated Vermont's racial and ethnic minority population to be about 2%, and to be 2.5% by 2000, with great diversity in language and representation from many different racial, ethnic, and cultural groups. We were unable to conduct meaningful population-based analyses of minority health issues because of the total size of these populations and their diversity, so we devised another strategy. We created advisory committees, lead by senior health department managers to identify health priorities of our largest minority communities. This contributed greatly to our overarching goal to eliminate health disparities. Access to health care was a theme common to all, but health needs and priorities were diverse and covered many areas of public health. And while we worked to refine our ability to collect data, we collected information from these advisory groups that could be used to help set priorities for all Vermonters.[1]

Outcomes are the bottom line for public health. They tell you where you are, where you have been, where you need to go, and how to use your precious resources to focus attention on health. They provide a framework for accountability, not only for the governmental public health system, the "backbone" of public health,[13] but for the collective work of all the involved groups and organizations that have a stake in these issues. Outcomes can be used for our nation, our states, and our communities. Impacting health outcomes requires us to look at the data and provide an unflinching picture of where we are no matter how difficult, uncomfortable, or sometimes unpopular. Measuring outcomes requires data, but doesn't require elaborate and expensive new data systems. Using measurable goals and objectives provides room for flexibility and new approaches. This approach provides a focus for public education and facilitates efforts for ongoing work with legislators, communities, the press, groups, organizations, and individual citizens. A focus on measurable results promotes efficiency, and allows us to discard strategies (no matter how old and familiar) that don't work. This approach provides accountability and fuels public expectations that can contribute to changing our culture to promote health. Outcomes allow us the opportunity, if we persist, to develop multidisciplinary public health approaches that are needed to see measurable health improvements become reality. They are the glue to facilitate progress for this century, by linking groups and organizations in health priorities. Outcomes can help us improve public health.

REFERENCES

1. Vermont Department of Health. *Healthy Vermonters 2010*. Burlington, Vt: Vermont Department of Health; September 2000.
2. U.S. Department of Health and Human Services (DHHS). *Healthy People 2010: National Health Promotion and Disease Prevention Objectives*. Washington, DC: DHHS; 2000. Available at http://www.healthypeople. gov. Accessed June 9, 2005.
3. Institute of Medicine. *The Future of Public Health*. Washington, DC: National Academy Press; 1988.
4. Better choices for life [Editorial]. *Burlington Free Press*. October 16, 2000; 4A.
5. Blueprint for Better Health [Editorial]. *Burlington Free Press*. February 18, 2001; 7E.
6. Nelson DE, Bland S, Powell-Griner E, et al. State trends in health risk factors and receipt of clinical preventive services among U.S. adults during the 1990s. *JAMA*. 2002;287:2659–2667.
7. McGinnis JM. Health in America—the sum of its parts. *JAMA*. 2002;287:2711–2712.
8. McGuiness JM, Foege WH. Actual causes of death in the United States. *JAMA*. 1993;270:2207–2212.
9. Mokdad AH, Marks JS, Stroup DF, Gerberding JL. Actual causes of death in the United States, 2000. *JAMA*. 2004;291:1238–1245.
10. Mokdad AH. Correction: actual causes of death in the United States, 2000. *JAMA*. 2005;293:293–294.
11. Vermont Department of Health. Health Status Report '02. Burlington, Vt: Vermont Department of Health; 2002.
12. Allen AW. Health Department: Northern Vermont needs a diet. *Rutland Herald*. July 23, 2002.
13. Institute of Medicine. *The Future of the Public's Health in the 21st Century*. Washington, DC: National Academies Press; 2003.

52

We Must Always be Prepared

After September 11, 2001, the world was different, and public health was propelled into an intense effort for preparedness. We had worked with the Centers for Disease Control and Prevention (CDC) and other organizations in Vermont, using a small amount of federal funding, to begin preliminary efforts, but the urgent need was clearly felt after September 11. Like many other states, we were inundated with white powder scares, all with the knowledge that they could be real, as was the case of powders found in the offices of national news media, the United States Senate, and in postal facilities.

A special issue of *The Disease Control Bulletin* was sent to health professionals throughout the state in October, alerting them of the signs and symptoms that should prompt a call to the health department. This publication was widely distributed and was an additional attempt to raise awareness about the common signs and symptoms of diseases caused by potential bioterrorism agents, symptoms that were not unlike those caused by many common medical conditions. Such signs and symptoms needed a higher index of suspicion among health care professionals in Vermont, most of whom had never seen or diagnosed these conditions.[1] Health department epidemiologists had already published an overview of bioterrorism (BT) agents in *The Disease Control Bulletin,* the most widely read health department epidemiology publication.[2] Information for health care professionals and the public was updated as Vermont increased its preparedness efforts.

In addition to responding to white powder scares and developing a distribution plan for potassium iodide (KI) for those living and working in close proximity to Vemont's nuclear power plant, work was also underway to develop a plan to prepare against the use of smallpox as a BT agent. The CDC had focused on agents of particular concern as *Bacillus anthracis* (anthrax), smallpox virus, *Yersinia pestis* (plague), *Clostridium botulinum* toxin and *Francisella tularensis* (tularemia), because symptoms would be initially nonspecific and might not be initially recognized.[2]

Routine smallpox vaccination was discontinued in 1972, leaving a large and potentially vulnerable population. This created a public health vulnerability due to smallpox's contagiousness and a high mortality rate, estimated at 30%.[3] Experts from the CDC warned of the possibility of bioterrorism attacks,[4] and reiterated that they had been working to strengthen state and local public health planning, education, and laboratory efforts. Another academic expert talked about the ease with which terrorists could spread smallpox,[4] and the consensus was that despite stockpiling, education, and planning, as of the end of September 2001, we were not prepared.[4]

The CDC was developing its smallpox plans, and in addition to near immediate review by state health officials, these efforts received much national public attention.[5] Under this initial plan, more than 100 members of epidemiologic teams were vaccinated to be sent to areas immediately when suspicion of smallpox was found. However, this approach, in our opinion was not enough, and possibly too slow. We concluded that we needed our own team, and that even a 12-hour delay was too long. The governor wrote to the CDC with Vermont's concerns,[6] including the need for more laboratory ability to confirm such events. We were concerned, as were other states and academic experts, that if something like this were to happen, it could happen simultaneously in many locations, making state and local advanced preparedness essential. When we received the CDC's draft, we provided constructive comments to make sure we, as other states, were heard, and that final plans would be the product of the most expert and practical thinking.

Meanwhile federal funds were becoming more available, and we had to brief legislative committees in order to gain support for additional funding. Representatives from state agencies or departments of public safety, emergency management, and other administration representatives, including myself, briefed the senate appropriations committee.[7] Although the state had emergency procedures in place, in particular, plans related to the nuclear power plant, these needed to be enhanced, particularly with the addition of preparedness for potential BT threats. After much testimony, a joint legislative committee signed off on our plan.[8] This was particularly difficult due to the juxtaposition of budget reductions and the elimination of some positions in state government. The health department was poised to get additional staff, and the state police was to receive more protective and testing equipment.[8] However, despite the national and state urgency that we felt to enhance our preparedness efforts, this was still quite difficult to implement, and the administration's unwavering support was critical to gaining the legislative committee's support.

Planning and educational efforts continued. Epidemiologists and other health department staff worked with physicians, nurses, emergency medical providers, hospitals, and health department public health nurses to develop a core response, called Phase 1, throughout the state. In December 2002, the health department filed its plan with the CDC and announced the plans.[9] The pre-event vaccination to prepare public health and medical response teams in four areas of the state included as a first priority those who might be in first contact with a patient with smallpox. A separate plan that detailed how Vermont would respond to a case of smallpox being discovered was also sent to CDC.[9] The press carried the news along with information for the public about smallpox.[10,11] The goal of these efforts was to make sure that Vermont's public health teams could rapidly respond anywhere in the state. Along with planning efforts, information was also available through the health department Web page.

In February 2003, the first smallpox vaccination clinic vaccinated 14 workers; 6 public health nurses had already been vaccinated in January. Vermont, along with Connecticut, Nebraska, and California, were the first states to receive doses of the smallpox vaccine.[12] Nationally, 1043 people had been vaccinated, far fewer than the 450,000 planned by the CDC. Elsewhere local health departments said such preparedness efforts could mean cuts in other areas of public health; in some cases, local health departments would have to struggle to carry out the first phase of these preparedness efforts against smallpox threats.[13] States varied in their abilities to carry out preparedness efforts; in some locations skepticism remained about the need for these intense efforts, given other competing public health priorities. The Council of State and Territorial Epidemiologists (CSTE) evaluated terrorism preparedness in health departments,[14] noting that federal funding for state public health preparedness efforts had increased from $67 million in FY2001 to about $1 billion in FY2002, and found that although there had been an increase in epidemiologists, nearly 200 additional epidemiologists were still needed for terrorism preparedness efforts. In addition, as this group looked at funding sources for those epidemiologists working in terrorism and emergency preparedness, they observed that more than a third were paid with state or other funds, indicating that resources had been redirected to meet these preparedness requirements.[14]

Although preliminary efforts were underway in states, the events of September 11, 2001, necessitated acceleration, with an increase in funds, to prepare for diseases caused by potential BT agents. As intense scrutiny focused on federal agencies, particularly the CDC, states struggled with efforts to provide rapid, credible, and effective means to be prepared for disease most of us had only read about. In Vermont, there were many challenges. There was a need to coordinate state agency efforts, including public health, public safety, and emergency management, at the state and local levels. There was a need to educate and train health professionals so that they could work side by side with epidemiologists and public health nurses in BT preparedness, working relationships that were already solid and firmly in place. Despite an influx of federal resources, applying these to their intended programs was not easy, given the fiscal pressures and other strains on state budgets, and there was a reluctance to giving any state agency many additional positions in such a fiscally frugal environment. The administration was solidly behind our efforts, contributing to a stronger effort to receive the funds and begin our needed activities.

The Institute of Medicine notes that lessons can be learned from our national smallpox vaccination effort—though it concluded that our nation's readiness is "indeterminate"[15] and recommended regular assessments of our preparedness. The institute also emphasized the importance of "clear and authoritative scientific information communicated by a credible source" and the importance of "open communication."[15] For us, such accelerated planning started at a time when the public was still uneasy and concerned about health and safety following September 11, 2001. At that time, our strategies were simple: get plans in place as quickly as possible and make them public. The fact that we were one of the first states to receive vaccines (as well as to begin efforts to distribute potassium iodide in the radius of the nuclear power plant) was not a coincidence, but a result of a conscious strategy to gain and maintain public confidence at a frightening time in our public health history.

REFERENCES

1. Vermont Department of Health. Bioterrorism: Detection and Response. Disease Control Bulletin, Special Issue. October 2001. Available at http://www. healthyvermonters.info. Accessed November 14, 2005.

2. Vermont Department of Health. Bioterrorism: a public health issue Disease control bulletin. 1999; 1(4). Available at http://www. healthyvermonters.info. Accessed June 17, 2005.

3. Henderson DA, Inglesby TV, Bartlett JG, et al. Smallpox as a biological weapon: medical and public health management: consensus statement. *JAMA.* 1999;281:2127–2137.

4. Haney D. Country not prepared for bioterrorism, experts say. *Rutland Herald.* September 27, 2000. Available at http://www.rutlandherald.com. Accessed May 7, 2005.

5. Altman LK. U.S. develops plan to deal with smallpox. *New York Times.* November 4, 2001. Available at http://www.rutlandherald.com. Accessed May 7, 2005.

6. Ring W. Smallpox planning a concern to Dean. *Rutland Herald.* January 4, 2002. Available at http://www.rutlandherald.com. Accessed May 7, 2005.

7. Ring W. Senate panel briefed on state's response to bioterrorism. *Rutland Herald.* April 4, 2002. Available at http://www.rutlandherald.com. Accessed May 7, 2005.

8. Mace D. State committee signs off on terrorism spending. *Rutland Herald.* September 17, 2002. Available at http://www.rutlandherald.com. Accessed May 7, 2005.

9. Vermont Department of Health. Vermont plans for vaccinating smallpox response teams [News release]. Burlington, Vt: Vermont Department of Health; December 6, 2002. Available at http://www. healthyvermonters.info. Accessed November 13, 2005.

10. Dritschilo F. Smallpox shots going first to health care workers. *Rutland Herald.* December 11, 2002. Available at http://www.rutlandherald.com. Accessed May 7, 2005.

11. Associated Press. State makes vaccine plan for smallpox. *Burlington Free Press.* December 7, 2002; 1B.

12. Associated Press. First smallpox clinic vaccinates 14 in state. *Rutland Herald.* February 13, 2003. Available at http://www.rutlandherald.com. Accessed May 7, 2005.

13. Altman LK, O'Connor A. Vaccine plan could force health cuts. *New York Times.* January 5, 2003.

14. CDC. Brief Report: Terrorism and Emergency Preparedness in State and Territorial Public Health Departments–United States, 2004. *MMWR.* 2005;54:459–460.

15. Institute of Medicine. Future BT preparedness can be improved through lessons from the national smallpox vaccine effort [News release]. Washington, DC: The National Academies; March 3, 2005. Available at http://www4.nas.edu/news. nsf. Accessed April 8, 2005.

53

Make Partnerships How You Do Business—Preventive Health Care for Children and Adolescents

In the Vermont Department of Health, the division of community public health and staff from the maternal and child health programs worked closely with the state Medicaid office, located in another department in the state government, to determine the Early Periodic Screening, Diagnosis, and Treatment (EPSDT) requirements. Part of this meant setting standards and developing protocols for health care services for children eligible for Medicaid. Eligibility for Medicaid for children had been dramatically expanded in the early 1990s during the statewide efforts to improve access to prenatal care and care for mothers and young children. Eligibility for children was expanded again in the late 1990s to ensure that nearly all Vermont children would have access to health care. Part of the federal requirements in developing these standards that guided preventive care for children, required consultation with medical and dental health care organizations involved in health care. As many Vermont children were potentially eligible for these EPSDT services, health department staff saw this as an opportunity to have a broad impact on Vermont children by trying to update these standards and protocols using the latest available science and recommendations by professional groups.[1] In previous years, the Department had used the national American Academy of Pediatrics schedule for these services. But there was potential for more benefit with a more comprehensive review from all national groups who recommended preventive services for children and adolescents. It would also be better to convene health professionals and others in Vermont to develop a schedule for these preventive services that was Vermont's own. Such a process, if successful, could provide a simpler, more uniform message about preventive care for all Vermont children, not only for health professionals, but also for children, adolescents, and parents, which was essential to our efforts to effectively communicate and promote health. There was also a climate of slightly expanded managed care, though not the largest factor, and it was felt that such a standardized roster of preventive care services, developed and supported by health providers, government payers, public health, and others, would be the strongest leverage with other insurance companies and types of health payers, by focusing on evidence-based, consensus-driven, uniform recommendations.

The history of working together in partnership in Vermont was already strong—collaborations between the health department and health providers, physicians, nurses, hospitals, and others had shown results in many other areas: improving access to prenatal care, preventing childhood lead poisoning, and ensuring that Vermont consistently was a leader in immunizing young children. Many new recommendations had been made in recent years before: *Bright Futures,* the American Medical Association's guide for adolescent preventive services (GAPS); and revised recommendations from the United States Preventive Services Task Force, and The American Academy of Family Physicians.

Health department staff convened a group of experts and stakeholders and performed a comprehensive review and comparison of all the recommendations for preventive care for children and adolescents from the different national organizations. Health department staff also included public health goals and objectives for Vermont, *Healthy Vermonters 2010,* in areas where improved public health outcomes for children related directly to clinical health care by physicians or nurses.[1] Such a focus on public health outcomes had potential to further strengthen partnerships between medicine, health care, and public health; link clinical health care to population-based prevention; and set the stage for future quality initiatives to improve health outcomes.

Collaborators on the panel of experts and stakeholders included representation from the Academy of Family Practice in Vermont, dental providers, school nurses, the Vermont chapter of the American Academy of Pediatrics, the Vermont Medicaid program, mental health providers, and the health department. The group met, utilized the comparison data, and made decisions by consensus. I advised a key health department leader involved in the process about the need to make this a "zero-sum" game, because if the absolute number of services that the group recommended grew too large, meaning much more clinical care would be recommended, the cost increases might be seen as potentially too great, and the recommendations would never get implemented. She agreed and tried her best to have the group understand the practical constraints and government concerns about budgets, and tried to use an "add one, subtract one" type of thinking in the discussions. For example, if you added a visit for adolescents, a great idea given the risks of smoking, alcohol and drug use, the need for advice about nutrition and physical activity advice, and so on, perhaps there could be a urinalysis recommendation dropped at an earlier age. The committee got the idea and worked hard, side by side with health department staff, to come up with recommendations that were something they could each endorse and would use in their practices, yet were practical and able to be implemented in a government climate of concern for increased health expenditures. Although it would have been easy, and very tempting, to shift costs to the Medicaid program, we felt that our responsibility for the long term was to maintain this practical approach, looking for recommendations that could be used for all Vermont children and improve health care and public health outcomes for the year 2010.

After meetings and discussions, the group came up with consensus recommendations that incorporated different recommendations into one set of preventive services recommended for Vermont children. It was called a periodicity schedule,[1,2] and listed the recommendations for health screening, vision, hearing, oral health, anemia, counseling for risk behaviors, and all other aspects of preventive health care for children and adolescents. The recommendations were put into a small poster, or large wall chart, that could be placed in the office. Services were listed, such as hearing screening, comprehensive physical exam, height and weight, blood pressure, lead screening, hematocrit, immunizations, and others preventive services, from newborn to age 20. There were simple codes for what was routine, or not, and references for background information, should health professionals want additional information.

In addition to the poster, a "toolkit" was developed, which looked like a rectangular briefcase, with a plastic handle, that could be carried to different places in offices, schools, or clinics, and had laminated page-sized cards in individual areas such as adolescent smoking cessation guidelines, and guidelines for screening and counseling and referral for alcohol and other substance use. These could be updated and replaced and new cards added to the toolkit as the recommendations changed or public health issues made it urgent to have counseling and screening information at the health provider or school nurse's fingertips. One of our goals was to take a detailed chart that gave preventive health recommendations in all areas at different ages and make it easy and efficient to use, depending on the age of the patient or health area of concern.[1]

Both the schedule and toolkits were distributed to family practitioners, pediatricians, nurse practitioners, school nurses, health department district offices, and others. They were well received and distributed all over the entire state. Records were kept of distribution to allow easy distribution of updated recommendations.[1] This collaborative work was further strengthened through innovative quality improvement efforts across Vermont by the Vermont Child Health Improvement Program at the University of Vermont College of Medicine.[3,4]

These successful partnerships strengthened public health and health care partnerships in areas such as immunizations, lead screening, counseling about tobacco, screening for alcohol and drug use, and many other areas. The process to develop the recommendations started with children eligible for Medicaid, but resulted in recommendations that could be used for all children. The use of science and evidence-based guidelines, a focus on broad collaboration and consensus, common sense about rising health care costs, and efforts aimed at linking these clinical efforts to public health outcomes, along with communication strategy, enabled the development and implementation of uniform recommendations to provide preventive health care for Vermont children and adolescents.

Make partnerships how you do business. It is the only way to tackle complex and challenging public health issues. Sometimes in public health, the usual partnerships—with doctors, nurses, hospitals, and schools—are comfortable. But to address the range and variety of typical public health issues requires being flexible, such as our partnerships with housing agencies to prevent childhood lead poisoning, something that was an effective strategy in Vermont; and our partnerships with business to maximize opportunities to reduce health risks in workplace settings as well as promote positive behaviors in an environment where people spend many hours per week. The Institute of Medicine's publication *Future of the Public's Health in the 21st Century*, cites partnerships as a crucial area to best address the health issues of this century. The document cites the importance of "building a generation of intersectoral partnerships" as one of six rec-ommended areas for action.[5] Public health agencies, government agencies, state and local health departments, through creativity and systematic thinking about ways to build and strengthen partnerships with a wide range of groups and indi-viduals, not only fulfill their own mission, but have the potential to reach their public health goals.

REFERENCES

1. Carney JK, Berry P. Providers' toolkit of health screening recommendations: Vermont's collaborative efforts to ensure comprehensive health care for children and adolescents. Abstract presented at the American Public Health Association 130th Annual Meeting, Philadelphia, PA, November 2002.
2. Vermont Department of Health. Health screening recommendations for children and adolescents. Burlington, Vt: Vermont Department of Health; 1998.
3. Vermont Child Health Improvement Program. The University of Vermont College of Medicine. Vermont Youth Health Improvement Initiative. Available at http://www.med.uvm.edu/vchip. Accessed February 28, 2005.
4. National Institute for Health Care Management (NIHCM) Foundation. Perspectives on Implementing Bright Futures. Action brief. December 2001;10–11. Available at www.nihcm.org/AB8.pdf. Accessed November 14, 2005.
5. Institute of Medicine. *The Future of the Public's Health in the 21st Century.* Washington, DC: The National Academies Press; 2003:1–18.

54

It Will Take All of Us to Keep the Public Healthy

In the fall of 2004, we began teaching public health to medical students in a new way. An entire class of medical students left the University of Vermont College of Medicine and went to work on public health projects in the local community as part of their second year courses.[1] Students had to figure out how to best use their limited time to devise practical strategies to approach the complex challenges of access to quality health care, health communication, and nutrition and physical activity, all listed in *Healthy People 2010*,[2] and driven by public health needs articulated by local community agencies. The students saw public health issues of many types, in many different settings, and some of the broader determinants and barriers to health. They worked in groups with different agencies, and over several months they developed innovative and practical ways to improve health. They became actively involved in public health.

They worked with focus groups of young women to identify barriers to accessing health care and devised a pocket-sized card that gave cues to these women about how to ask questions, get complete information, and become empowered during their brief and sometimes intimidating health care visits. The students worked with the community food shelf to develop lists of foods suitable for patients with diabetes, high blood pressure, and heart disease, and organized the lists by price and brand name. Students listed which local grocery store products could be used by the food shelf during food drives in order to obtain food donations that were healthier. The students made house calls with visiting nurses to understand practical ways to help nurses and patients prevent medication errors in patients in their homes and to develop pilot strategies that could be more formally tested in the future. They worked with refugee families to ensure that new families to Vermont understood how to prevent childhood lead poisoning and other environmental health concerns. The students developed a system to help patients and employees of a nursing home achieve high rates of influenza immunization and developed lists for patients with chronic conditions to help them more easily navigate their brief doctor visits and better communicate with health professionals. The students shared their results with their peers, teachers, and the community.[1]

Can these strategies teach students public health and improve the health of the community? Although answering these questions may take several years, such approaches, linking our academic efforts to communities and starting with community needs as the first priority, are feasible ways to teach public health. These methods can be incorporated into an already busy medical school curriculum and can cover many broad and timely areas of public health, such as those defined in *Healthy People 2010* (e.g., diabetes, health communication, access to quality health services, mental health, environmental health, nutrition, physical activity, and immunizations and infectious diseases).[2] Community agencies felt that our students' work benefited the communities and populations they served and wanted to continue to work with us. Such community–academic partnerships produced pilot data for public health practice and community-based participatory research. These partnerships can build relationships and have real and practical potential to improve the health of our local communities.[1]

Although medical students face a growing list of public health issues during their careers, such as preventing childhood obesity and emerging infectious diseases, plus the challenges of preventing and caring for chronic conditions in an aging population, in many medical schools, there is no assurance that students will fully understand the community context of individual patients, the need to prevent as well as treat illness, using interventions both inside and outside the doctor's office, and that many of the determinants of health include education and literacy, social and economic factors, environmental factors, and habits and behaviors (many with roots in childhood and adolescence), as well as genetic and individual factors.

The redesign and integration of the medical school curriculum at the University of Vermont College of Medicine provided a unique opportunity for us to look ahead, envision what students would need to be the best possible physicians, and test some new ways to teach these concepts, including public health. Defining competencies for student learning in all areas of medicine, including prevention and public health, set a foundation for best educating our future physicians. This new curriculum, called the Vermont Integrated Curriculum (VIC), integrates sciences and clinical medicine, develops skills for life-long learning, and includes public health competencies. Its development was the result of an extensive faculty process to define areas and reshape what and how these areas were taught.[3]

From the first week of medical school, students worked in groups of seven or eight learning about those skills, tasks, and knowledge areas not encompassed in a biochemical formula or metabolic pathway. The students went to the art museum to sharpen their powers of observation; they struggled with a rationing exercise to determine who would get an organ transplant. They learned how to approach a task and try to crystallize amorphous concepts and resolve conflicts in addressing complex health problems. They were introduced to public health on the second day of medical school and learned the basics of epidemiology and population-based concepts of public health in their first two weeks. The idea was to train them from the very start in population-based concepts alongside their training in focusing on individual patients. It was hoped this effort would avoid public health, population-based learning, and preventive medicine being considered secondary to the diagnosis and treatment of individual patients. We did not want medical students to treat public health like a foreign language. In their second year, the students went out to the community to work in partnership with local community agencies to undertake public health projects.

The idea that the students might learn public health by doing, seeing, and experiencing community health needs seemed better than a series of classroom lectures. This gave them an opportunity to see the scope of public health and the determinants of health. Public health is not a discipline that is either easy or intuitive to understand; it is more abstract than renal physiology or the function of the immune system, but it is necessary to better understand and impact health needs of patients. Linking the academic setting to public health issues in communities requires understanding and addressing these issues from a community perspective. In designing student learning projects, we felt that a "community first" mindset might be a good starting place, and began by asking for proposals from community agencies and organizations working in health and health care areas, in any of the issue areas covered in *Healthy People 2010*. Projects developed through this route put the community needs first but framed them in a way that defined a public health issue and incorporated research methods and strategies. Such community-based participatory research has the potential to improve community health and contribute to our knowledge base in public health practice.[4]

Current and emerging public health issues intersect with clinical medicine at many levels, seemingly more now than in the past, and students in the health professions, including medicine, need to learn about current and emerging public health issues and how specifically public health interfaces with health care. Preventing childhood obesity can be aided by physicians in clinical offices, but given the rapid increase of the obesity epidemic in young children all across our nation, more leverage is needed; we must promote nutrition and physical activity in schools, communities, and households.[5] If we fail to better prevent diseases and make improvements in their risk factors, the consequences will be to see health professionals treating more and more patients with diabetes and associated complications, superimposed on an already aging population. It is not enough for physicians just to treat growing numbers of younger people with diabetes, physicians must also understand what we know about how and why our population has been increasing in weight and sedentary behavior, and what we know (and don't know) about how to help focus community efforts to prevent these problems in the first place.

Similarly, physician's advice to children and adolescents about not smoking is essential to efforts to prevent young people from starting to smoke, but must be understood in the context of peer-led efforts in schools; science-based school curriculum in middle-school aged children to prevent smoking, alcohol, and drug use; media efforts aimed at creating realistic perceptions about the declining percentage of young people smoking; policy initiatives to prevent illegal sales of tobacco and raise the price of tobacco products; and efforts to encourage and support the attempts of adults to quit smoking. Such efforts to help better prevent disease are important in the education of health professionals. The critical role of health department, community agencies in public health, and the partnerships needed to improve public health are critical elements of educational efforts to teach medical students and other health professionals about public health.

It will take all of us to keep the public healthy, and if we are going to directly face the large and complex challenges of public health, we need to create new partnerships,[6] pursue new areas of teaching and research, and teach public health to students in a wide range of professional disciplines, including medicine, nursing, and allied health services, as well as making it more available to undergraduates—all this in addition to the critical role of the research and teaching in schools and programs in public health. Recent recommendations reinforce changes in traditional areas of public health: epidemiology and biostatistics, environmental health, health services administration, and social and behavioral sciences should also include such new areas as informatics, genomics, communication, cultural competence, community-based participatory research, policy and law, global health and ethics.[4] Academic health centers are called to lead the way in making the changes needed to maintain health in this century.[7] It has been recommended that all medical students receive "basic public health training in the population-based prevention approaches to health," and recommendations for schools of public health, nursing, and undergraduate levels have also been made, broadening the access to public health education to include the undergraduate level.[4] This only makes sense, if you think about the type of complex public health problems that characterize the work of public health, and the many types of individuals, disciplines, and skills to collectively address these issues, whether through teaching, research, or practice. If we are to be successful, public health must become a way of thinking that is incorporated into these curricula, rather than separate content areas with a few narrow examples. Collaborations and systematic linkages, including communities and public health groups and organizations, are needed to practically implement these concepts.

These broad challenges and concepts must be made operational, practical, and relevant, both to educational institutions and communities, if these ideas are to take root and produce both knowledge and measurable impacts that improve the public's health. Such approaches to training health professionals have implications for schools of medicine, nursing, allied health services, and undergraduate education. The key challenges will be finding creative and practical ways to engage communities, teach students, and articulate why it is essential to broaden the focus of professional education to ensure health professionals are fully trained to improve health. It will take all of us to keep the public healthy.

REFERENCES

1. Carney JK, Walrath D, Pigeon Y. Community-academic partnerships: Teaching medical students public health. Abstract presented at the American Public Health Association annual meeting. Washington, DC. November 2004.
2. U.S. Department of Health and Human Services. *Healthy People 2010.* Available at: http://www.healthypeople.gov. Accessed June 9, 2005.
3. Vermont Integrated Curriculum (VIC) at the University of Vermont College of Medicine. Available at http://www.med.uvm.edu. Accessed November 7, 2005.

4. Institute of Medicine. *Who will keep the Public Healthy? Educating Public Health Professionals for the 21st Century.* Washington, DC: National Academies Press; 2003:1–26.
5. Institute of Medicine. *Preventing Childhood Obesity, Health in the Balance.* Washington, DC: National Academies Press; 2005:1.
6. Institute of Medicine. *The Future of the Public's Health in the 21st Century.* Washington, DC: National Academics Press; 2003:1–18, 33.
7. Institute of Medicine. *Academic Health Centers, Leading Change in the 21st Century.* Washington, DC: National Academies Press; 2004:5–6.

PR (Public Relations) Is Not the Same as PH (Public Health)

After work I was scheduled to attend a Vermont Expos baseball game. I was to briefly appear with the governor and agriculture commissioner at a promotion for Vermont apples, an effort of the agriculture department. The agriculture commissioner was there to promote Vermont apples, and I was there to help by promoting health, after all "an apple a day" or "five fruits and vegetables a day" was a key recommendation for better health. Before the real game started, the governor would pitch a couple of apples, and the agriculture commissioner would hit one. I was the catcher and borrowed a catcher's mitt from a team member. Rolled up sleeves, jeans, and a fruit and vegetable t-shirt (mine) were the uniform of the day. We took our positions on the field. The first apple pitch was low and outside. I whispered to the agriculture commissioner that he had better hit the next one, no matter where it went, or his job was on the line. All I had to do was catch it. The second pitch became applesauce after a big and accurate swing by the Ag chief. Our job was done, and we went off the field after a short but fun event.

Was this public health? No, it was public relations. But for years after, every time we found ourselves in another health and agriculture joint issue (the toughest ones involving maple syrup) the agriculture commissioner and I would joke that we would rather be out on the ball field. We had a good working relationship. My list of such events, though enjoyable, was pretty short, and it was important to distinguish them and their role from communication strategies in public health.

One of the six areas of action and change recommended by the Institute of Medicine is in the area of communication, with recommendations to improve communication both within the public health system and between public health and the community. This area had been identified as a "critical core competency" in public health practice.[1] It is also necessary for such information to fit with literacy levels and be culturally appropriate.[1] There are strong ties between education and health outcomes and growing evidence linking limitations in health literacy to health outcomes and health behaviors.[2] In the areas where public health and health care intersect, clear communication is also critically important. For information related to health care, it has been estimated that 90 million adults in the United States who have limited health literacy are unable to benefit and act from available health and health care information.[2] Health communication has the potential to impact prevention at the individual and population level, can raise awareness about health, and impact attitudes about health.[3] Communication strategies can help facilitate positive health behavior through positive cultural changes and help distribute health messages on a broad scale.[3]

In addition to improving health outcomes, systematically improved health communication in the public health system has the potential to extend such skills to health care and link population-based communication strategies to those currently serving individual patients. Improvements in health indicators have been seen in public health areas more related to clinical services, such as adult immunizations and screening mammograms. Tremendous challenges remain in the effort to change those behaviors associated with the leading causes of death, such as smoking, poor diet, physical activity, and misuse of alcohol.[4] Achieving improvements in many public health areas relies, at least in part, on health communication strategies.[3] Challenges related to the increasing complexity of the communication environment, both in terms of numbers of channels and competition among health issues,[3] as well as the breadth of needs and interventions necessary to improve current levels of health literacy,[2] are huge and will take sustained and multidisciplinary efforts to address them.

We adopted many communication strategies in public health. Because of limited resources, we focused our efforts on educating targeted groups on specific issues, such as HIV prevention, women getting mammograms, prenatal care, accessing the state's health insurance programs, or preventing smoking in children. Larger efforts required planning and development, sometimes focus groups, and a comprehensive strategy, to develop and match messages with targeted populations, as well as to find a funding source. Some media campaigns were funded though public–private partnerships, some through federal grants, and some with funding from the tobacco master settlement agreement. Evaluation efforts, both formal and informal, were often practical: the number of calls to a toll-free hotline publicized through a campaign was one example. Ultimately, process and health outcome indicators from the usual data sources were also used to evaluate our efforts. It was not always easy to determine the precise impact of all these efforts, as they were sometimes done as part of a multidisciplinary or public health approach to addressing a problem, such as youth smoking or access to health care, but we worked hard to follow best practices in their development, implementation, and evaluation, no matter how small our budget.

Communication in public health has been integrated in other ways as well. Strategies to educate the public about public health, as a way to focus public attention on health and health issues was done through the development of easy-to-understand reports and documents that used our best information, science, and best practices about public health issues. Taking technical and scientific information and presenting it in a way that was clear and easily understandable was immensely challenging, but in everything—mercury levels in fish from Vermont waters, the incidence of the most common forms of cancer in Vermont, summaries of our health behaviors from the Behavioral Risk Factor surveys, women's health, men's health, cutting smoking in half by the year 2010, and preventing alcohol and drug abuse in Vermont—communicating health information in a systematic way, one that emphasized the "public" in public health, was essential to improving public health and reaching 2010 goals. Reports on health status were ways to highlight relative priorities, both short and long term, and reiterate important health recommendations.

Although the Institute of Medicine talked about how people understand public health and the difficulty of communicating its content,[5] we always found that it was most important to give people information in a way that they would most likely use it, while still focusing on the issues. People were interested in mercury, lead, smoking, alcohol and drugs, obesity, diabetes, HIV, cancer, and heart disease. So it was less important that the public understood what "assessment," "policy development," and "assurance" meant or that they valued the importance of "population health," than it was to ensure preventive care for infants and immunizations for children and adults. We needed to communicate the importance of not smoking, being more active, and understanding the causes of lead poisoning.

PR (public relations) is not the same as PH (public health), and it is essential to understand the difference. Catching apples at a promotion (although fun) is not a substitute for creating partnerships and communication strategies to improve the nutritional health of the population. Every public health official needs a strategy to talk and communicate about public health, one that is comfortable and will help systematically address the difficult challenges of changing behaviors that collectively have a huge impact on health and also represent critical leverage points for disease prevention. Public health practitioners must integrate health communication strategies into their short-term and long-term efforts. Public health, if successful in our efforts to improve health communication, has the potential to improve health knowledge, health behaviors, and ultimately health outcomes.

REFERENCES

1. Institute of Medicine. *The Future of the Public's Health in the 21st Century.* Washington, DC: National Academies Press; 2003:4–7.
2. Institute of Medicine. *Health Literacy: A Prescription to End Confusion.* Washington, DC: National Academies Press; 2004:5–8.
3. U.S. Department of Health and Human Services. Chapter 11 Health communication. In: *Healthy People 2010.* Washington, DC: USDHHS;2000. Available at http://www.healthypeople.gov/document/HTML/Volume1/11HealthCom.htm. Accessed June 30, 2005.
4. McGinnis JM. Health in America–the sum of its parts. *JAMA.* 2002;87: 2711–2712.
5. Institute of Medicine. *The Future of Public Health.* Washington, DC: National Academy Press; 1988.

56

CHAPTER

Consider Every Day an Adventure

The phone is ringing, the newspaper carries an article about a new health claim, an advocacy group writes the governor to ask you to pay more attention to their cause. Your staff is tired. The CDC has issued a new report. The legislature is asking why you haven't put more money in a certain area. What are you doing about obesity, smoking, alcohol, drugs, the infections that can't be cured with antibiotics, insufficient vaccines for children, and potassium iodide pills for citizens around the nuclear power plant?

How can you possibly keep your priorities straight when everyone is calling, writing, demanding, needing, asking, and pleading for you to do something about the long and growing and changing list of public health issues that are important to them, whether they are citizens, your bosses, the legislature, advocacy groups, or your own staff?

The good news is health gets more and more attention. The bad news is that health agencies, in getting so much attention, find themselves reacting more to day-to-day concerns and less to taking care of the problems that affect the most people, are the most serious, and could be prevented. How can you reconcile the core duties of public health and their broad responsibilities in an environment in which every day a new aspect of health and health care gathers public attention? There are no simple answers, but there are strategies that can help.

In an environment where we had tremendous responsibility to implement public health programs such as the Women, Infants and Children's (WIC) program, provide direct health care services for children with special health care needs, oversee state programs such as those promoting healthy indoor air in school environments, and respond to day-to-day challenges, there were many demands on the finite resources of the department. Your research into an overall strategy to address and prevent hepatitis C could be interrupted by investigating a disease outbreak. An unpredicted natural disaster, such as a flood or ice storm, could draw attention from the day-to-day activities. The question of a cancer cluster could put a discussion around health planning on hold. So in all this, how do you keep your priorities straight?

The first strategy is to know your core duties. Many organizations call them essential public health services, core services, and other terms, but the bottom line is that public health agencies have a short list of core responsibilities that form a backdrop for public health activities. These core responsibilities include preventing epidemics, promoting health in the environment, monitoring the health of the population, promoting healthy behaviors, responding to disas-

258

ters, linking populations to services when needed, providing direct health services when needed, providing public health policy and planning, and on some lists, assuring the quality and accessibility of medical care. Each of these are tall, comprehensive orders, and some of these, such as assuring access to quality health services, are national challenges in which public health is one of many participants. In addition, sometimes state law defines both general and specific program responsibilities in public health.

But despite the fact that health departments have varying structures, resources, statutory responsibilities and personnel, being conscious of these core responsibilities is still important because it keeps your focus on the key elements needed to protect and improve public health. In some places and at certain times, the provision of direct health care services, with the factors contributing to the demand and costs, can be nearly overwhelming and a drain on the resources for public health. We made a conscious policy decision to build and link our efforts for many health care services (particularly for primary and preventive care for children) to both academic and community health professionals, such that our role in this was different, but together we could fill this core responsibility.

Another strategy to keep priorities focused, not just today, tomorrow, and next week, but next month, next year, and for five or more years, is to outline the measurable goals and objectives needed to protect and improve public health. Nationally, *Healthy People 2000* and *Healthy People 2010,* were instrumental in helping states pick and choose those priorities for public health that were most pressing. In Vermont, *Healthy Vermonters 2000* and *Healthy Vermonters 2010* were essential to focusing attention on measurable outcomes. They helped us keep our own focus. They served as a frame of reference. No matter what else was happening in our immediate environment, in the day-to-day, and sometimes moment-to-moment chaos, we had targets set out in front of us that we knew we had to continue to reach for. Such measurable outcomes also provided an opportunity to educate the public about the issues, both urgent and enduring, that comprise the scope of public health.

Of course, you must also respond to immediate priorities. Somewhere in the chaos may be an opportunity to help others for the future. Tragic deaths of young Vermonters driving under the influence (DUI) propelled public and legislative discussion, making it not a distant goal, but an urgent priority, and part of larger efforts to reduce the negative impact of alcohol use among young people. Making sure a large department can be flexible enough to respond when one area on your list of priorities has the public's attention is a challenge to organizational cultures, including public health. But a quick and successful response has potential to help such tragedies in the future and improve public health in such a large and complex area.

There are many huge and complex challenges in public health, and part of our approach must include how we think about them in the day-to-day environment of our work. There are always limited resources, and in public health agencies, the expectation that you provide leadership and are always able to help in any issue even remotely related to health, is ever present. The ability to continue to look forward, use the data and measurable goals to highlight goals and priorities, while having the flexibility to respond to urgent day-to-day issues, requires an attitude on the part of staff, as well as a leadership and management tone, that is not distracted by new issues and even emergencies, but views them as part of their job. Putting science into practice, while at the same time being mindful of opportunities to educate the public and policy makers about public health, and being able to take immediate circumstances and connect them to priorities is incredibly challenging. But in the end, it also brings great rewards. How you look at and think about these seemingly competing priorities, the short term and long term, and your attitude, makes all the difference. In public health, consider every day an adventure.

CHAPTER 57

Skate to Where the Puck Will Be

In Vermont, during the winter, you can't turn on sports news without seeing ice hockey. Imagine a college hockey game, where the teams are playing for a spot in the NCAA national tournament. The pace of the game is so fast, that if you are momentarily distracted, the play may have gone to the other end of the rink by the time you look back. The play is faster than fast, the competition intense, and the difference in winning or losing is often split-second instinct, a single movement, an exact placement, and anticipating what could happen next. A defenseman anticipates a pass, intercepts, and skates forward, starting a break for his own team. A player skates into a vacant space, receives a pass, and shoots, seemingly all in one motion, and hits a corner of the goal. Players coming onto the ice, pick up the same pace, looking ahead, anticipating their next opportunity. In the fast pace of the game, successful players anticipate where the next pass will be and are already heading in that direction, to outskate their opponent and head for their goal.

Consultants, managers, the National Science Foundation, a U.S. secretary of education, as well as hockey coaches who teach hockey fundamentals have often been heard or quoted as using a phrase similar to "Skate to where the puck is going, not to where it is." This phrase has been used in teaching basic hockey skills in children as well as a bigger analogy in the business world, academics, and government. The exact origin of the quote, and the words used, are even a point of controversy, the phrase often attributed to hockey great Wayne Gretsky, has attributed it to his father Walter.[1] Our dean at the University of Vermont College of Medicine used this concept at a faculty meeting to emphasize his vision and direction for leadership.[2] It was a perfect fit for the future of medicine, and it also relates to the challenges of public health. No matter who first said it and what the exact words were, this phrase, as you visualize the pace of an ice hockey game and compare it to the pace of business, medical research, or public health, gives an image that links the challenges of today to the future.

Anticipating where our next issues will be and taking steps in those directions are some of the most difficult tasks in public health. The events of September 2001 and the anthrax and white powder investigations were nearly overwhelming for many public health departments. And those of us working during those months remember the previous efforts of the Centers for Disease Control and Prevention (CDC) to think of potential bioterrorism threats and begin preparedness before September 11 and before we had responded to even a single white powder incident.

Public health must deal with short-term and longer-term issues. On a day-to-day basis, public health agencies are challenged to operate in a way that is proactive and anticipates public health issues before they become crises. We have all seen organizations that operate in a "crisis" mode: they scramble to address an issue, often with much confusion, sometimes with conflicting messages and changes in direction, and they don't engender confidence in their organization's ability to manage difficult problems. They further appear "slow," because they are responding, rather than anticipating situations. In Vermont, we knew raccoon rabies was heading up the East Coast, and we started to lay a tremendous groundwork for collaboration between state and federal agencies, physicians and veterinarians, and to educate the public about steps they should take to protect their pets, themselves, and their families.

However, many public health issues aren't as systematic; they erupt rather than evolve. To be proactive, you must anticipate the issues and management of the organization to ensure you have capacity to carry out core responsibilities and to ensure the ability to skate in a new direction.

How can we anticipate the next public health crisis, epidemic, or chronic condition? How can we, as a matter of routine, start to skate where the puck will be? For some events, we can't, and we can't predict the future with absolute certainty, but for many areas of public health, we can anticipate the issues that will face us before they become imminent. We can look ahead, looking at demographics and scientific knowledge and anticipate issues that will challenge us in the years ahead. The other requirement is strong leadership and management and working to put partnerships in place that not only bring resources to the table as we focus on improving health outcomes but also begin to add all the pieces needed to develop sustained and comprehensive approaches to complex problems. In addition, we must broaden our day-to-day view of health, making sure to include those factors such as habits, behaviors, and social, economic, and environmental conditions that closely relate to root causes and potential strategies for improvement.

Trends in actual causes of death show that tobacco, diet, physical activity levels, and alcohol are still major contributors to preventable deaths in our country.[3] The prevalence of obesity and diabetes continues to rise in adults, calling for a national focus to improve activity levels and nutrition.[4] The increases in these two conditions among adults have been noted in all ages, races, and educational levels,[5] reinforcing the need for stronger prevention efforts across our nation. In the past 30 years, the rate of obesity in children has doubled for children ages 2 to 19 years; in children aged 6 to 11 years the rate has tripled. Prevention of obesity in children is now a national priority for public health.[6]

Despite periods of economic growth in our country, more than 40 million Americans—adults and children—are without health insurance, putting them at risk for worse health through reduced access to health care services. Recent reports highlight principles to guide the difficult and complex discussions about how to make improvements.[7] In addition, it is estimated that almost half of adults in the United States struggle to understand and utilize health information,[8] further compounding the difficulty in accessing health care. In addition, much literature is available showing that access to routine medical procedures and quality of health services are lower among racial and ethnic minorities than among white Americans and that comprehensive strategies are needed to reduce and eliminate such disparities.[9] Our measurable goals and objectives in public health for the nation for the year 2010, *Healthy People 2010,* includes increasing the span of healthy life and eliminating health disparities as overarching goals in its vision of healthy people in healthy communities, reflecting the increasing age and diversity in our population.[10]

Although much recent focus has been on bioterrorism preparedness, SARS, risks of pandemic influenza, zoonotic infections, the global impact of HIV, and a broad spectrum of microbial threats continue to challenge our capacity to respond, and experts recommend increasing our local, state, and national capacity as well as our ability to respond to global threats, emphasizing surveillance, diagnostic tests, vaccines, and need for new antimicrobial drugs.[11]

It has been estimated that more than 90% of health spending goes toward medical care and related research,[12] despite research showing that the majority of preventable deaths relate to behavioral and environmental factors.[13] Recent reports recommend adopting a broader view of public health that also includes the multiple determinants impacting health of individuals and communities.[14] Much of our future work to improve the public's health will take place outside the doctor's office, but include strong links to health care and health care professionals.

As I sat in front of legislative committees, I often thought about how best to educate those senators and representatives who were making decisions about the resources available for public health for the entire state, so that we could have a mix of support for current crises and future issues. In the small Senate appropriations committee room, sitting at the table, while giving a terse presentation about budget changes from the previous year, I was tremendously hard pressed to interject these issues into a discussion of case load and federal grant policy. It was much easier to garner support for funding the immunization of children than for efforts to decrease the effects of risk factors such as poor nutrition, physical inactivity, tobacco use, and alcohol use, on elementary school children and the diseases that would follow years and decades later. Our work to set 10-year priorities with measurable goals and objectives was a helpful framework during times of budget crises, prison overcrowding, human service needs, and environmental priorities. Because we had developed a framework for longer-term thinking, one that set priorities but still left us nimble enough to deal with short-term emergencies, we had a better chance of addressing longer-term chronic issues. Looking at the data to see where we were, where we had been, and where we needed to go, provided opportunities to discuss the issues. The challenges of educating policy makers who have to make difficult and urgent decisions about policy and funding priorities gave us an opportunity to enter the discussion.

In addition to using our best available science and best practices, we can also benefit from our own successes and failures. How can you apply those strategies that have been successful in your own public health setting to other public health issues? Despite the fact that there are immense differences in health issues, there are also similarities in some aspects of their approach, particularly those regarding measuring outcomes, using comprehensive and multidisciplinary (public health) approaches, and health communication strategies. Utilizing health outcomes, measurable goals, and objectives, provide a focus for public education and helps bring resources to the issues through partnerships and shared health priorities.

Progress in reducing tobacco use in Vermont was helped by a framework of legislative steps and laws that helped lay a foundation for cultural change. The realizations that prevention efforts must start earlier, with young children, and change perceptions to one that supported not smoking as the norm were key. The benefit of other states' experiences and the expertise of the CDC to develop a science-based, Vermont-specific comprehensive effort were key elements to reducing smoking.

Successes in decreasing infectious diseases in Vermont, a cornerstone of public health efforts, were characterized by a rapid response, formal and informal surveillance systems, and efforts to communicate with the public while serious and urgent events unfolded, such as in the anthrax scares following September 11, 2001, and to outbreaks of Legionnaires' disease. Strong support for high rates of immunization, for both children and adults, was also essential.

In the area of preventing childhood lead poisoning, a Vermont study was needed to initially convince health professionals that this was a priority. Laws were put into place, public health had to deliver lead screening services, and public education was the cornerstone of prevention efforts. New partners in housing who made this a similar priority made a comprehensive and sustained approach possible.

Access to health care continues to be a challenge, attempting to balance costs, access, and quality. Although progress has been extensive, particularly in ensuring access to health care for children, barriers such as health literacy, fragility of primary care supply in some rural areas, and transportation in many parts of the state make comprehensive efforts particularly challenging particularly in light of the changing demographics of our population.

The demographics of our population also give us tremendous clues as to emerging issues. The fact that our population continues to age and live longer has implications for all diseases and chronic conditions that become more common as people get older. Public health officials have data, knowledge, and experience that cumulatively could help us anticipate and prevent many of the health conditions that we will face in the future. However, in order for momentum, focus, and resources to be applied, the issues must be agreed upon and explained in such a way that they are widely understood and supported. Such a systematic approach could save countless lives, prevent illness, and improve the quality of our lives. If we are to improve our collective health, we must stop chasing the puck and learn to skate where it will be. This mindset, whether you are a hockey fan or not, and whether you are dealing with a month ahead, a year ahead, or a decade ahead, will help you more effectively improve health.

REFERENCES

1. Rosenfeld J. Consultant debunking unit (CDU) to Gretsky: the puck stops here! *Fast Company Magazine.* 2000;36(July):60. Available at http://pf.fastcompany.com/magazine/36/cdu.html. Accessed March 15, 2005.
2. Leading by example. *Vermont Medicine.* 2004; Fall:23–25.
3. McGinnis JM, Foege WH. The immediate vs the important. *JAMA.* 2004;291:1263–1264.
4. Mokdad AH, Bowman BA, Ford ES, Vinicor F, Marks JS, Koplan JP. The Continuing epidemic of obesity and diabetes in the United States. *JAMA.* 2001;286:1195–1200.
5. Mokdad AH, Ford ES, Bowman BA, Dietz WH, Vinivor F, Bales VS, JS Marks. Prevalence of obesity, diabetes, and obesity-related health risk factors, 2001. *JAMA.* 2003;289:76–79.
6. Institute of Medicine. *Preventing Childhood Obesity, Health in the Balance.* Washington, DC: National Academies Press; 2005:1–5.
7. Institute of Medicine. *Insuring America's Health.* Washington, DC: National Academies Press; 2004:1–14.
8. Institute of Medicine. *Health Literacy, A Prescription to End Confusion.* Washington, DC: National Academies Press; 2004:1.
9. Institute of Medicine. *Unequal Treatment, Confronting Racial and Ethnic Disparities in Health Care.* Washington, DC: National Academies Press; 2003:1–2.
10. U.S. Department of Health and Human Services. *Healthy People 2010.* Available at: http://www.healthypeople.gov. Accessed June 9, 2005.
11. Institute of Medicine. *Microbial Threats to Health, Emergence, Detection, and Response.* Washington, DC: National Academies Press; 2003:7–15.
12. McGinnis JM, Williams-Russo P, Knickman JR. The case for more active policy attention to health promotion. *Health Affairs.* 2002;21:78–93.
13. McGinnis JM, Foege WH. Actual causes of death in the United States. *JAMA.* 1993;270:2207–2212.
14. Institute of Medicine. *The Future of the Public's Health in the 21st Century.* Washington, DC: National Academies Press; 2003:4, 20–23.

Two Words—*Public Health*

During the time when Vermont first worked to expand access to health care by expanding health insurance and ensuring a supply of primary care providers to care for people in all areas of our rural state, policy makers made efforts to understand the components of the health care "system" and all those working to improve health. There was some confusion in legislative committees about population-based health. Couldn't managed care just do this? What was public health? Why do we need to spend money on this?

During this time we worked to explain, using the clearest examples we could find, the responsibilities of public health from a state health department perspective, and used concrete examples to illustrate. In one of our publications, a rural health newsletter, I wrote a short editorial, called "Two Words," about our efforts to define the public's need for primary care and other rural health issues. Those two words—*public health*—are still our most important way to think about health.

A long time ago Hippocrates noted that "Protecting and developing health must rank even above that of restoring it when it is impaired."[1] Surgeons general have focused on public health issues, such as tobacco, preventing obesity, improving levels of physical activity, and addressing mental health issues, and tried to reinforce that prevention is our best investment in health.[2] But in public health we continue to struggle with balancing growing care needs with prevention, and urgent issues with chronic conditions, as our population ages and health disparities persist. We have not yet systematized our efforts to put those two words—*public health*—into practice. Although we are making tremendous strides in some areas, particularly those that connect to clinical services,[3] we vary in our efforts to improve health outcomes in those areas critical to preventing disease in the future, such as smoking, poor nutrition, lack of physical activity, and alcohol misuse, that are risks for a list of diseases already all too prevalent in our society.

Many of the remedies for these will come from outside the doctor's office, outside the health care delivery system (although health care is an essential partner). Public health efforts, through population-based strategies, public health education, science-based community prevention, and leadership, must all be strengthened to improve health. Public health must do this all at the same time urgent problems are imminent, such as emerging infectious diseases and the need to be prepared, whether against pandemic influenza or potential bioterrorism threats. Identifying and filling research gaps, and just as important, systematizing our efforts, and teaching our peers our best current strategies for putting science into practice, are needed.

Think about what public health has already achieved in such areas as immunizations, drinking water, lead poisoning, cancer screening, infectious diseases, and tobacco, and think about the opportunities to achieve even more, prevent even more, and see a much healthier population in the future. If we even make a small difference in a public health issue, something in health that is common, serious, and potentially preventable, it translates to health benefits for many people. The people in those populations, the *public* in *public health,* can be our neighbors, our families, and our friends—they can be our towns and our cities; they can be our counties and our state. Who knows how far we can get if we focus on those two words—*public health.*

Think about those two words, *public health,* and what images they bring to mind. It would not be at all surprising if the pictures painted were different, depending on whether you are in public health, in health care, in business, the media, education, academics, or a member of the public. And that is part of the problem. We need additional clarity, more examples, more clearly articulated images of what public health is and what public health does, and why it is urgently needed. Those working in public health may picture a system that promotes health and prevents disease, all using the most current scientific basis, and measuring our results. We may know the intricacies of surveillance systems for infectious diseases, the early warning systems that may still seem invisible to the public when they are doing their day-to-day job, unless there is an outbreak or epidemic. The notion that populations are distant groups of people with problems sometimes seemingly too remote to grasp our immediate attention may put up a barrier of understanding for the need for public health. We must emphasize that *populations are groups of people,* not just statistics. Population health is public health, and *we* are the public.

If we want to improve health, we must focus on it. In our efforts to improve access to health care, we must improve health. We need to think about and work to actively remove all barriers to health in the process. This broader view of health, one that recognizes that many public health issues have deep roots and many causes, will require us to better demonstrate to many audiences the links between social, economic, and cultural factors and health outcomes, as we work to improve our years of healthy life and eliminate health disparities, the overarching goals of our national framework.

As we struggle to keep up and stay ahead of immediate challenges, we have to address the chronic ones, determine how to systematically put science into practice, and better explain how and why public health is so important. To make our population healthier in the future, we must prevent chronic diseases as we work to care best for those conditions already so common, and in many cases increasing. Preventing diseases is not an option; it *must* be an essential part of what we collectively do to improve health.

Public health may be the least talked about component of our health care system, because it is the hardest to talk about. We must overcome this hurdle if we want to realize the potential improvements in health that we are capable of achieving. We need to work to make what we do, and how we do it, clearer to all those groups, organizations, constituencies, and the public, who are all participants in a public health approach. In any conversation about health, two words—*public health*—will make all the difference.

REFERENCES

1. McGinnis JM, Foege WH. The immediate vs. the important. *JAMA.* 2004; 291:1263–1264.
2. Satcher D, Hull FL. The weight of an ounce. *JAMA.* 1995;273: 1149–1150.
3. McGinnis JM. Health in America–The sum of its parts. *JAMA.* 2002; 287:2711–2712.

INDEX

Page numbers followed by t denotes tables